DATE DUE

NOV 03 1993	
GAYLORD	PRINTED IN U.S.A.

The Cross-Cultural Approach
to Health Behavior

The Cross-Cultural Approach to Health Behavior

L. RIDDICK LYNCH, *Editor*

Rutherford • Madison • Teaneck
Fairleigh Dickinson University Press

Associated University Presses, Inc.

Cranbury, New Jersey 08512

SBN: 8386 7439 9

Printed in the United States of America

In memory of my mother,
Mrs. Rosa B. Riddick,
whose life's work as an elementary school
teacher was not spectacular, but whose
wholesome character, ideals, hope, and
encouragement were instrumental in
making this work a reality.

Contributors

John Adair, Professor of Anthropology, San Francisco State College

Don Adams, Director, Center for Development Education, Syracuse University

Ethel J. Alpenfels, Professor of Anthropology, New York University

Flora L. Bailey, Supervisor of Physical Education, K-VI Schools, South Orange, New Jersey

F. John Bennett, Acting Head, Department of Preventive Medicine, Makerere University College, Kampala, Uganda

Richard Currier, Department of Anthropology, University of California, Berkeley

William A. Darity, Professor of Public Health, University of Massachusetts, Amherst

Kurt W. Deuschle, Chairman and Professor, Department of Community Medicine, Mount Sinai School of Medicine, New York, New York

Charles John Erasmus, Professor of Anthropology, University of California, Santa Barbara

George H. Fathauer, Professor of Sociology and Anthropology, Miami University, Ohio

Hugh Fulmer, Professor of Community Medicine, University of Massachusetts School of Medicine, Worcester

Michael Gelfand, University College of Rodesia, Salisbury

Luther P. Gerlach, Professor of Anthropology, University of Minnesota, Minneapolis

Nancie L. Solien Gonzalez, University of New Mexico

Harold A. Gould, Professor of Anthropology, University of Pittsburgh

Gordon W. Hewes, Professor of Anthropology, University of Colorado, Boulder

Derrick B. Jelliffe, Director, Caribbean Food & Nutrition Institute, Kingston, Jamaica

Bernice W. Loughlin, Field Health Nursing Services, Gallup Field Health Station, Gallup, New Mexico

Margaret Mead, Curator of Ethnology, American Museum of Natural History, New York, New York

Walsh McDermott, Department of Public Health, Cornell University Medical College, New York, New York

Benjamin D. Paul, Professor of Anthropology, Stanford University, Stanford, California

Arthur J. Rubel, The Ford Foundation, Mexico 5, D.F. (formerly

(Continued on page 8)

of Department of Sociology and Anthropology, University of
Notre Dame, South Bend, Indiana)

Lyle Saunders, Professor of Medicine and Public Health, University
of Colorado, Denver

Ozzie G. Simmons, Program Adviser, The Ford Foundation, Santiago,
Chile (formerly of School of Public Health, Harvard University,
Cambridge, Massachusetts

Melford E. Spiro, Professor of Anthropology, University of Chicago

Annie D. Wauneka, Division of Indian Health, U.S. Public Health
Service, Window Rock, Arizona

Robert J. Wolff, Professor, School of Public Health, University of
Hawaii

Contents

Foreword

Few people have an opportunity to become sufficiently acquainted with people from other cultures—or even subcultures within their own—to fully understand the uniqueness that distinguish groups. It is easy to believe that customs, values, attitudes, and behaviors of others are much like one's own. Yet, study reveals that there are sharp differences in the group characteristics of men, and that these are strong determinants of behavior.

In this volume, the author is concerned with the interrelationships between socio-cultural background and health behavior. She has made a careful selection of articles that throw light on the question of how the culture in which people live affects their attitudes, values, and beliefs about health. Included are a variety of readings that describe highly diverse health practices, from the use of health services to eating patterns.

Mrs. Lynch, a teacher with great appreciation for the need for anthropological material related to health, has provided a most useful volume for use by graduate and undergraduate students in their quest to help people improve the quality of living. It can be said with confidence that it will be a useful supplement in a variety of formal and informal health education programs.

Marian V. Hamburg

11

Preface

This volume, *The Cross-Cultural Approach to Health Behavior*, is a compilation of twenty-four separate research studies and articles representing cultural groups from various areas throughout the world, including the Americas, Africa, Asia, and island groups in the South Pacific.

As one whose chief concern is in the area of public health, the editor is convinced that studying the cultures of various peoples enables one to look beyond the horizon of a particular society and perceive custom as the basis for thought and action. The findings of the works included in this volume lends credence to this conviction.

While the research in no way attempts to reveal a complete study of the behavior of any single society, it provides enough information to enable professional personnel in health and health-related activities to have greater insight into factors that affect behavior. It presents evidence to reinforce the contention that persons born into a particular society are conditioned and molded by the customs that comprise the cultural heritage of that society. Likewise, the findings recorded here enable presons to understand that cultural factors determine the health patterns of a society and ultimately the health behavior of the individuals comprising that society. Furthermore, they point out that programs in public health often have limited appeal when offered to people whose cultural heritage differs from that of those offering the program. Often one experiences indifference to, and sometimes total rejection of, new health programs if application of the new threatens to destroy or alter the existing customs and thought of the recipients. It was with this in mind that these studies were compiled. For those who might refer to this volume, the information has been organized into sections I through VIII. This organization should be interesting and helpful. Part I is presented as guidelines for the application of anthropological perspectives to public-health practices. Studies that concern themselves with ethnic groups indigenous to the Americas are to be found in Parts II and III. Attempts also have been made in Parts IV and V to include studies of cultural groups in some Pacific Islands and South East Asia. The Middle East and Africa are represented in Part VI. Part VII offers the primitive concept of medicine and health and folk medicine, while Part VIII is considered a conclusion.

The editor especially feels indebted to Professor Ethel J. Alpenfels for the encouragement and many helpful suggestions given for the organization of materials. It was while studying The Child in Contemporary Culture under Professor Alpenfels that the idea for this volume had its inception.

Also particular gratitude is offered my colleagues of Jersey City State College, whose interest and assistance helped make this volume a reality. I am especially grateful to Miss Barbara Bochis, Mrs. Pauline Garrett, and Mr. Frank G. French for their encouragement and advice in securing materials, and to Miss Dolores Kruk for her excellent secretarial assistance.

Acknowledgments

This book was made possible by the numerous research activities sponsored by private foundations, public institutions, university groups, and individuals. I wish to convey my sincere thanks and appreciation to all.

For permission to reproduce previously published articles, I wish to express my thanks to all their authors and to the following organizations:

1. "Anthropological Perspectives on Medicine and Public Health"
   by Benjamin D. Paul
     Reprinted from the *Annals* of the American Academy of Political and Social Science 346, March, 1963, pp. 34–43. (Courtesy of the American Academy of Political and Social Science)
2. "Cultural Problems in Technical Assistance"
   by Derrick B. Jelliffe and F. John Bennett
     Reprinted from *Children* 9:5, September–October, 1962, pp. 171–177. (Courtesy of the Children's Bureau, U.S. Department of Health, Education, and Welfare, Social Security Administration)
3. "Food Habits—An Anthropologist's View"
   by George Fathauer
     Reprinted from the Journal of the American Dietetic Association 37:4, October, 1960, pp. 335–338. (Courtesy of the American Dietetic Association)
4. "Cancer in Situ of the Cervix—Cultural Clues to Reactions"
   by Ethel J. Alpenfels
     Reprinted from American Journal of Nursing 64:4, April, 1964, pp. 83–86. (Courtesy of The American Journal of Nursing Company)
5. "Patterns of Health and Disease Among the Navaho"

54:10, October, 1964, pp. 1726–1734. (Courtesy of the American Public Health Association, Inc.)

12. "Popular and Modern Medicine in Mestizo Communities of Coastal Peru and Chile"
by Ozzie G. Simmons
Reprinted from the *Journal of American Folklore* 68:1, January, 1955, pp. 57–71. (Courtesy of American Folklore Society)

13. "The Hot-Cold Syndrome and Symbolic Balance in Mexican and Spanish American Folk Medicine"
by Richard L. Currier
Reprinted from *Ethnology* 3:3, July, 1966, pp. 251–263. (Courtesy of the Department of Anthropology, University of Pittsburgh)

14. "Ghosts, Ifaluk, and Teleological Functionalism"
by Melford E. Spiro
Reprinted from *American Anthropologist* 54:4, October–December, 1952, pp. 497–503. (Courtesy of American Anthropological Association)

15. "Social Culture and Nutrition—Cultural Blocks and Protein Malnutrition in Early Childhood in Rural West Bengal"
by Derrick B. Jelliffe
Reprinted from *Pediatrics* 20, 1957, pp. 128–138. (Courtesy of American Academy of Pediatrics)

16. "Modern Medicine and Folk Cognition in Rural India"
by Harold A. Gould
Reprinted from *Human Organization* 24:3, Fall, 1965, pp. 201–208. (Courtesy of The Society for Applied Anthropology)

17. "Modern Medicine and Traditional Culture: Confrontation on the Malay Peninsula"
by Robert J. Wolff
Reprinted from *Human Organization* 24:4, Winter, 1965, pp. 339–345. (Courtesy of The Society for Applied Anthropology)

18. "Some Sociocultural Factors in the Administration of

The Cross-Cultural Approach
to Health Behavior

Part I

GUIDELINES FOR THE APPLICATION OF ANTHROPOLOGICAL
PERSPECTIVES TO PUBLIC HEALTH PRACTICES

Introduction

In their health-related research, cultural anthropologists seem to offer the general consensus that anthropology has demonstrated a definite usefulness in public health programs. They further contend that a wider use of the anthropologist's point of view in combination with the knowledge and technical skill of the health personnel would bring about increased effectiveness of the total public health effort in any community. The research herein included as *Guidelines* offers a description of the findings and suggestions of experts in the fields of social science and medical science. The progression of the findings goes from general overall guidelines to specific plans for developing effective programs in various areas of public health, i.e., maternal and child care, nutrition, and chronic disease.

In his anthropological perspectives, Paul suggests the need for recognition of certain gaps by public health personnel, especially the public health administrators. These gaps, which have been found to be impediments to health progress, are referred to as (1) the cultural gap (between members of a community and between the community and the health worker), (2) the status gap, and (3) the urban adjustment gap.

Paul's findings are corroborated by Foster in "Use of Anthropological Methods and Data in Planning an Operation."[1]

---

1. George M. Foster, *"Use of Anthropological Methods and Data in Planning and Operation,"* Public Health Reports, *68, no. 9, September 1953, pp. 841–56.*

Though excellence in medical knowledge and practice is necessary for success in any health program, Foster found that the socio-economic potential of an area is also a major factor. In addition, the cultural problems that arose in the Bilateral Health Programs' evaluation came about not only because of ineffective human relations but also from the difference between the way of life of the programs' donors and the way of life of the programs' recipients. The following broad categorical list of essential cultural data is proposed by Foster for any who might attempt to promote or enhance the effectiveness of any health program.

1. Folk medicine and native curing practices
2. Social organization of the families
3. Education and literacy
4. Political organization
5. Religion
6. Basic value system
7. Other types of data—credit facilities and money usages, labor division within the family, time utilization, working and eating schedules, cooking and dietary practices, etc.[2]

Jelliffe and Bennett, concentrating their effort on maternal and child health services, further reinforced previously recorded findings. In giving technical assistance in maternal and child care, the donors' cultural conditioning was as much a factor in the problems encountered as was the recipients' culture. In addition to the language barrier, problem areas recorded are: problem evaluation and statistical recording, personnel provision and training, organization and operation of maternal and child health services, nutrition education, and health education. Like former researchers, Jelliffe and Bennett conclude that cultural factors shape the health and disease patterns of a community; therefore, these factors (community structure, family function, attitude toward innovation, etc.)

---

2. Ibid., *p. 856.*

should be given major consideration when determining "the work, the personnel, and the emphasis of maternal and child health services." Generally, these findings are those considered to be prerequisite to effective planning for any public health program.

In his discussion of food habits, Fathauer reemphasizes the necessity for inclusion of facts about cultures in the overall education of food specialists. To achieve appreciable success, according to him, food specialists need to understand the extent to which food culture relates to such factors as the individual's socio-economic status, values, attitudes, and the reasons for food consumption other than hunger—the symbolic aspects of food.

Alpenfels refers to *cultural clues to reactions to disease of Americans,* a future-oriented society. As a possible cause of their resistance to early cancer detection and prevention, she stresses modesty feelings that are developed early in childhood training. Such modesty feelings, she states, might be the foremost cause of failure to submit to periodical cancer detection examinations even among professionals—nurses and other health-oriented persons.

Summarizing the implications of culture for public health as recorded by the anthropologists, Edward Wellins suggests that a community's culture might be considered to have implications for public health in that it (1) influences the prevailing ecology of health and disease, (2) creates its own definition and reaction toward disease, and (3) influences the effectiveness (or lack of effectiveness) of the health program because response to a situation is in terms of concepts that, in turn, are based on cultural values. In this light, knowledge of the local culture together with knowledge of the cultural differences between the community constituents and the health team are of inestimable value in interpreting local culture in terms useful to health programs.[3]

3. *Edward Wellins, "Implication of Local Culture for Public Health,"* Human Organization, *16, no. 4 (Winter 1958), pp. 16–18.*

1

Anthropological Perspectives on Medicine and Public Health

Benjamin D. Paul

Benjamin D. Paul, Ph.D., is Professor of Anthropology and Director of the Program in Medicine and the Behavioral Sciences at Stanford University, California. He was formerly Director of the Social Science Program and Professor of Anthropology at Harvard University, School of Public Health. In addition to his anthropological field work among the Maja-speaking Indians of Highland Guatemala, he is distinguished for his interest, research, and writings in the area of ethnography, anthropological method, and social-science aspects of public health. His publications include: (editor) Health, Culture, and Community, *Russell Sage, (1955); (co-author)* Trigger for Community Conflict: The Case of Fluoridation, *(1961); and "Changing Marriage Patterns in a Highland Guatemalan Community,"* Southwestern Journal of Anthropology, *(Summer 1963). "Anthropological Perspectives on Medicine and Public Health" is reprinted with the permission of the author and of The American Academy of Political and Social Science from* The Annals, *Vol. 346, (March 1963), pp. 34–43.*

ABSTRACT: Some cultural anthropologists, when they do health-related research, investigate the role of sociocultural factors in the origin and prevalence of specific disease entities, particularly among ethnic minorities and people of divergent cultures. Others study the effect of cultural and social differences on the outcome of public-health programs carried out in intercultural settings. Directors of health programs, as agents of social change and community development, should

26

understand the nature of certain gaps that recurrently impede realization of program objectives. One is the cultural gap, which complicates communication and leads to the selective acceptance of offered innovations, owing to differences in cultural values and in culturally conditioned assumptions about the cause of illness. Another is the status gap between the health team and the public and between the ruling elites and their people. Still another is the urban-adjustment gap created by the influx of rural population into the cities. Compared to the sums of money spent on basic medical research and program operations in the field, the amount available for studying the human aspects of health-improvement programs and other phases of community development is disappointingly small. This imbalance constitutes the research gap.

Because man is not only a social but also a cultural animal, it scarcely surprises us to be told that cultural as well as social factors often play a significant role in man's susceptibility and response to illness. Broadly speaking, culture is a group's design for living, a shared set of socially transmitted assumptions about the nature of the physical and social world, the goals of life, and the appropriate means of achieving them. These things we know; we also know that cultures vary considerably from group to group within and between nations. But, without special effort, we cannot readily know just how given cultures differ from others and how these differences influence behavior in regard to specific illnesses and to specific programs of medical care. Anthropologists have not been the only behavioral scientists to study variations of this kind, but, as students of comparative cultures, anthropologists attracted to the field of medicine have naturally tended to fix their attention on the cultural contexts in which health, illness, and therapy are framed.

In publishing their ethnographic reports on Eskimo, Navaho, Polynesian, or other communities, anthropologists have usually included a sizable section on sickness and curing, but these reports, mainly written for the benefit of academic insiders, have had little impact on members of the medical and public-health professions. During the last decade, however, a number of anthropologists have begun to collaborate with medical teams and organizations and to select research problems pertinent to research physicians and other health workers. These might be called "medical anthropologists," for their activities are linked to those of the health professions, although the term is not in common usage—as is the term "medical sociologists"— and its members are not a group in any organizational sense.

Medical anthropologists generally are of two kinds, those who investigate cultural components in the etiology and incidence of illness and those who analyze popular reactions to programs of health maintenance and health improvement. Investigators in the first category study how cultural patterns mediate between conditions of climate, economy, sanitation, diet, child rearing, daily routines, and social contact, on the one hand, and death, disability, and disease, on the other.

Although mortality and morbidity rates tend to be inversely related to economic and nutritional status the effect is often modified by cultural practices. A good example is kwashiorkor —a children's disease due to nutritional, particularly protein, deficiency—prevalent in many technologically underdeveloped areas. Two populations living in the same general environment with equally limited food resources may differ in their weaning practices and culturally conditioned assumptions about the kinds and quantities of nutriments suitable during the postweaning period. In consequence, the extent of kwashiorkor among children one to five years of age may vary appreciably as between the two populations. It is an open question whether psychological factors such as parental solicitude or indifference are also involved, but, if they are, these dispositions, too, are partly a product of cultural conditioning.

Rates of venereal disease, tuberculosis, and other communicable illnesses are affected by conditions of crowding and social contact. These conditions are influenced in turn by cultural standards, which differ from one group to another. Psychological components subsumed under the catch-all concept of "stress" are often thought to play a part in the origin and persistence of noncontagious chronic diseases and the so-called psychosomatic ailments. The presence and degree of stress, a subjective experience, are notoriously governed by varying cultural expectations and definitions.[1]

The second and larger category of medical anthropologists have been concerned not with the determinants of disease and its prevalence but with the behavior of people in the face of sickness and in the presence of medical and other community resources for maintaining health and coping with illness. While sociologists have taken the lead in studying social class as a variable in medical behavior, some of the anthropologists working with segments of our own society have selected ethnicity as a variable. Comparative studies designed to disclose subcultural variations do indeed reveal characteristic group differences among "Old Yankees," Irish, Italians, Jews, Spanish Americans, and others with respect to a variety of circumstances—for example, responses to pain and to programs of physical rehabilitation, drinking behavior and alcoholism, deciding to seek medical care, tolerance of mentally retarded children in the home, reaction to mental illness.

Perhaps the kind of health-related research for which cultural anthropologists are especially qualified by temperament and training is the study of popular reactions to programs of public health carried out in foreign cultural settings. Personnel of action programs generally strive to measure the success of their efforts in such terms as number of mothers attending clinics, quantity of latrines installed, or extent of altered dietary practice. But usually they are not in a good position to ascertain the reasons why parts of the message are lost or transformed, why certain parts of the program work and others not, or why certain segments of the target population accept the assistance offered while others do not. Without this knowledge of the dynamics that intervene between action and outcome, it is difficult to profit from experience, avoiding past mistakes and repeating past successes.

It is here that the anthropologist can help. For he is accustomed to work in alien settings, patiently establishing his role as an interested but detached observer, developing relationships with reliable informants, slowly building up a picture of the local culture by watching, listening, making inquiries, and collecting incidents, cases, and statistics.

In most general terms the (anthropological) field worker aims to gather and relate two sets of data, a description of the situation as he sees it, looking from the outside in, and a description of the situation as the native sees it, looking from the inside out. The first comprises the visible world of objects and actions: the people in their material and environmental setting, their groupings and interactions, their techniques and activities. This objective frame of reference the ethnographer shares with the human geographer, the economist, and the natural historian. The subjective frame of reference embraces the world view of the people, the pattern of assumptions that guides their perceptions, the network of meanings that binds their percepts into the semblance of a system, the hierarchy of values animating their actions. The student of culture cannot ignore the objective situation, but it is the subjective view that constitutes his distinctive concern. He needs to know the what and the how, but he also wants to know the cultural wherefore.[2]

By this method, anthropologists in recent years have produced a fair number of instructive case studies of interaction between health teams and local populations. A pioneer report of this kind was an analysis of the operation of bilateral health projects in several Latin-American countries by George M. Foster and his anthropological colleagues.[3] Additional detailed case studies based on programs in Africa, Asia, the Pacific, Latin America, and North America have since been assembled in a volume prepared primarily to assist teaching in schools of public health.[4] In a very useful essay, Foster has summarized some of the recurrent problems and processes encountered in intercultural health programs.[5] Another anthropologist, Steven Polgar, has published an organized and comprehensive review of the literature on health and human behavior generally.[6]

Intercultural Health Programs

The profession of public health prides itself on being in the forefront of the campaign to increase the productivity of peoples and nations and to elevate their standard of living. Sick and undernourished people cannot work efficiently; improved health is often a precondition for economic improvement. Of all forms of technical aid, health programs, if soundly conceived, are most likely to be welcomed and least likely to be feared as forms of political or economic interference. Of course, programs of health improvement can proceed only so far without parallel development in agriculture, transportation, education, public administration, and general economic development. Moreover, mortality reduction, if not accompanied by per capita economic growth, will only increase pressure on the food supply.

Despite the generally uncontroversial nature of public health aid, it should be recognized that new modes of behavior, whether they concern health or anything else, are seldom accepted simply on their intrinsic merits. The success or failure of a health program is largely governed by the way in which it fits the modes of thought and action of the recipient population. Thus, public-health workers, like other agents of social change, need to understand the nature of sociocultural patterns, what purposes they serve, why they persist, and how they change. In their planning and in their approach, health experts need to be particularly aware of four gaps which often impede realization of program aims: the cultural gap, the status gap, the urban-adjustment gap, and the research gap.

The Cultural Gap

There frequently exists a considerable gap or difference between the culture of the beneficiary population and that of the action team. What seems obvious, feasible, and desirable to health personnel, looking at the world with their own culturally tinted glasses, may seem quite otherwise to the people they serve.

Cultural gaps complicate the problem of elementary communication. Caudill provides an amusing example from Japan. He writes:[7]

> If one wants to refer rather roughly and familiarly to one's own mother, one may use the word *ofukuro*. This word, without the prefix "o" which is honorific, means "bag" or "sack." If a Japanese patient working with an English-speaking [psychoanalyst] were to refer to his mother as an "honorable bag" I expect the pattern of the analyst's emotional associations with this would go off in directions other than those of the patient's. The term has invidious connotations in English that it does not have in Japanese.

The cultural gap can also impede the acceptance of new health services. People of other societies often find the new modes incompatible with their own notions of illness and curing, and it is therefore practical, not to say considerate, to understand their beliefs and practices before trying to change them. Anthropological field work on folk medicine yields several generalizations. One is that local disease taxonomies, though seldom explicit and varying greatly from culture to culture, are often as orderly and systematic as they are complex. This has been well documented, for example, by Adams for a rural community in Guatemala[8] and by Frake for a pagan group in the southern Philippines.[9]

Another generalization about folk medicine is that the local population tends to divide afflictions into two great classes: those that respond to folk methods of treatment and those amenable to scientific medication, although the dividing line may shift from one culture to another. Drawing on field material from northern India, Gould asserts that the inhabitants view village medicine as applying mainly to chronic nonincapacitating ailments such as arthritis, while modern medicine is seen as applying to critical incapacitatng dysfunctons such as acute appendicitis.[10] Of course, people who repeatedly fail to find relief under one type of medicine will often try the other type as a desperate last resort.

Still another proposition is that local concepts of etiology and curing serve more purposes than the technical one of maintaining physical health. Within the context of their culture, they may also serve psychological as well as expressive and symbolic needs, although these functions are seldom made explicit.[11] But perhaps the most important of the latent purposes is that of social control, namely, providing sanction or support for the moral and social system. Rubel describes "evil eye" and several other folk illnesses which remain firmly embedded in the sociocultural matrix of a Mexican-American border community, despite the introduction of an alternative system of belief and ways of healing, because they function "to sustain some of the dominant values of the Mexican-American culture, those which prescribe the maintenance of the solidarity of the small, bilateral family unit, and others which prescribe the appropriate role behavior of males and females, of older and younger individuals."[12] Here, as elsewhere, diseases interpreted as punishment for violation of social norms are usually held to fall outside the ken or competence of the technically trained physician. However, health workers who have taken the trouble to master the rationale of the native system of medical concepts have usually gained greater acceptance of their own.

Cultures are layered. What we call customs rest on top and are most apparent. Deepest and least apparent are the cultural values that give meaning and direction to life. Values influence people's perceptions of needs and their choice between perceived alternative courses of action. Although sound health is everywhere appreciated, a deliberate quest for good health as such does not rank equally high in the hierarchy of every society's value system. Concern for health may be masked by a quest for merit, virtue, or staying in harmony with the moral and cosmic order.

Cleanliness for its own sake, apart from its role in reducing infection, occupies a high place in the scale of values implicit in the culture of the American middle class, but this is not always the case in other cultures. Although the Japanese likewise place high value on cleanliness, they are less dedicated to the cluster of values which Americans, invoking democratic ideals, often try to export via health promotion and other improvement programs. With America as a model, health workers have tried to stimulate group discussion as a method of achieving health education in rural areas of Japan, but group discussion does not come easily where respect for authority is a built-in value and where the concepts of voluntarism, self-help, and citizen participation are still alien to the basic value system.

Appeals to pride or invitations to gain prestige or excitation of other strong motives outside the sphere of health can sometimes stimulate people to implement new health measures. To start a program of rural sanitation in a demonstration village in Thailand, Textor appealed to the head priest to enlist the aid of lay citizens in building latrines at the Buddhist temple for the use of temple priests, citizens coming to sleep at the temple on holy days, and children attending school on temple grounds. The latrine-construction project was completed in two days not because the volunteer laborers valued improved sanitation but because they were willing to earn religious merit by performing good works for the temple, an important value in their culture.[13] Whether or not this kind of approach yields favorable long-run results is a matter for empirical investigation; whether or not it is warranted is a question of policy and a legitimate subject for debate.

The public-health approach rightly stresses the prevention

of illness and the promotion of good health habits, not just the cure of illness. Some positive measures can be carried out—such as malaria control—without enlisting the active involvement of the beneficiary population; others require their participation. The latter kind, which depends for its successful implementation on engaging and sustaining human motivation, obviously demands much effort, patience, and ingenuity.

But even the former type of program, which asks only for passive acceptance, can arouse unexpected resistance, as many supervisors of DDT campaigns can ruefully attest, because the people affected may bring to the situation culturally conditioned expectations and interpretations at variance with those held by public-health specialists. In North Borneo, delegations from the countryside petitioned the government to stop antimalarial teams from spraying their houses, complaining that they disliked having strangers enter their homes, that their religion forbade them to allow any toxic substance in their houses, that their farm animals and even children were being killed by the poison, and that they were prepared to go to jail rather than submit to the spraying. In Peru, antitriatoma spraying brought Chagas' disease under control according to plan, but the citizens mistakenly assumed that the aim was to eliminate bothersome flies. Judging the campaign a fly-control fiasco, they drew up a resolution, submitted it to the national congress in Lima, and forced the health officer responsible for the project to answer charges of malfeasance.

Although programs of prevention are justifiable from the standpoint of long-run efficiency, they are frequently difficult to implement for several interrelated reasons. One is the relatively low salience of health as a value among some groups, as already indicated; able-bodied people are often disposed to leave well enough alone rather than worry continuously about keeping fit. A second reason is the difficulty of perceiving the connection between a given action and its beneficial effect. Thus, people in tropical areas may readily accept antibotic treatment of yaws because the effect is rapid and visible but hesitate to use latrines designed to break the invisible cycle of infection from feces to water to mouth.

A third reason is the limited future-time orientation of people in most technologically underdeveloped areas. Accustomed mainly to short-term planning, they find long-run goals unrealistic and uncompelling. A fourth reason is the existence in the local culture of competing "preventive" measures, namely, the dos and don'ts of proper behavior which are supposed to forestall sickness and other types of misfortune.

This array of possible impediments does not mean that preventive medicine programs are doomed to failure. It means that they should be shaped to fit the cultural profile, as well as the health profile, of the population involved. It also implies that long-range goals stand a better chance of being implemented if they are combined with measures to meet immediate needs. For medical programs this usually means offering curative along with preventive services. A mother who receives attention for a sick child by that token will be a little more disposed to heed advice about how to prevent the illness of a healthy child. Folk medicine and folk practitioners may be trusted, but they do not always provide relief, and at least some of the disappointed sufferers will be impelled to seek help elsewhere, especially if the new services are not too inconsistent with existing conditions and expectations.

The Status Gap

In any social system, there are likely to be gradations of classes and social statuses. In many technologically underdeveloped areas, the status gap between the educate elite and the bulk of the population is apt to be particularly marked. The difference between the "felt needs" of these divergent social strata has important implications for health programing and other forms of technical co-operation. The people-to-people approach is laudable enough, but usually it is neither prudent nor possible to bypass the ruling elite, whose vested interest may discourage reforms essential to improving the lot of the common man. However, this is not always the case, especially where leadership is based on education rather than land ownership.

Let us assume that the elite are genuinely eager to assist the masses, a condition that exists in some newly emerging states such as India. The problem here is the divergence of outlook and aspiration between the peasantry and the city-bred elite, coupled with the inability or unwillingness of the elite to acknowledge this gap. While the peasants are reluctant to abandon time-tested ways, the elite of technologically under-developed countries are eager to bring their nations, overnight if possible, up to the level of the well-developed nations.

Ruling elites understandably lay claim to knowing the people of their own country. But, as Freedman points out on the basis of his experience as a health consultant in Asia:[14]

> I am impressed by three kinds of error which spring from [this unwarranted claim]. The first of these is the error of supposing that within a given political territory all local communities conform to a standard pattern of social organization. The second error is to confuse the legislated pattern of rural life with the actual pattern. The third error is to entertain a view of rural life which I can only call romantic; in this view—and it is a common one—the inhabitants of rural communities are credited with powers of spontaneous cooperation and harmonious co-existence to the extent that they resemble no human community which has ever been studied.

There is often status gap enough in the United States between physicians and other health personnel, as well as between physicians and patients. But the status gaps are greater in Latin-America and other countries where physicians usually come from the upper class (rather than middle class, as in the United States), nurses from less privileged strata, and patients in public clinics from the lowest level. In these circumstances, as Simmons[15] and others have shown, the health "team" may in fact be a hierarchy of command, mistrust may mark the relations between the team and clientele, and teams made up of American and local physicians may operate under strain due to conflicting social postures vis-à-vis the public.

The Urban-Adjustment Gap

In many places, the population surge from rural and tribal areas into the cities creates unhealthful conditions of over-crowding, poor sanitation, and malnutrition. Uprooted from familiar surroundings and not yet assimilated into city life, the migrants often face difficult problems of adjustment. How traumatic this experience actually proves to be depends on the particular combination of material, social, and psychological factors, as anthropological studies of slum conditions in different countries are beginning to show.

In an effort to assess the role of social factors in the etiology of hypertension, Scotch compared African Zulus situated at different points on the rural-urban continuum. Blocked by a policy of apartheid, destitute Zulus from rural reservations who live in squatter settlements near Durban suffer degradation and other forms of frustration which seem to exact a heavy toll in antisocial behavior and psychosomatic illness, particularly among the young men, who bear the brunt of the strain. With few opportunities to express their resentments directly against the whites, African men apparently seek displaced targets, venting their hostility on wives (higher rate of broken homes), other Africans (increased rates of bewitchment and accusations of sorcery), and against themselves (alcoholism and markedly increased essential hypertension).[16]

On the other hand, Mangin found little evidence of psychological stress or social disorganization among low-status mountain people who migrated to Lima, Peru. They, too, move into squatter settlements which are often crowded, with flimsy houses, poor sewage disposal, and no water supply. The new residents feel themselves under attack, and they experience a sense of separateness from the city. Nevertheless, for most migrants, the new environment represents progress in terms of housing and income, and urban residence spells improvement over the semifeudal life of the Indian or lower-class mestizo in the Andean hinterland.[17] Thus, the precise effect of the urban-adjustment gap often depends on more factors than meet the eye on first inspection.

The Research Gap

As detached observers of interaction between representatives of different cultures (the health team and the beneficiary population), anthropologists can add insight into social processes activated by intercultural health programs. But, so far, they have been able to provide only a modest amount of assistance to program administrators. Too few anthropologists have yet had an opportunity to become familiar with the field of health and the subculture of its practitioners, and too few public-health administrators know enough about the way anthropologists work. These deficiencies are diminishing as case studies of health and culture accumulate and as anthropologists are added to the faculties of medical and public-health schools. These are encouraging signs, but they are not enough.

Compared to the sums of money spent on basic medical research to generate new technical knowledge and on program operations in the field, the amount of money available for studying the human aspects of community development, including health improvement, is disappointingly small. In their report to the International Cooperation Administration (ICA) on community development programs in India. Pakistan, and the Philippines, submitted in 1955, Adams, Foster, and Taylor found:[18]

> Recognition of the potential usefulness of scientific research in the broad fields of social and economic development generally is conspicuous by its absence. . . . The United States supports research in agronomy, animal husbandry, medicine and education in many countries as parts of development programs, but contributes very little to the research that will promote more effective utilization of the fruits of these technical investigations. . . . There is almost no exploitation of the rich research possibilities inherent in community development programs. . . . We believe that, until such time as social science research techniques and knowledge are utilized much more fully in planning and operations, community development programs will not realize their full potential.

The research gap that impressed Adams, Foster, and Taylor in 1955 is no longer so wide and so disheartening. There is growing awareness of the problem, and steps are being taken to do something about it. Narrowing the research gap would help bridge the other gaps—the cultural, status, and urban-adjustment gaps already reviewed.

Social scientists should not aim merely to facilitate the implementation of predetermined plans and policies. Questions of *how* to induce response to a program should be set in the larger frame of *whether* to promote a given program at all. Although not directing his remarks specifically at work in the health field, Ralph Beals expresses this concern when he criticizes "the view that the basic problem is how someone can do something to other people tacitly understood as inferior or subordinate. . . . It is time some emphasis of applied anthropology should be on determining what people want and aiding them to get it rather than how they can best be persuaded to do what people in another culture think is best for them. The latter too often is a rationalization really concealing what is thought best for the dominant culture."[19]

References

1. The literature on the role of sociocultural factors in the etiology of disease has been critically reviewed recently by an anthropologist working with a physician: see Norman A. Scotch and H. Jack Geiger, "The Epidemiology of Rheumatoid Arthritis," *Journal of Chronic Diseases,* Vol. 15 (1962), pp. 1037–1067. Also see "The Epidemiology of Essential Hypertension" by the same authors, as well as "Sociocultural Factors in the Epidemiology of Schizophrenia," by Elliot G. Mishler and Norman A. Scotch, both mimeographed, Harvard School of Public Health, 1962.

2. Benjamin D. Paul, "Interview Techniques and Field Relationships," *Anthropology Today,* ed. A. L. Kroeber (Chicago: University of Chicago Press, 1953), p. 442.

3. George M. Foster and others, "A Cross-cultural Anthropological Analysis of a Technical Aid Program" (mimeographed; Washington, D.C.: Smithsonian Institution, 1951).

4. Benjamin D. Paul and Walter B. Miller (eds.), *Health, Culture, and Community: Case Studies of Public Reactions to Health Programs* (New York: Russell Sage Foundation, 1955).

5. George M. Foster, *Problems in Intercultural Health Practice,* Social Science Research Council, Pamphlet no. 12, 1958.

6. Steven Polgar, "Health and Human Behavior: Areas of Interest Common to the Social and Medical Sciences," *Current Anthropology,* Vol. 3, No. 2 (April 1962), pp. 159–205.

7. William Caudill, "Some Problems in Transcultural Communication (Japan-U.S.)," *Application of Psychiatric Insights to Cross-Cultural Communication* (New York: Group for the Advancement of Psychiatry, 1961), p. 420.

8. Richard N. Adams, *An Analysis of Medical Beliefs and Practices in a Guatemalan Indian Town* (Guatemala City: Pan American Sanitary Bureau, 1953).

9. Charles O. Frake, "The Diagnosis of Disease Among the Subanun of Mindanao," *American Anthropologist* 63 (1961), pp. 113–32.

10. Harold A. Gould, "The Implications of Technological Change for Folk and Scientific Medicine," *American Anthropologist,* 59 (1957), pp. 507–16.

11. Benjamin D. Paul, "The Cultural Context of Health Education," *Symposium Proceedings, School of Social Work* (University of Pittsburgh, 1953), pp. 31–38.

12. Arthur J. Rubel, "Concepts of Disease in Mexican-American Culture," *American Anthropologist,* Vol. 62 (1960), pp. 795–814.

13. Robert B. Textor and Others, *Manual for the Community Health Worker in Thailand* (Thailand: Ministry of Public Health, 1958).

14. Maurice Freedman, "Health Education and Self-Education," *Health Education Journal*, 15 (May 1957), p. 79.

15. Ozzie G. Simmons, *Social Status and Public Health*, Social Science Research Council, Pamphlet no. 13, 1958.

16. Norman Scotch, "A Preliminary Report on the Relation of Sociocultural Factors to Hypertension among the Zulu," *Annals of the New York Academy of Science*, 84 (1960), pp. 1000–9.

17. William Mangin, "Mental Health and Migration to Cities: A Peruvian Case," *Annals of the New York Academy of Science*, 84 (1960), pp. 911–17.

18. Harold Adams, George Foster, and Paul S. Taylor, *Report on Community Development Programs in India, Pakistan and the Philippines* (Washington, D.C.: International Cooperative Administration, 1955), pp. 41–42.

19. Sol Tax and Others, eds., *An Appraisal of Anthropology Today* (Chicago: University of Chicago Press, 1952), p. 189.

2

Cultural Problems in Technical Assistance

Derrick B. Jelliffe, M.D. and F. John Bennett, M.B.

Derrick B. Jelliffe, M.D., is Director of the Caribbean Food and Nutrition Institute, University of the West Indies, Kingston, Jamaica. He was formerly UNICEF Professor of Child Health at Makerere University College Medical School, Kampala, Uganda. Dr. Jelliffe's extended research has been chiefly in the area of maternal and child health (especially nutrition of the mother and child). He is co-author with Dr. John Bennett, and others, of many articles in this area. Outstanding among his latest publications are "Education for Child Health Workers in Developing Regions," Postgraduate Medical Journal, London, (February 1962); and (editor) Child Health in the Tropics, Edward Arnold, London, 1962.

F. John Bennett, M.D., is Acting Head of Department of Preventive Medicine Makerere University College of Medicine, Kampala, Uganda. He has made a tremendous research contribution in the area of maternal and child health. He is co-author with Dr. Derrick B. Jelliffe of numerous articles in this area. Among the outstanding ones are: "Worldwide Care of the Mother and Newborn Child," Clinical Obstetrics and Gynecology, (March 1962); "Cultural and Anthropological Factors in Infant and Maternal Nutrition," Federation Proceedings, London, (March 1961).

"Cultural Problems in Technical Assistance" is reproduced with permission of the authors and of the U.S. Department of Health, Education, and Welfare, Social Security Administration, from Children *9:5 (September-October) 1962, pp. 171–177.*

Of the numerous definitions of "culture," we tend to use one which fits our thesis best. In this article we use the word to refer to the whole way of life of a group of people—including the artifacts produced; the adaptation to the environment; the shared mosaic of belief, feeling, and behavior; and the patterns of relationship between individuals.

Many of the cultural problems of giving technical aid in the field of maternal and child health in developing regions arise from the donor's Western-based scientific cultural conditioning rather than from the recipient culture.[1-3] In tropical countries these problems arise in connection with five major aspects of maternal and child health, or as we usually say, MCH work:

1. The evaluation of the country's health problems and the establishment of health statistics.

2. The provision and training of personnel.

3. The organization and operation of maternal and child health services.

4. Nutrition education.

5. Health education.

In most underdeveloped countries there are no accurate vital statistics relating to illness and death among mothers and children. Usually even census figures, showing the proportion of children of different ages in the population, are not available. The maternal and child health worker is thus faced with an imperfect knowledge of his major problems and no baseline from which to gauge progress. Moreover, he lacks one of the most effective weapons for overcoming public and administrative inertia.

One of the commonest difficulties in carrying out a census in newly developing countries lies in the fact that many people do not like to have their children counted. This reluctance is sometimes due to a general mistrust of strangers, sometimes to a suspicion that the process is related to tax registration, and sometimes, as among the Baganda in Africa, that it is tempting providence to draw attention to family size. At Makerere College Health Center in Uganda, it has taken over two years to obtain an approximate census of a relatively small area. The process was additionally handicapped by the lack of villages or groupings of dwellings in the area, and by the local custom of sending children to live with relatives, who maintain they are their own.

In many developing regions, as among the Zulus, the maintenance of census figures around a health center is further hampered by the continuous movement of men, women, and children between towns and rural areas. Similar problems are present to an even greater extent among such nomadic peoples as the Karamojong cattle raisers of Uganda or the Hadza hunters of northern Tanganyika.

Attempts to receive notification of births, deaths, and illnesses may also meet with little success owing to a general fear that the information might be used for ulterior motives, especially taxation, and also because of local concepts of the cause and significance of these events. For example, death of a newborn may be considered a result of a mother's promiscuity, and so a cause of shame which should not be revealed.

Inaccuracies in health statistics may also result from a variety of other cultural concepts and practices. In some communities, births, and in others deaths, are accompanied by much obvious ceremonial, which may lead to overreporting on the part of field observers. In parts of southeast Asia problems arise from the belief that the death of a baby is of little consequence since he had not yet been initiated into his community, and to the superstition that it is inauspicious to reveal the name or sex of a newborn.[4]

Rituals, Taboos, and Disease

Hospital statistics in some underdeveloped areas may be subject to even greater bias because people believe that certain diseases are not amenable to modern scientific medicine, and, therefore, do not present themselves for treatment. For example, among the Zulus, important communicable diseases, such as tuberculosis and syphilis, are thought to be forms of poisoning and bewitchment, best treated by indigenous practitioners. Especially where concepts of causation include the transgression of social taboos are people likely to think that such diseases only occur among themselves and therefore cannot be understood or treated by the foreign-trained.

Statistical bias can also occur in hospital and clinic practice in relation to certain age groups. Thus, in New Guinea, the incident of neonatal tetanus seemed to be much less than might have been expected. This, however, was not because the disease was not widespread, but because mothers and newborns were kept in ritual postnatal seclusion during which many babies died without ever being seen.[5] Similar situations probably exist elsewhere, as in India where postnatal seclusion is customary.

Yet another factor making precise diagnosis and hence precise statistics hard to achieve in hospital work, particularly in Moslem societies, is the great difficulty in obtaining autopsies, especially on children. Moreover, in most tropical countries where the fear of witchcraft is widespread, the removal of pathological specimens at post mortems is viewed with much suspicion. The use of human tissue, whether nails, hair, or flesh, is a basic maneuver in many magical processes, such as the potent *borfirma* (charm) of the Leopard Men of Sierra Leone, an essential ingredient of which is human omental fat.

Much so-called "buried disease" exists among children in the tropics including illnesses that do not reach the attention of the pediatrician, who is apt to be preoccupied with the constant battle against such overwhelming problems as protein-calorie malnutrition and diarrheal disease. Even Western-labeled "behavior problems" may occur, but, as they are not recognized as constituting problems at all in a different cultural nexus, they are not reported. Since bed wetting among Baganda children is a source of pride as it portends great fertility and potency, a Baganda peasant mother would certainly not consider it as something to mention to the doctor. Nevertheless, it might occur under exactly the same conditions as in European and American children.

In spite of these difficulties, prevalence studies are extremely helpful for the MCH worker in an underdeveloped country, for they not only acquaint him with the relative commonness of disease in the community itself, but also help him learn something of the causative environmental and cultural factors responsible. Surveys of this type, in which students participate as "teaching safaris,"[6] are carried out by the Department of Child Health and of Preventive Medicine at Makerere Medical School as a continuing series of community studies in child health in east Africa.[7]

Certain maneuvers employed in such field studies may create difficulties because of cultural misinterpretation. The sucking up of blood into a pipette to obtain a specimen may be thought to be blood drinking for magical reasons, an idea that is reinforced if the staff member concerned is a woman wearing red lipstick. Again the weighing of children may be regarded as tempting providence, or the collection of stool specimens feared, lest they be used for bewitchment.

Wherever a high incidence of some particular disease is discovered, whether by survey or by clinic notification, it is, of course, necessary for applying preventive measures logically to determine etiologic "molding forces." These often lie as much in the field of human behavior as in the environment alone. Before attempting the investigation of etiologic factors, the MCH worker must acquire as much knowledge as possible of the local culture pattern. Otherwise he will have little idea even where to begin to seek the complex factors making up the mosaic of causation. Hours spent on reading anthropological literature and on discussions with local people about their lives are, in fact, hours spent on gaining medical insight.

Only after such preliminary exploration can the form, scope, and aims of technical aid in MCH programs best be determined and deployed. In fact, an evaluation of problems and their causes is a most urgent research project for developing countries.

Orientation courses conducted by anthropologists, sociologists, and members of the recipient community could well form part of the training of new foreign recruits to underdeveloped areas.

Provision and Training of Personnel

Foreign personnel often work with many disadvantages which prevent them from being as valuable to a country lacking technical experts as they otherwise might be. In Africa, for example, many foreign workers have personal feelings of not belonging, of being unable to identify themselves with the people for whom they are working, or of disillusionment arising from their discovery of the hugeness of some of the problems the countries face and of the smallness of any immediate contribution that they themselves can make.

One of the greatest problems in technical assistance is the language barrier. Without knowledge of the local language, the MCH worker is always one step removed from his patient. Yet few consultants can spare the time to learn one or more new languages while, at the same time, having to learn so much else about the local situation and to deal with the flood of other problems inherent in their work.

To overcome the handicap of his foreignness, the technical assistant must adjust himself as quickly as possible to the culture and society in which he is working. He must make genuine friends among the local people and must try to cast off the blinders imposed by his own culture. He must rid himself of the "Jehovah complex"—the feeling that he unaided can make immense improvements—and must realize that his greatest contribution will be in the degree to which he stimulates the local population to recognize and solve their own problems, and to which he encourages and teaches local colleagues.

The training of local personnel to carry out maternal and child health work is a top priority of technical aid programs in underdeveloped countries. The tutors are often foreigners or local persons who have been trained overseas. Above all they should not teach out of their foreign culture, but should clothe the scientific bones of their instruction with flesh and muscle of the local culture pattern. Often one still finds locally trained workers repeating the "orange juice and bottle-feeding" information that they have unnecessarily and dangerously been taught.[8]

In most developing areas, little money, few teachers, and very few candidates are available with suitable basic qualifications for training to the professional level. Auxiliaries, therefore, have to be trained at lower levels to supplement the work of the few professional workers. The relationship between professional and auxiliary must be both supervisory and advisory— the greater the gap in qualifications, the more emphasis being placed on supervision. Many foreign professionals, however, have never worked with auxiliaries, and so teamwork suffers. Training often has to be radically different than in the teacher's own country and material for teaching, including textbooks, may have to be prepared for the local culture, perhaps even in the vernacular.[9]

The selection and stimulation of local individuals to specialize in pediatrics, once regarded simply as procedures of providing scholarships to Britain, the United States, or elsewhere, are not so simple when viewed from within the country concerned.[6] Does postgraduate training in a highly advanced country equip a person suitably for tackling problems which may have their origin in a cassava and plantain diet? Is not higher education in Europe and America too bound up in Western culture to fit the MCH worker for practice in a totally different society?

The contribution of modern scientific training to the personnel problems of the tropics would be much greater if attention were paid to variations among cultures and societies.

MCH Services

Antenatal care in many societies consists of the use of medicines to prevent the fetus from being harmed by bewitchment or other noxious influences, and of the observance of certain rituals and taboos.[10] Sometimes these practices may be directly harmful in themselves; more frequently they exert an indirect deleterious effect by preventing the mother from seeking modern antenatal care.

Scientific maternity care, no matter how well distributed, may have little appeal to people if it does not cater to traditional beliefs, such as those regarding importance of the way the umbilical cord is cut or the disposal of the placenta. In some societies the person conducting the delivery has traditional duties in connection wtih the care of the home or of the mother during her period of ritual seclusion, which a foreign-trained midwife does not fulfill. Scientific midwifery, therefore, in its techniques, its equipment, and its personnel, may be at variance with local customs and traditions, and unless it can make the necessary adjustments it will probably not be fully utilized.

Some seemingly trivial customs in the immediate postnatal period can have far-reaching consequences. In some societies the tradition of placing cow dung on the baby's umbilical stump is responsible for a high incidence of neonatal tetanus. In others, failure to tie the cord, common among the Baganda, results in hemorrhage and neonatal anemia in the newborn, necessitating emergency transfusion. Understanding of such dangers has to be transmitted through health education to expectant mothers who are going to be delivered at home and through the training courses to the midwives.

In the care of premature babies, special attention has to be paid to keeping up lactation, for failure of the mother to produce breast milk is usually a death sentence for a baby among poor people in tropical regions[11] where hygienic bottle feeding is almost impossible to achieve. Difficulties can arise if the person in charge of a premature unit does not understand the need to encourage mothers to express breast milk until their infants can suckle for themselves.

Infant welfare clinics can rarely limit their clientele to well babies in tropical areas where a procession of sicknesses of one degree or another is the fate of the majority of young children. Failure to understand this is a common Western-based cultural difficulty in MCH assistance, as many workers have tried to make their clinics approximate the streamlined weighing, counseling, and immunizing sessions of North America and Europe.

Tropical hospitals usually have to make arrangements for the admission of a mother with her child. This represents an extremely valuable opportunity for health education and is, of course, imperative for the continued breast feeding of the younger child. But it also leads to a slight change in the nurse's role in the hospital, for the mother does much of the actual nursing of the child such as feeding and bathing, while the nurse mostly supervises and performs more technical tasks such as giving injections.

Many predominantly rural countries have developed a system of health centers, each with a team of medical, nursing, health education, and sanitation workers, combining their efforts to improve the health of the surrounding community. Knowledge of the maternal culture (such as housing, methods of disposal of excreta, water supplies, and available foods), the beliefs and values of the people, and their family structure is vital for the success of this teamwork as it is in all aspects of MCH work.

The provision of medical services sometimes has to be adapted drastically to the way of life of the community. For example, to reach the pastoral Masai in Kenya mobile health centers have been established which sometimes have to concentrate their activities around communal waterholes.

In no other aspect of child health is intimate knowledge of the local culture so absolutely vital for MCH workers as in nutrition; for the nutrition of a community depends not only on the production of foodstuffs, but also on the methods of food storage and food preparation and on the attitudes of the people to foods.

In some tropical regions, as in Buganda in east Africa, sufficient nutrients are available to prevent malnutrition, but despite this, protein-calorie malnutrition of early childhood is common because people do not make full use of the nutritious foods available. [12, 13] This failure to use what is available is often due to the idea that one type of food only is really food, and that other items are of no consequence. These cultural "superfoods" include steamed plantain (*matoke*) in Buganda, rice in much of southeast Asia, and maize in Central America. Also in some places certain types of food are prohibited to the whole community sometimes for elaborate cultural reasons, but sometimes merely because the particular item is not regarded as food.

Man everywhere, even under adverse conditions, eats only part of the actually edible material available. Even the nutritionally hard-pressed Hadza hunters of Tanganyika will not eat the blood of animals and meticulously discard the apex of the hearts of animals they have shot. Moreover, in almost every country there are prevalent concepts regarding the suitability of certain foods for certain people, especially children. Sometimes these ideas are nutritionally harmful, as in Malaya where fish, the main souce of animal protein, is forbidden to children until they are two years old as it is believed that if eaten by a younger child he will get worms.[14] Similarly, in parts of India the age-old *tridosha* (humoral) concept of body physiology means that a "hot" food, such as milk, must not be given to a person euffering from a "hot" illness such as diarrhea, even during recovery. This can have nutritionally ill consequences in a previously subnourished infant.

In many places the ideas that young children need specially prepared foods and three or four meals a day are practically unheard of; people do not make the Westerner's customary association between growth and food, between the qualities of different foods, and between malnutrition and a lack of certain foods. Thus kwashiorkor, although widespread in many tropical regions, is rarely equated with nutrition. Under these circumstances nutrition education is especially difficult, as the people are not motivated to make innovations in their food habits except in times of famine.

There is a widespread belief that eating well during pregnancy is undesirable since this might result in an overlarge fetus with consequent difficulty in labor. In Burma a customary maternal diet of small amounts of boiled polished rice means that the neonate has little stored thiamine. This contributes to infantile beriberi.[15]

However, in some tropical communities the pregnant woman is given a more nutritious diet than usual. Thus among the Basuto in South Africa, pregnant women eat porridge made of sorghum, which is more nutritious than the usual maize. When such a beneficial custom exists, it should be encouraged and incorporated into nutrition education.

Because a people's use of foods is usually so bound up with their whole way of life, dietary custom is one of the most difficult areas of behavior in which to achieve any fundamental change. Small modifications based on indigenous practice are the most likely to be accepted. In Buganda mothers are being encouraged to use the traditional plantain leaf packets for preparing special high-protein meals for babies.[16]

For the majority of infants in tropical countries, breast milk is the *only* food given until the child develops one or two teeth. Thereafter, throughout infancy, breast feeding is continued, providing a small but significant protein supplement as the more digestible and nutritious portions of the available diet—protein foods both of animal and vegetable origin—are gradually added. However, among some tropical people such as the Bemba of Northern Rhodesia, breast milk is not regarded as food and other items are added early to the baby's diet, often leading to gastroenteritis.

Milk powder issued freely in child health clinics tends to encourage mothers to abandon breast feeding in favor of bottle feeding, unless the firm policy is adopted of mixing the powder directly with local foods.

The practice of direct distribution of the powder and the

high-powered advertisement by milk-powder firms are potent
factors in the falling off in breast feeding occurring at the
present day in tropical regions. Among the unfortunate results is an increased incidence of gastroenteritis caused by
pollution of the feeding through unsanitary methods of preparation and of nutritional marasmus caused by overdilution of
the formula.[17]

The causative factors behind protein-calorie malnutrition—
the major nutritional problem of underdeveloped areas—are
rarely entirely nutritional. In Buganda, for example, the high
incidence of kwashiorkor is undoubtedly correlated with the
increasing tendency to stop breast feeding at even earlier ages
and the reliance on a diet of steamed plantain. At the time
of weaning, children are often sent away to relatives, especially
a grandparent, and thus are subjected to emotional as well as
nutritional deprivation.[18] One reason for this geographical
separation at weaning is the belief that one form of kwashiorkor (obwosi) is due to the heat from a mother's pregnant
uterus.

This practice of sending children away often delays treatment of the sick child as an older relative is more likely to
hold the local concept of etiology and to rely on indigenous
methods of treatment. Moreover, if modern therapy is not
rapidly and obviously effective, the child is often removed
from the hospital for herbal treatment at home. In Uganda
a large proportion of milk powder is wasted because people are
not prepared to persist with modern methods of treatment
that take several weeks to produce a cure.

In planning health education, not only do the beliefs, attitudes, and behavior underlying the disease pattern have to be
understood in order to formulate adequate educational objectives, but the structure of the society has to be understood also
to enable the best use to be made of situations and personnel.
Methods and media of communication have to fit in with what
people know and can understand and accept.

In Buganda one of the major diseases of children is hookworm anemia, which lowers hemoglobin levels to a point necessitating emergency blood transfusions. Investigation carried out recently showed that while many adults used adequate pit latrines, children were sent to small, very shallow pits, or perhaps to just a defecating area in the plantain grove. The reason usually given for this practice were that children if permitted to use the adults' latrine would soil it, or fall in, or would see their parents defecating; but another reason seemed to be a general feeling that the feces of younger and older generations should not mix.

Buganda parents of children with hookworm did not notice the pallor of their children's mucous membranes, nor did they attribute the disease to worms. The only intestinal helminths the parents did recognize were roundworms (thought to be due to the mother's unfaithfulness and, therefore, not usually reported), tapeworms, and pinworms. They were aware of a skin disease suffered after working in the fields, which was probably "the ground itch" due to the penetration of the skin by the hookworm larvae, but they tended to confuse the edema of severe hookworm anemia with the similar picture of kwashiorkor for which they had indigenous ideas of causation and treatment. Most peasant families could not afford to buy shoes for their children, who in any case probably gave the larvae plenty of opportunity to penetrate through the back, buttocks, and thighs.

When this information was gathered, pediatricians and other health workers were immediately struck by the unsuitability of their program of health education. They had been placing emphasis on the details of the offending organism's life cycle, using diagrams of the course of the larvae through the lungs and blood vessels—none of which could be understood by the local people. The health education program was, therefore, redrafted to put emphasis on the transmission of the organism from feces on the ground to the human body through the skin, thus producing "ground itch" and the eventual result of loss of blood from the bowel. As visual aids, actual worms expelled from a patient were exhibited, together with before-and-after color photographs of the patient's mucous membranes. The chief emphasis was laid on ways of recognizing anemia and on the necessity of building latrines for children with the hole surrounded by an impervious material. All the old visual aids with dragon-size hookworms, anatomical line drawings, and emphasis on shoes and adult latrines were discarded.

With rapid culture changes and urbanization in most developing areas, new problems of health education have arisen, and will do so increasingly in the future. We have already noted one of the most serious, the abandonment of breast feeding. The difficulty in propagandizing against bottle feeding is that many members of the elite do not breast-feed their children. Efforts to persuade the poor to feed through the breast rather than bottles are apt to be interpreted as efforts to withhold something from the masses. Moreover, campaigns to encourage breast feeding are likely to make mothers self-conscious about it and so interfere with the complex psychological reflexes which seem to require that the whole process be taken for granted if it is to function naturally.

In Conclusion

Thus we see that a society's traditional food habits, child-rearing practices, and habits of personal hygiene along with other cultural factors shape the disease patterns of a community. The structure of the community, the functioning of the family and its attitudes toward innovation, the beliefs and attitudes of the people in regard to childbearing, disease causation, and food must all be taken into account in determining the work, the personnel, and the emphases of child health services. There must also be an awareness that the changes induced by the agents of modern scientific medicine are themselves not always beneficial, so that potential deleterious effects can be anticipated, and, if possible, prevented in advance rather than regretted later.

Cultural inexperience is expensive and wasteful. One million pounds of milk powder or a corps of experts may make no impression whatsoever on a problem, if the local culture pattern is ignored.

References

1. Foster, G. M.: "Guidelines to community development programs." *Public Health Reports,* January 1955.

2. ————: Relationship between theoretical and applied anthropology; a public health program analysis. *Human Organisation,* Fall 1952.

3. Paul, B. D. (ed.) : *Health, culture, and community.* Russell Sage Foundation, New York. 1955.

4. Edge, P. G.: *Vital statistics and public health work in the tropics.* Ballière, Tindall & Cox, London, England. 1947.

5. Schofield, F. D.; Tucker, V. M.; Westbrook, G. R.: "Neonatal tetanus in New Guinea." *British Medical Journal,* September 1961.

6. Jelliffe, D. B.: "Education for child health workers in developing regions." *Postgraduate Medical Journal (London),* February 1962.

7. Jelliffe, D. B.; Bennett, F. J.; Stroud, E. C.; Novotny, N.; Karrach, K.; Musoke, L. K.; Jelliffe, E. F. P.: "The health of Bachiga children." *American Journal of Tropical Medicine and Hygiene,* May 1961.

8. Jelliffe, D. B.: *Infant nutrition in the subtropics and tropics.* WHO Monograph Series No. 29, Geneva, 1955.

9. ———— (ed.) : *Child health in the tropics.* Edward Arnold, London, England. 1962.

10. Jelliffe, D. B.; Bennett, F. J.: "Worldwide care of the mother and newborn child." *Clinical Obstetrics and Gynecology,* March 1962.

11. Yankauer, Alfred: "Intercultural communication in technical consultation." *Children,* September-October 1959.

12. Jelliffe, D. B.: "Cultural blocks and protein malnutrition in early childhood in rural West Bengal." *Pediatrics,* July 1957.

13. Jelliffe, D. B.; Bennett, F. J.: "Cultural and anthropological factors in infant and maternal nutrition." *Federation Proceedings,* March 1961.

14. Dean, R. F.: "Kwashiorkor in Malaya; the clinical evidence" (Part II). *Journal of Tropical Pediatrics and African Child Health (Kampala),* September 1961.

15. Foll, C. V.: "An account of some of the beliefs and superstitions about pregnancy, parturition, and infant health in Burma."

Journal of Tropical Pediatrics and African Child Health (*Kampala*), September 1959.

16. Jelliffe, D. B.; Morton, C.; Nansubuga, G.: *"Ettu* pastes in infant feeding in Buganda." *Journal of Tropical Medicine and Hygiene* (*London*), February 1962.

17. Welbourn, H. F.: "Bottle-feeding problem of civilization." *Journal of Tropical Pediatrics and African Child Health* (*Kampala*), March 1958.

18. Geber, M.; Dean, R. F.: "The psychological changes accompanying kwashiorkor." *Courrier,* December 1957.

3

Food Habits—An Anthropologist's Views

George H. Fathauer, Ph.D.

George H. Fathauer, Ph.D., is Professor of Anthropology, Miami University (Ohio). His interest and research has been in social anthropology, especially among the Mohave Indians. His most recent publications include the following: "Mohave Ghost Doctor," American Anthropologist; *"Structure and Causation of Mohave Warfare,"* Southwestern Journal of Anthropology; *and "Triobriand,"* Matrilineal Kinship. *Dr. Fathauer's article "Food Habits—An Anthropologist's View" is reprinted with his permission and that of the* Journal of the American Dietetic Association *from the* Journal, *Vol. 37 (October, 1960), pp. 335–338.*

In one of the oil-rich countries of the Middle East, an American company became concerned about the inadequate nutrition of its Arab workers. As a means of increasing efficiency, but also with praiseworthy interest in improving the lot of the inhabitants of the country, the company decided to provide one nutritious meal for each worker on the job, at a nominal charge, far below the cost of the meal. A well-equipped cafeteria was built, and the program was inaugurated. The company felt, at the very least, that it would gain the good will of the workers. To its dismay, the result was the direct opposite. The workers expressed extreme displeasure over the arrangements, maintaining that this was another example of insulting American behavior—an expression of the belief that the workers were inferiors who need not be treated

with dignity. Dismayed by this reaction, the company investigated to find out what had gone wrong. The answer proved
to be the cafeteria pattern of providing the food. In this country, only beggars stood in line to be fed. Asking the workers
to pass through the cafeteria line was insulting them by imply-
ing that they were beggars, without self-respect, dependent
on the company for a handout.

Another illustration of Arab attitudes toward food is the
rather amusing story of a newly arrived diplomat from one
of the Middle Eastern countries who attended an elaborate
Washington dinner. After the affair was over, the man implored another Arab who was familiar with the United States
to take him someplace where he could eat; he was famished.
The experienced Arab laughed and said, "Don't you know
that when you say 'no, thank you,' Americans assume that you
do not want what has been offered." It is good manners for a
guest at an Arab dinner to refuse the food offered to him while
the host implores him again and again to eat. Finally, the
guest succumbs to the host's pleading. The Arab had refused
each course at the banquet, as his code of manners dictated,
only to find that it was removed by the waiters who accepted
his refusal as final.[2]

Next I should like to describe two incidents involving public health projects. As part of a program for improving health
in the underdeveloped countries, some American educational
films were sent abroad. One film showing how to bathe a baby
in a bathinette horrified a group of mothers in India who
maintained that American parents were guilty of cruelty for
bathing infants in stagnant water instead of in running water.
A UNESCO publication *Cultural Patterns and Technical
Change*,[3] edited by Margaret Mead, describes the following
experience of a public health nurse who had been attempting
to persuade a group of Mexican immigrant mothers in the
United States to abandon their customary diet and to feed
their babies milk. She had been violently condemning their
traditional diet, but finally, when she discovered that she was

making no progress, she suggested that they feed their babies the water in which their beans were cooked. The babies began to thrive, and when the nurse later pointed out to the mothers the supposed effects of the bean-water, they replied: "Oh, but we are feeding them milk now, too. We have followed your advice about the milk ever since you stopped calling our own food bad."

Understanding and Respecting Others' Cultures

All of these incidents are tied together by a common thread. They all involve misunderstandings based on the failure to understand and respect a different way of life. Anthropologists call such a way of life a "culture." They have devoted many years of study to describing hundreds of distinct cultures throughout all the continents. One conclusion of all this research may be simply summarized by saying that the people of different societies live, to some degree, in separate cultural worlds. This statement, i.e., there are tremendous gulfs separating people, tends to be resisted by many, especially Americans, who want to believe that "people are pretty much alike wherever you find them."

Recognizing the significance of cultural differences, for one thing, means that much effort must be made to understand the other fellow. It is much easier to react to values and attitudes that do not agree with ours by classifying such behavior as "crazy," "illogical," or "stupid." If people are different, it is because they have misunderstood reality. Our own view, of course, is the "correct" version of the real situation. This attitude is characteristic of most people in almost all societies, but the study of anthropology seems to indicate that it is responsible for many failures in intercultural relations.

Let us briefly summarize some anthropologic conclusions about culture. It consists of values, attitudes, habits, and customs that are acquired by learning. This learning starts with the earliest experiences of the child. Much of it is not deliberately taught by anyone. Some of it is largely unconscious because it is so thoroughly internalized. Culture, the anthropologist believes, goes deep.

There are certain general similarities in all cultures because all human beings must solve certain fundamental problems of existence. They all must eat, drink, protect themselves from the elements, cooperate—minimally at least—with others, face the terrors of illness and death, and so on. The ways in which these needs are met, however, may vary greatly from one culture to another.

The fact that culture is learned means that it is subject to change, and this is the most optimistic fact about human behavior. Some relatively superficial aspects of culture change readily; other parts, especially basic values and beliefs, change more slowly and sometimes only with great difficulty. Many people who see American Indians working in varied occupations, speaking English and wearing standard clothing, are surprised to read anthropologic testimony to the effect that many of the basic values and beliefs of their Indian heritage have remained intact to this day, and in some cases are growing stronger. Public attention recently has been directed to a revival of their ancient religious practices by several Indian groups.

Problems in Changing Cultures

Much effort in the modern world is being devoted to attempts to deliberately change certain patterns of culture. The anthropologist recognizes that this can be done successfully, but he insists that it is a mistake to think that mere good intentions are enough to do the job. If we desire to introduce change in people's behavior, we will be wise to study carefully the existing cultural beliefs before undertaking the project. One should not be surprised to encounter opposition. To successfully introduce significant cultural changes increasingly demands special training and a willingness to do research—a kind of "social engineering" as it has been called. Without this, disillusionment and failure are likely to result.

One further comment of a general sort should be made. Many people who accept the significance of cultural differences among distinct societies will balk at recognizing the same principle within one society. Social research has demonstrated the existence of many significant cultural differences within modern American society. These subcultural variations may be regional, religious, rural as contrasted with urban, occupational, or based on social class differences, to name only a few of the most important. Thus the necessity of considering cultural differences when trying to bring about a change of behavior within our own society is as pressing as when we are dealing with a foreign society.

Food Habits—A Part of Culture

Let us now turn directly to the subject of food habits viewed as part of culture. "Food" is always defined culturally. The same plant may be defined as edible by one society, inedible by another. The pig is clearly not a food animal in a Jewish or Moslem country. Increasing the supply of cattle in Hindu territory will not improve the diet of the people. These definitions of food, of course, have no reference to the nutritional value of the material. It seems likely that all societies ignore certain plants or animals in their environment that possess nutritional value. Even our own science-based society ignores certain items having nutritional value that are eaten by other societies. The point seems obvious: food is primarily a matter of cultural definition for most people, with the possible exception of specialists in the nutritional area. Nutritional studies may overlook certain items of diet having important food value because the cultural background of the expert does not include them.

The cultural aspects of food do not merely involve definition as such. There is also a considerable symbolism associated with particular items of the diet. Mead has said: "In most societies, food is the focus of emotional associations, a channel for interpersonal relations, for the communication of love or discrimination or disapproval; it usually has a symbolic reference."[3] Food habits apparently become quite deeply imbedded in the personalities of people raised in a particular cultural pattern. One evidence of this is the sacred symbolism frequently associated with food; almost all religions of the world have certain rituals involving special foods. The sharing of food almost universally symbolizes a rather high degree of social intimacy and acceptance. In many simple societies, the climax of the wedding ceremony comes when the bride and groom jointly eat certain special foods. Eating together is a widespread social lubricant in our own society in all classes and regions.

Food in Family Relationships

One reason for the tenacity of food habits is their association with family sentiments. Food is one of the basic media through which attitudes and sentiments are communicated to the child. Mother receives her definition for the child in association with feeding experiences. The family meal situation is one of the most important events in producing morale or a sense of unity. The roles of close relatives, father, brother, sister, grandmother are clearly illustrated for the child as the family eats together. Certain foods eaten early in life become associated with these family sentiments, thereby acquiring the power to trigger a flood of affectionate childhood memories. The family eating together, in privacy, also becomes a major value in some societies. Late in World War II, after the liberation of Greece, some direct food relief was provided for the inhabitants. It was observed that most residents of Athens preferred to eat cold food in their unheated houses than hot food in warm soup kitchens.[3]

The point, I think, is clear. Some foods in all societies become the focus of deep and persistent sentiments that have little connection with nutritional value. When we condemn a person's undesirable food habits, we may be degrading his mother's memory and his nostalgic vision of his childhood family. Such symbolism attaches not only to specific foods, but to certain meals as well.

Food may be eaten at certain times of the day primarily for satisfying hunger; other meals have a strong symbolic content. The family sentiment associated with "dinner" in our society is much stronger than that associated with "lunch" for most people. The pattern of dinner is more complex; the symbolism is more obvious. If we wish to understand fully the dietary culture of any group, we must study the patterning of meals and the meaning of each meal in the life of the people. The patterns of choosing, preparing, and consuming food must be fitted into the total pattern of the culture.

Significance of Culture to Food Specialists

What is the significance of all this for modern food specialists? Science and its method are a part of our culture. The development of a science of foods has meant rapid growth in our knowledge of the nutritional requirements for health. Since health is a major value of our culture, dietitians feel that it is their duty to transfer this knowledge to people who lack an optimal diet. The achievement of this objective frequently involves a change in food habits. Let us attempt to connect up the previous comments on culture with attempts to introduce dietary change.

If members of our own group have certain deficiencies in their usual diet, it may be relatively easy to bring about improvement. If the people concerned are middle-class, urban Americans who have been reared to respect science and accept its results, there may be little difficulty in introducing a new food into their diet. The problem may be merely a tactical one: what means of communication—radio, television, or magazines—should be used to achieve the desired results? We are dealing, in this case, with people who share to a substantial degree the dietitian's own set of values and attitudes toward food and health.

However, the problem of changing food habits becomes more complex when the values of the people to be influenced are different from those of the dietitian. Americans of lower socio-economic class or recent immigrants of diverse ethnic backgrounds may not have familiarity with, or respect for, science. Other values may be more important than good diet. The bare announcement that changing certain food habits will improve health may not carry much weight. When workers who traditionally ate a diet of beans and pork, when available, obtained jobs in war industry at the end of the Great Depression, their increased affluence did not automatically lead to a better diet, even if educational programs were developed to inform them. A radio or a flashy used car frequently had a higher priority in their scheme of values than a healthful diet. We may disagree with such a set of values, but criticism will not yield the desired result. If we wish to improve diet in this kind of situation, we must attempt to understand the food culture of the people involved.

Symbolism of Food

What is the symbolism associated with important foods? What qualities of these foods have value for the people who consume them? Much effort has been expended in certain parts of Asia trying to correct the dietary deficiency resulting from overwhelming reliance on polished rice. The attempt has largely failed because the *whiteness* of the rice is highly valued, leading to a rejection of much more healthful unpolished rice. Similarly, introducing wheat in the form of dark bread leads to rejection, while white bread is accepted in these areas. Recognition of the cultural value of whiteness can lead to experimentation which may produce an acceptable type of rice which still contains the vital nutritional values. The general conclusion to be drawn from hundreds of such examples from different countries, as well as from different classes or ethnic groups in the United States, is that it is important to try to bring about changes that are in keeping with the established food habits of the people and which are acceptable within the framework of their value system. A corollary proposition is: criticism of the nutritionally inadequate foods is likely to arouse stubborn opposition based on deep-rooted sentiments associated with such foods, which will compound the difficulty of introducing change. The aim of the dietitian should be to set up a situation in which people will pleasantly and easily eat the right foods.

Introducing change in food habits may also require an understanding of the symbolic aspects of the different meals. Change probably can be more easily introduced in a meal which is not the focus of deep family sentiments than in one which is. In urban areas, lunch may be a more opportune time to introduce dietary improvements than dinner. In rural areas, where the main family meal is sometimes served at noon, supper may offer the least resistance. The patterning of one meal may be significant. If one type of food is traditionally regarded as of major importance, change can probably be more easily introduced in the subsidiary elements of the meal.

Use Caution in Changing Cultural Factors

Anthropologists who have studied numerous cases of cultural change would add a word of caution, even where modifications are successfully introduced. There is always danger that the expert will introduce changes largely on the basis of his own cultural experiences. This may lead to a failure to recognize the total patterning of the culture which is being modified. As a consequence, a change introduced to produce improvement may result in unforeseen difficulties. A quotation from the UNESCO publication previously mentioned illustrates the point:[3] "We upset dietary balance by persuading Spanish-American school children in New Mexico to eat white bread instead of cold corn *tortillas,* when their main source of calcium came from the limewater in which the corn of the *tortillas* had been soaked. We persuaded their mothers to substitute canned spinach for wild greens, and, when there was no money to buy spinach, the children went without greens." To emphasize the point again: every culture has pattern of organization, and unless we understand the cultural context of food habits, we may, with the best of intentions, introduce harmful disruptions.

Summary

My assignment has been to discuss food habits in general rather than concrete terms. I have no special competence in the area of dietetics. I have been using the approach that an anthropologist would take to any aspect of culture. Dietitians are confronted by diverse food habits in concrete terms. You are faced with the important task of improving the dietary practices of the American public. I hope that my remarks, which are not intended to tell you how to solve specific problems, may be useful in giving you something to think about— a point of view.

Trying to help people for their own good may sometimes be a frustrating business. They may stubbornly oppose efforts made for their benefit. Familiarity with the facts of culture helps one to avoid disillusionment. Change is possible, but it is frequently not accomplished easily. Human beings are exasperating creatures. The anthropologist is convinced, however, that their apparently illogical behavior is understandable when we become familiar with their cultural assumptions. Stupid, illogical *individuals* may resist our attempts to improve them in *all* cultures, but *groups* of people are never stupid or illogical. If we encounter group opposition to change, it is because a cultural difference is involved which demands an objective attempt to understand rather than condemn.

References

1. Presented before the Ohio Dietetic Association in Cincinnati, on May 6, 1960.
2. Hall, E. T., Jr., Orientation and Training in Government for Work Overseas. Human Organization 15, no. 1, 1956.
3. World Federation for Mental Health, *Cultural Patterns and Technical Change*. Mead, M., ed. Tensions and Tech. Ser. no. 8. Paris, France: UNESCO, 1953. (Available in U.S. from: Intl. Documents Serv., Columbia Univ. Press, N. Y. 27) .

4

Cancer in Situ of the Cervix
Cultural Clues to Reactions

By Ethel J. Alpenfels

Ethel J. Alpenfels, Sc.D., is Professor of Anthropology, New York University, School of Education. She is a nationally known lecturer and authority on social behavior. She has carried out a three year study, "Will Facts Change Attitudes?," under the auspices of the National Conference of Christians and Jews. She has served as Fellow of the Encyclopedia Britanica and edited the one-million word section on Anthropology. Recently, she served as Chairman, New York University Solar Stove Project to India, sponsored by the Ford Foundation. Her writings and publications are many. Among her latest are her new audio-visual series on Anthropology: Man on The Move, *Miller-Brody, 1969 and* Japan: A Study in Depth, *Warren Schloats, 1968. "Cancer in Situ of the Cervix: Cultural Clues to Reactions" is reprinted with permission of the author and of the American Journal of Nursing Company from* The American Journal of Nursing, *Vol. 4, April, 1964, pp. 83–86.*

An eminent physician recently proposed marriage between the field of medicine and that of anthropology. Some members of both families have long hoped for a public announcement but, whether or not the offer is accepted, it is high time that the two disciplines concerned with the study of man begin "to go steady." For the solution of a number of medical problems, perhaps including those clustering around cancer, depends not only on technical skill but on early detection and rehabilitation. These rest, in turn, on improved health attitudes and health habits of the American public.[1]

This gap between knowledge and action has been a pivotal problem for all health practitioners and investigators, especially the public health educator. What people *know* about illness and disease and what people *do* about programs aimed at detection and prevention may be as important as the technical problems of illness and its prognosis. Personal and social factors do affect the organism, as every nurse knows, and the social dynamics of illness calls for an immediate and shared attack through the collaboration of medicine and social science.[2] Can the miracle of modern medicine, in either its theoretical or applied aspects, provide complete answers to disease causation if the concepts of the behavioral sciences which bear directly on such problems are ignored?

Whatever answers may be given to this question, the crucial fact is that there is need for a closer relationship between these two disciplines which are equally involved, in their special ways, with the behavior problems of man.[3] This collaboration, furthermore, is made easier by the number of areas of concern they hold in common. Such factors as individual attitudes toward pain or illness, as trained observers in both fields have pointed out, may interfere with therapy and well-being sometimes as effectively as the disease process itself.[4] Likewise, human relationships fermenting within the context of the group pressures within a society may evoke responses which are not conducive to good health habits.

Response to Disease

There is, indeed, a growing body of literature on the variety of ways in which the individual or a group may respond to a disease threat. In the communicable diseases, a number of social factors, among them social class conformity or the stresses arising out of the competitive nature of American society, have been identified. Likewise in the chronic degenerative diseases, especially those which develop after many symptomless years, clues have been discovered to the kinds of cultural barriers which interfere with early detection. Public response to programs of cancer screening as well as findings on response to public health preventive measures for tuberculosis, rheumatic fever, influenza, and poliomyelitis demonstrate the network of conflicting social pressures which smother individual action.[1, 5-9]

Thus, it is obvious that medical researchers and medical practitioners have not neglected the social environment of illness. Rather they have tended to ignore the methods and the conceptual framework of those disciples whose major area of research is man in his social and cultural environment. They have done this primarily because, explicitly and implicitly, they feel that the behavioral sciences lack verifiable substance and that they are, at the present, inadequate to meet the strict requirements of medical science. Whether this belief is true or untrue, there are central concepts, tentative formulations, and methodological tools which bear directly on medical problems.

On the other hand, social scientists must also bear their share of the responsibility. Interested as the social scientist is in group processes, he must also be aware of the goals of the medical profession. Only then will his research be relevant and able to provide answers to important questions which medical science is asking.

The nurse, meanwhile, has been trapped between the two factions. Perhaps more than either of them, the nurse is not only made aware of the special concerns of medicine but, through day-by-day experience, knows the hospital as a social institution. She lives within the hierarchy of precedent, deals daily with the personal and social factors which bear on illness and, finally, comes to know the individual patient in a way that neither the doctor nor the social scientist can. The cultural milieu of the hospital with all of its dos and don'ts, all of its unique folkways and mores, results in a laboratory population for the nurse.

Such a laboratory is useless if it is unrecognized. This population then becomes simply another community of persons bound together by their common escape from a larger society unless the technical, the organic, and the social understandings in medicine are brought into focus. Even in illness, the individual is not free from his cultural pressures or social environment. He reacts, as anthropologists perceive the individual, as an *organism* in his physical habitat, as a *group member* in his society, and as a *person* in his culture.[10] It is with the person that anthropology as a discipline is primarily concerned: how the value orientations of American culture permeate behavior and perceptions in the hospital and to what extent these values take the place of what has long been called human nature.

Where to Look

We do not know to what extent nor exactly how an individual is able to resist programs of prevention and detection of disease. We know only that he does. Why, in a society that all authorities tell us is "future-oriented," does the individual refuse to act on the findings of the most future-oriented science for personal well-being, medicine and health education? The cultural barriers are often higher than most of us recognize. If they are neglected or negated, therapy in fact cannot occur. Where can one look for clues?

Talcott Parsons, in his classic article on illness, put his finger on a neglected institution, even though it is the most talked about unit, the American family.[11] Of special relevance here is his concern with the hospital as a home-away-from-home, even though the two differ in very fundamental respects. Certain analogies will occur immediately to the reader. Dr. Parsons' sensitive analysis of the child in the family and the sick person in the hospital, however, raises the question of why we, alone among the societies of the world, "are so ready to send our sick outside the family to special medical institutions." Dr. Parsons writes:

Illness is an escape from the pressures of ordinary life. In a society such as our own, illness is a very strategic expression of deviance; first, because our culture enforces an unusually high level of activity, independence and responsibility on the average individual; and second, because it connects so closely with the residua of childhood dependency. . . . From the point of view of the stability of the social system, therefore, too frequent resort to this avenue of escape presents a serious danger. This is the primary context in which we think of illness as an institutionalized role and its relation to therapy as an important mechanism of social control.[11]

Modesty's Roots

If one thinks of disease as a form of deviant behavior and if it connects so closely with childhood learning patterns, as Dr. Parsons indicates, a crucial area to examine for roots of resistance is the cultural conditioning of children.

One of the deeply rooted patterns of childhood training is that of feelings grouped around modesty. Immediately at birth and with economy of training, as Ruth Benedict has written:

We waste no time in clothing the baby, and, in contrast to many societies where the child runs naked till it is ceremoniously given its skirt or its pubic sheath at adolescence the child's training fits it precisely for adult convention.[12]

One is rarely aware of how deep and with what precision feelings of modesty are embedded in our culture until we see and feel the response of students in a classroom to films of other cultures in which the skin is worn unadorned well into the teens. False modesty on the ward can be an irritant to the patients' recovery and to the nurses' nerves. But modesty is taught in childhood, and such deeply embedded patterns of childhood can and do surface. This is what the nurse sees.

We recognize patterns of modesty in other societies and even among our various ethnic groups in the United States. Often, however, the professional does not act on his knowledge. Mac-

Gregor reports the case of a pregnant Italian woman about to have a pelvic examination who angered the gynecologist because of her tears and behavior.[13] Finally, the physician threw down his gloves and stamped out of the room. "She must be crazy," he said. "She has had six children and puts up a fuss over a simple examination." The nurse, left with the patient, discovered that all of her children had been delivered by a midwife in Sicily. She had expected to be examined by a woman doctor and was horrified when a male physician walked into the room.

We are learning to recognize modesty among various ethnic groups but, at the same time, we fail to recognize an equally deep commitment to modesty by the much-studied middle class. Modesty may be one of the key factors in resistance to cervical examination in cancer detection programs. It is also a key factor which may help to explain the reluctance of nurses and other health-oriented professionals to be examined at regular periods?

Embedded Feelings

Perhaps the point about the strength of conditioning may be made more clearly if, for a moment, we consider another habit of conditioning the child for later life. It is a habit we talk about more than modesty but it has relevance as well for hospital life: conditioning to eat three meals a day. As Benedict writes, ". . . the training begins at birth, and no crying of the child and no inconvenience to the mother is allowed to interfere." By two years of age, the child is on the adult feeding schedule. By the time he reaches adolescence, he is eating six meals a day—for the coffee break has become a national institution. By young adulthood, we learn "that the way to a man's heart is through his stomach." Our national defense, likewise, depends on three meals a day for "our army marches on its stomach." Our emotions find their outlet there for we "feel things in the pit of our stomachs," and the condemned man is always given his choice of a "last meal" and newspapers faithfully record his choice. And, what is more talked about, complained over, and reported than what we eat and how and why?

These areas of conditioning show how deeply feelings become embedded. Other areas may be less obvious. Early conditioning needs to be examined in specific areas relating to cancer. How, for example, do Americans really handle fear? How do nurses deal with the fears engendered around terminal cancer patients? As with modesty and three meals a day, there are deeply hidden fears about life and death, about the realities of living, about such words as "cancer" itself, that are difficult enough for the physician dealing with technical problems. How about health preventive measures? How difficult for the nurse who must face them daily on the ward?

Each culture has its own unique attitudes toward life and death. In a society that can spend so much money on outer space or electronic computers, there is urgent need for equal amounts on what motivates human behavior in illness. If the computers are not to give both the questions *and* the answers to man, all disciplines concerned must begin to talk and work together.

References

1. Kelly, Janet S., and Thomson, Isabella C. *Anthropology, A Catalyst in Health Promotion.* New York, New York University, 1963. (Unpublished paper)

2. Simmons, L. W., and Wolff, H. G. *Social Science in Medicine.* New York, Russell Sage Foundation, 1954.

3. *Ibid,* pp. 194–201.

4. Zborowski, Mark. Cultural components in response to pain. *J. Soc. Issues* 8: (4)16–30, 1952.

5. Conference on Behavioral Sciences in Cancer Control. *Papers presented at . . . Johns Hopkins University, March 2–3, 1962.*

6. U.S. Public Health Service. *Public Participation in Medical Screening Programs; A Socio-Psychological Study,* by G. M. Hochbaum. (Publication No. 572) Washington, D.C., U.S. Government Printing Office, 1958.

7. Heinzelmann, Fredrich. Factors inffuencing prophylaxis behavior with respect to rheumatic fever. *J. Health Hum. Behav.* 3:73, Summer 1962.

8. U.S. Public Health Service. *The Impact of Asian influenza on Community Life; A Study in Five Cities,* by I. M. Rosenstock and others. (Publication No. 776) Washington, D.C., U.S. Government Printing Office, 1960.

9. Rosenstock, I. M., et al., Why people fail to seek poliomyelitis vaccination. *Public Health Rep.* 74:98–103, Feb. 1959.

10. Simmons and Wolff, pp. 50–82.

11. Parsons, Talcott, and Rox, Renée. Illness, therapy and the modern urban American family. *J. Soc. Issues* 8: (4) 31–55, 1952.

12. Benedict, Ruth. Continuities and discontinuities in cultural conditioning. *Psychiatry* 1:161–167, May 1938.

13. MacGregor, Frances, M. C. *Social Science in Nursing.* New York, Russell Sage Foundation, 1960, p. 236.

Part II

AMERICANS—INDIANS, MEXICAN AMERICANS

Introduction

Though the tremendous promise of anthropology in public health has too seldom been realized, recent research with population groups indigenous to the United States indicates that an amalgamation of anthropology and medical science in public health care might prove to be a most effective and foremost inroad to acculturation.

In the main, the research that follows was selected to show contrast between the health behavior of the more primitive groups and the more advanced ethnic groups in the culture and to indicate the impact religion or religio-magical belief has on health behavior. A second aim was to show that the technically less advanced groups tend to accept professional health care when the methods and techniques are offered with recognition of and respect for (and often in conjunction with) traditional ways.

The Navaho culture seems to be one that has judiciously extracted elements of other cultures—especially those elements shown to hold unlimited potentials for improvement of Navaho life. In a like manner, recent investigations by a Cornell University health team reveals that the Navaho's favorable reaction to modern medical and health practices might be owing to observed effectiveness in many instances. However, their recent acceptance of health programs is also directly related to (1) the increased tolerance and appreciation shown by health workers for the Navaho's way of life (including his spirit beliefs), and (2) a genuine effort on

81

the part of health workers to inject scientific methods into the Navaho's cultural framework.

In recording their experiences with the Navaho in maternal and child health care, Loughlin, Bailey, and Wauneka find that factors that influence Navaho acceptance of health education and medical procedures include: (1) increasing knowledge of, as well as a sensitivity to, cultural values and fears that serve as emotional blocks, (2) donors' establishment of rapport and identification with the recipients, (3) donors' capitalizing on any parallels between scientific medical practice and Navaho medical practice.

According to Ruebel, the Mexican-Americans, like the Navahos, evince changing concepts of health and disease; however, they hold to a belief that certain specific maladies are either within the realm of God or the realm of the devil. They further believe that these illnesses affect only people of Mexican extraction and are beyond the range of knowledge and treatment of the technically trained.

Further research by Hostetler with the Amish (not appearing here) offers some parallelism when compared with the Navahos and the Mexican-Americans. His findings show folk practitioners and quack healers very much in evidence; however, contrary to popular beliefs, modern medical practices have penetrated Amish life to an appreciable extent. According to Hostetler, there is evidence of a folk pragmatism—a selective principle that influences the choice of treatment methods.[1]

---

1. *Hostetler, John A. "Folk and Scientific Medicine in Amish Society,"* Human Organization, *22, no. 4 (Winter, 1963–1964), pp. 269–75.*

5

Patterns of Health and Disease Among the Navahos

John Adair, Kurt Deuschle, and Walsh McDermott

John Adair, Ph.D., is Professor of Anthropology, San Francisco State College. Previously, he served at Cornell University and the University of New Mexico. He has researched and written extensively in the area of Indian life and culture. His publications include: First Look at Strangers, *Rutgers University Press, 1959;* Navajo and Pueblo Silversmiths, *University of Oklahoma Press, 1954; (co-author),* People of the Middle Place: A Study of the Zuni Indians, *Human Relations Area Files, Inc., 1966; and (co-author)* Hastings to Culloden, *Dufour, 1964.*

Kurt W. Deuschle, M.D., is Chairman and Professor, Department of Community Medicine, Mount Sinai School of Medicine, New York. He was formerly affiliated with the Department of Public Health and Preventive Medicine, The New York Hospital-Cornell Medical Center, New York.

Dr. Walsh McDermott, M.D., is Livingston Farrand Professor, Department of Public Health, New York Hospital at Cornell University Medical Center. Among the professional organizations with which he is affiliated are the National Academy of Science, American Public Health Association, and the American Medical Association. He has been the recipient of the Lasker Award and the first recipient of the National Institutes of Health Lectureship Award, (1963). He is co-editor, Cecil-Loeb Textbook of Medicine, *(12th edition), Saunders, 1967.*

"Patterns of Health and Disease Among the Navahos" is reprinted with the permission of the authors and of The American Academy of Political and Social Science from The Annals, *Vol. 311 (May, 1957,) pp. 80–94.*

ABSTRACT: Community patterns of our Indian citizens range from ordinary American communities to ways of life more comparable with those seen in parts of Asia or South America. In each type the disease picture can be expected to be different and the ways of dealing with it must necessarily be somewhat different. The Navaho tribe is the largest Indian tribe, a group whose ways of life perhaps differ the most from the rest of the United States. The broad principles revealed in an analysis of Navaho health are applicable to other tribes, although the particular health situation of another tribe would depend on the circumstances of its tribal life.

It has long been recognized that the particular pattern of a community determines in large measure the particular diseases to which it is most subject. The community patterns of the United States Indian citizens range all the way from communities essentially the same as the rest of the United States to ways of life more comparable with those seen in many parts of Asia or South America. In each of these different types of community the disease picture can be expected to be different and the ways of dealing with it must necessarily be somewhat different. It has seemed reasonable, therefore, in attempting the present discussion of Indian health problems, to select a single tribe for primary consideration. The tribe so selected—the Navaho—represents by far the largest single tribe and is a group whose ways of life perhaps differ the most from the rest of the United States. It is believed that the broad principles revealed in an analysis of Navaho health are equally applicable to the other tribes, but the particulars of the health situation of another tribe would depend on the particular circumstances of the tribal life.

The Navaho Indians live in northern Arizona, New Mexico, and southern Utah on a reservation extending over 15,000,000 acres—an area as large as the state of West Virginia. In 1868, when the Navaho returned from their forced captivity at

Fort Sumner in eastern New Mexico, it was estimated that the tribe numbered around 10,000. It has expanded very rapidly in the last century, and today the population exceeds 80,000.

Large as their reservation is, it is no longer able to support the tribe; severe erosion has denuded much of the land and thousands of Navahoes have sought employment out of the area. They work as itinerant crop pickers, on the railroads all over the Western states, and at other jobs which for the most part require only unskilled labor.

The reservation is located on the southern edge of the Colorado Plateau at an altitude ranging from 4,500 feet to over 10,000 feet on the crest of the mountain range which roughly follows the New Mexico–Arizona border. The climate of this region, in contrast to that of the southern Arizona lowland desert, is temperate in the summer and cold in the winter, with a great range in the daily temperature the year round. There is little precipitation—from up to seven inches at the lower altitude to around twenty inches in a few mountain areas. However, during the last seven years the whole Southwest has been in severe drought and there has been only a fraction of even the customary small rainfall.

The Navaho are a Southern Athabaskan-speaking people closely related linguistically, but not culturally, to the Apache and more remotely to the Northern Athabaskan tribes of Alaska and Canada. Centuries ago the ancestors of the Navaho and the Apache migrated southward and reached the northern limit of their present range by the sixteenth century or earlier. The newcomers were hunters and gatherers; these occupations reflected a primitive way of life compared to that of the Pueblo Indians who already inhabited the more fertile regions of this plateau country. Even in the fourteenth century the Navahos were highly eclectic and adopted that which was to their advantage and rejected that for which they felt no need. They took over agriculture, pottery making, weaving, and other technologies from the town-dwelling Indians. But they rejected village living and the socioreligious structure of Pueblo society. The traits of Pueblo religion which they did borrow became modified to support a religion primarily concerned with curing practices rather than the fertility and rain-making goal of Pueblo ritual.

All of Navaho history has been a succession of judicious borrowing from other peoples with whom they came in contact. During the subsequent centuries they took over the idea of using horses, sheep, and cattle from the Spanish-speaking colonists in New Spain. As a result, their economic base shifted from primary dependence on agriculture to livestock raising and the raiding of settlements in the Southwest.

This history has a relevance to the present-day health picture, for the Navaho are still a changing people. Now, as earlier, they pick and choose what seems to "fit" with their way of life and pass up what does not. This process extends to their present-day attitude and behavior towards Western medicine, as well as to other aspects of twentieth-century civilization.

Navaho Culture

One of the remarkable features of Navaho life today is that the central core of Navaho culture, their religion, is still a vigorous and going concern. The Christian missionaries have not made the inroads they have made among Indian tribes in other parts of the United States.

The Navahos have also clung to certain other traditional ways; given their physical environment, these have proven very practical. For example, housing on most of the reservation is but a modification of the type of structure their ancestors brought with them from the North centuries ago. The hogan, a one-room log house (in some places built of stone) remains hemispherical in shape with a mud floor. Cradleboards are still used by most mothers as a convenient way of carrying their babies and providing a secure place for sleep. Sheep and goats are still their most prized material possession. The pastoral economy has shaped the land settlement pattern, determined the course of daily life within the family, and provided credit for the families at the trading posts. Today many families possess only a small number of sheep and fewer goats. This stands in contrast to the situation twenty years ago before the livestock reduction program was carried out by the Bureau of Indian Affairs in an attempt to conserve the markedly overgrazed and eroded land.

The Navahos have retained the use of their own language. Even in families in which both English and Navaho are spoken, the native tongue is apt to be the language of the home and the community and English is used only in talking with non-Nahavo people. A high percentage of the adults have no working knowledge of English, either spoken or written. This has been a major problem in rendering a good medical service, because it forces the doctors and nurses to depend on interpreters for effective communication with their patients.

In 1945, 6,543 of the 20,435 school-age children were in school. In 1955 there were 24,560 and only about 8 per cent were receiving no schooling.[1] This stepping up of the elementary education will, of course, have a tremendous effect on the tribe and will speed up the acculturation process. In addition, at the present time 246 Navahos are in universities and colleges. This tremendous drive for education in "the white man's ways" should bring about marked changes in medical attitudes as well as knowledge of good medical practice during the years to come.

The Navaho tribe consists of a series of matrilineal clans, some sixty in number. These are exogamous units which function primarily to regulate marriage because marriage within the clan is still considered incestuous. Residence is matrilocal—a husband goes to live with the family of his wife, but a separate household is established in a hogan not too distant from those of her mother and sisters.

The place of the woman in the Navaho family is central and remains so among most Navaho families. She has property rights—the sheep are usually passed down through the female line—and she has a great deal to say not only about family affairs but those of the community. Because the women tend to be retiring in public the government administrators (and non-Indians generally) have tended to bypass them, and many programs have suffered as a result. To be sure, the Navaho women do sit at the back of the room at public meetings and the men do most of the talking. But ultimately many decisions in Navaho society are made in the household, and there the men feel the force of their wives' opinions.

The trading post and the local school form a focus for community activity. Here too may be a chapter house, the community meeting place where local affairs are discussed by the Navaho from the surrounding area—a radius reaching out fifty or more miles on all sides. There duly elected officers preside, but the importance of the chapter organization and the frequency of meetings vary greatly from one community to the next.

Changes in Navaho Way of Life

The social organization, especially the structure of the family, is undergoing rapid change. On the edge of the reservation—where contacts with the outside are much more frequent—and in areas immediately surrounding such communities as Ganado, Tuba City, or Chinle (where there have been many years of contact with the "white" world through government or mission channels) the extended family is no longer the principal functioning unit. In these areas, more and more the life revolves around the biologic family. Dependence on and reciprocal relations with collateral relatives—those of differing generations: cousins, aunts, and uncles—are not as important as they once were. This means that the parents of the Navaho child, as in our society, have the sole responsibility for the family care of the younger generation; this pattern differs from the extended family system that used to be universal to all of Navaho society. Then there were many parent substitutes. Today there are not. The men are working off the reservation and far from home much of the time.

This change in parental pattern is causing strains within the family which are indicated by the growth of child neglect. This has become a problem in some of these most acculturated areas—by a greater incidence of drinking alcohol, and by other symptoms that may have a significant correlation with rapid culture change.

Problems of this sort would be classified in our society as those related to tension affecting mental health. But the Navaho traditionally makes no concrete distinction between his mental and his bodily health. He knows that he is ill and seeks the help of either his medicine man or the doctor. As somatic health may reflect such tensions, it is possible that the increased demand for medical service at hospitals and clinics may be related to this rapid series of changes in Navaho technology, social organization, and behavior.

In addition to the scattered local chapter organizations, the only other formal political groupings are on the tribal level. There is an elected Tribal Council, and an overall legislative body, which was established as recently as 1923. For many years it remained a "puppet government" in the eyes of many Navahos, established to rubber-stamp the actions of the Bureau of Indian Affairs. This was especially true during the last half of the 1930's and early 1940's, when the government was enforcing the livestock reduction program with which this body became identified in the eyes of its constituency.

This Council did not come into its own until after World War II and since that time has made rapid strides—perhaps the most outstanding example of development in self-government among any Indian group within the United States.

There are seventy-four councilmen chosen by the Navahos

from that number of voting districts on the reservation. The Chairman and the Vice Chairman of the Council are the presiding executive officers who are elected directly by the voters on the same secret ballot that is used in the case of the councilmen. Within the Council there is an Advisory Committee that meets once a month and proposes legislation, establishes tribal budget, and draws up the agenda for the quarterly meeting of the Council.

In recent years, as tribal responsibility for their own affairs has grown, a series of special committees from within the council has been established in such fields as law and order, administration, welfare, education, and health. The tribal health committee today takes an active part in meeting with United States Public Health Service, state and local health officers, as well as tuberculosis sanatorium administrators and physicians who advise them on the health needs of the Navaho people.

This rapid development in self-government has come about with the encouragement and the guidance of the Bureau of Indian Affairs administrators at Window Rock. The Navaho tribe has been fortunate in having a series of administrators who have placed first priority on encouraging the development of self-government, and who have worked very closely with the council on problems of tribal legislation, administration, and financial responsibility.

Today, unlike twenty years ago, there is a Nahavo political structure that can help the federal government in its public health programming. The Tribal Council and the health committee, if present trends are projected into the future, will play an ever increasing role in designing an effective health service that meets the needs of their own people. There is still much to be done in the development of communications between the federal government (United States Public Health Service) and the tribe, but with time these may be expected to grow more effective.

Health Facilities

The responsibility for providing medical services to the Navaho and the other United States Indian Tribes rested with the Bureau of Indian Affairs from its creation until July 1, 1955. On that date this responsibility was transferred to the United States Public Health Service as a result of congressional action.

In the decade from the close of World War II to the assumption of responsibility by the United States Public Health Service, the central hospital facility on the reservation consisted of a 115-bed general hospital and a 100-bed tuberculosis hospital at the "government town" of Fort Defiance, Arizona. In addition there were four 35-bed field hospitals situated respectively at Winslow and at Tuba City in Arizona, and at Shiprock and Crown Point in New Mexico. At Keams Canyon in the Hopi reservation (which lies within the Navaho reservation) there is another 35-bed hospital which in actuality served both tribes. In addition to these government hospitals there is the 88-bed general hospital of the Ganado Presbyterian Mission (Sage Memorial) approximately thirty-five miles from the government general hospital at Fort Defiance.

With two exceptions (Shiprock and Tuba City) these hospitals were of good modern construction and were well equipped. The professional personnel varied from well-trained highly dedicated physicians and nurses to poorly trained indifferent misfits. Of far greater importance, however, was the fact that the full complement of staff was seldom if ever filled and the turnover was constantly high. Sometimes it was necessary to supply a different physician on a fortnightly or monthly basis to serve as the chief and sole physician at one of the field hospitals. The supply of physicians was improved in part by the "doctor draft" of the Korean War. For, under the draft, some young physicians could be commissioned in the United States Public Health Service and assigned to the

Indian Medical Service of the Indian Bureau. Even with this additional "recruiting," however, the full complement of staff on the Navaho reservation was never filled. Some of these young men made the most of their opportunity and served their two years as perceptive, compassionate, and highly effective physicians. All too often, however, they were completely blind to the problems both of the government and the Navaho and rather quickly became embittered "time-servers."

This adequately equipped but chronically undermanned hospital system was connected together by roads which were frequent impassable. Indeed, a hard-surfaced road of entry was available only at Fort Defiance, Shiprock, and Winslow and the latter hospital was little used. As a consequence of the weather-induced impassability of the roads, a physician in his middle twenties might find himself marooned at one of the field hospitals, for example, Tuba City with a patient requiring some complicated surgical procedure far beyond his competence to perform. Even when the roads were not impassable, it was the common practice to transport such a seriously ill patient by ambulance over a bumpy dirt road for the 160 miles from Tuba City to the Medical Center at Fort Defiance. Only in 1954 was an airplane type of patient transfer organized for emergency cases.

The frequently washed-out roads in this semi-arid land played an even greater role in the usefulness of the hospital facilities to the sick Navaho. For example, in certain parts of the reservation, a patient with acute pneumonia or meningitis might have to be carried as far as 100 miles by horse-drawn vehicle or pickup truck before he could be admitted to one of the field hospitals. The prospect of this journey together with the universal human tendency to try to "sweat out" a beginning illness at home led to many delays. Not infrequently such delays would result in deaths, soon after hospital admission, from diseases which can be easily controlled if they are treated promptly. A less critically ill patient might make a 50 or 100 mile trip to seek medical care and arrive at 6 P.M. on a Friday afternoon and receive word to report back on Monday.

Formidable barriers, both cultural and geographic, thus existed between twentieth-century Western medicine on the one hand, and the Navaho stricken with illness in his remote canyon, on the other hand.

The obvious answer to this problem—an adequate field health service—did not really exist. It was not possible to find enough nurses and physicians for the hospitals much less to find personnel for a field service. Nevertheless, there were always a few clinically frustrated but dedicated field health nurses who tried to maintain some sort of a program—which had to be principally localized to the young children in the schools. With these people—some government servants, some medical missionaries—it was possible to maintain a few field clinics serving a few small areas.

A field program for tuberculosis case finding was out of the question because as late as January 1952 there were an estimated 2,000 active cases of tuberculosis on the reservation, and there were exactly 100 beds which could be used for the care of tuberculosis patients.[2] As late as 1954, one of these Field Health Nurses had a district of 10,000 square miles with a population of approximately 10,000 persons.

This then is the situation as it existed in the decade immediately preceding the transfer of responsibility for Indian health to the United States Public Health Service. It is of the greatest importance to realize that no wicked man or collection of such men were responsible. On the contrary, the Indian Bureau officials on the Navaho reservation constantly labored long and hard to do what they could, but the sheer magnitude of the problem and its high degree of complexity required far greater resources than were ever made available.

Before considering what has happened in the less than two years that the Public Health Service program has been in operation, it is appropriate to review certain aspects of the Navaho culture from the standpoint of health.

Navaho Concern with Health

The Navaho people are much concerned with their bodily health. In 1941 Drs. Alexander and Dorothea Leighton made a psycho-biological study of stresses and strains in Navaho life. They estimated from an analysis of their interviews with 6 per cent of a group of 600 Indians in the Ramah area, some 50 miles south of Gallup, N. M., that 60 per cent of the references "to overtly threatening events and situations" consisted of threats to bodily health including disease, accident, and injury. By contrast, only 21 per cent of the threats were concerned with subsistence.[3]

The Navaho conception of health is very different from ours. For him, health is symptomatic of a correct relationship between man and his environment: his supernatural "environment," the world around him, and his fellow man. Health is associated with good, blessing, and beauty—all that is positively valued in life. Illness, on the other hand, bears evidence that one has fallen out of this delicate balance; it is usually ascribed to the breaking of one of the taboos which guide the behavior of the Navahos, especially in the case of the conservative elders. Illness may also be due to contact with the ghosts of the dead, or even to the malevolence of another Navaho who has resorted to witchery.

In order to restore harmony with the environment, which results once evil is driven out from the body and good is restored, a *singer,* as he is known to the people in their own language, must perform an exactly prescribed ritual for the patient. Dr. Clyde Kluckhohn in his detailed study of religious behavior in the Ramah area estimated that in 1938 the Navaho men devoted from one-quarter to one-third of their time to such ceremonials, and the women only slightly less.[4] The Navaho does not make the distinction between religion and medicine that we do; for him, they are aspects of the same thing. This is an important cultural fact that many workers

in the health field have failed to realize; as a result, m̀
doctors and nurses have antagonized their patients.

Virtually all Navaho religious behavior is oriented towards
curing an individual. The patient, once he feels ill, consults
with his immediate family and they call in a diagnostician who
by various techniques (the most common method is by *motion-
in-the-hand,* an involuntary trembling of the diviner's hand
and arm) discovers the cause of the present illness. Possibly
when the patient was a child carried in his mother's womb
she had looked at a forbidden sand painting; or possibly the
patient had come in contact with a lightning-struck object,
and an evil that must be exorcised had entered his body; or
perhaps he had eaten a taboo food which brought on the
illness. Any one of these, or hundreds of other causes, might
have brought about the present illness which is manifested by
bodily pain or mental anguish. Then in order to bring back
the patient to the correct balance with nature a particular *sing*
is performed. Evil is driven out and beauty and health restored.

The individual who is sick does not act on his own. The
family is likely to take the matter into his own hands once
its members know that one of their number is sick. After
the diagnostician has indicated the root of the illness he
suggests what *sing* should be performed; the family then goes
off for a *singer* who knows the required ceremony, and they
arrange with him what the fee for the *sing* shall be. No ceremonies are performed free of charge; a payment is essential
for the efficacy of treatment.

Psychotherapeutic Effects of Sings

Furthermore, the family is all present while the *sing* is in
progress; it may last from one to nine nights, depending on
the nature of the illness for which the *sing* is given, the economic position of the family, and other factors. Relatives and
friends come to the ceremony and take part in the chants and

prayers directed by the medicine man and his assistant. By association they too receive positive benefits from the cure, and in turn the presence of the family and friends is assuring to the patient who feels they are all working to restore his health. Alexander and Dorothea Leighton have written of the psychotherapeutic effects of Navaho ceremonials:

> All these people are gathered, their attention focused on the patient, bringing their influence and expectations to bear on his illness, their very presence implying that power-ful forces are working for his well-being. The Singer, as the mouthpiece of the Holy Beings, speaks in their voice and tells the patient that all is well. In the height of the ceremonial the patient himself becomes one of the Beings, puts his feet in their moccasins, breathes in the strength of the sun. He comes into complete harmony with the infinite, and as such must, of course, be free of all ills and evils.[5]

There is no doubt that these curing ceremonies, in which the Navaho people have so much faith, have a psychothera-peutic effect on the "patient." There is also good evidence that the sweat bath sedative and the body massage that is used in some ceremonies may act as beneficial physiotherapy.[6] But while *sings* may be effective in curing disease of primarily a psychogenic order, such things have been less successful and often positively harmful in the treatment of contagious dis-eases, appendicitis, and gall bladder attacks. The Navaho who has an acute case of such a disease may be sung over for many days—often if one *sing* does not cure the patient, he is taken to another *singer* for treatment—by the time the family decides to take him to the doctor, it is frequently too late for the physician's treatment to be effective.

Until the recent past, it was not always appreciated by the health workers that the *singer* is a respected man in the Navaho community, and often a leader. He may know only a few of the shorter *sings* or he may be one of those who have learned one of the nine night ceremonies, in which case he has considerable status in Navaho society. These men were traditionally the "intellectuals" of the tribe; it takes many years to learn the required set of songs, procedures, myths, and sand paintings that must all be exactly controlled, otherwise the *sing* will not be effective.

Again, we must couch all of this in terms of the dynamic change that is affecting the culture of the Navaho people. Today, unlike in the old days, very few men are learning these *sings*. The economic life of the people has changed because of population growth, denudation of the land, and other factors. Present-day cash economy and the values of the dominant society "compete" with these Navaho religious values for the time of every individual who may have an interest in becoming a *singer*. There are no longer months on end to concentrate on such learning of ceremonials.

This does not mean that Navaho ceremonial life, and the religious values that go with it, will change overnight. But it probably does mean that the ceremonies will become briefer; less time-consuming to learn, perform, and attend; and that many of the less valued *sings* will no longer be handed down. the *blessing-way* and certain other important ceremonials may very well last for generations to come.

What is the meaning of all of this for modern medicine? For one thing, as Navaho *singers* grow fewer in number, the laity will increasingly depend on the medical services that our physicians and eventually physicians among their own tribesmen, as they develop such a professional group in the years to come, have to offer. Because of their cultural "predisposition" which places such a high value on health, the Navaho may demand an availability of service on a level not deemed necessary by less health-conscious Indians in the Southwest.

Health Problems Among the Navahos

If one took into consideration only those physical factors which exist on the Navaho reservation, the disease pattern could be predicted whether it be a Navaho or a white population group. For example: the poor roads, and long distances from medical facilities being what they are, it follows that even a highly intelligent, well-educated non-Navaho would have his problems in this environment. The non-Navaho might come into a medical center with an advanced case of pneumonia or ruptured appendix or severely dehydrated from an acute diarrhea. The severe problems of transportation and delays mentioned previously might result in a more advanced state of disease regardless of whether the patient were Navaho or non-Navaho.

The fact that a Navaho might first seek attention from a medicine man and thus delay his treatment further might complicate the medical problem. Many of the Navahos have only meager health knowledge and are ill-informed as to the needs for early treatment in a clinic or hospital.

There is also the further problem of the communication barrier due to the language difference. The medical history which the physician might obtain is distorted by an incompetent interpreter. This problem, of course, can be magnified in reverse if the interpreter cannot place into appropriate Navaho the English which is presented to him by the physician. The problem involved is not simply one of translation of words, but translation of the ideas and concepts of bodily health and disease which are expressed by the patient and by the physician.

The economy of the people must also be considered in summing up the various determinants of the pattern of disease on the Navaho. While it is true that the Navaho tribal organization has recently come into large sums of money through contracts for uranium, oil, gas, and lumber, the economy of the individual or family remains substandard, with the per capita income less than $500 per year. Navaho housing, which is culturally valued, results in overcrowding and poor ventilation. Sanitary facilities and plumbing are not commonly available. Since water is scarce and must be hauled to the hogan long distances over bad roads, there is a major problem in personal and family sanitation. The problem is not that the water used for drinking or washing is contaminated—it is that there is so little of it.

In these crowded and unsanitary family surroundings, one would expect to have infections and communicable diseases as the outstanding medical problems; and indeed this is the case. It might be said that the disease pattern of the Navaho is comparable with that of the general United States population fifty to one hundred years ago.

What are the facts about the health status of the Navaho Indians? How reliable are the medical statistics which are

TABLE 1—Ten Leading Causes of Death Among Navahos and Comparative U.S. General Population Rates, 1954[a]

Causes	Rates per 100,000 Population		Per cent of Total Deaths	
	Navahos	U.S. General	Navahos	U.S. General
1. Pneumonia	123.5	23.7	16.2	2.6
2. Gastritis, Duodenitis, Enteritis, Colitis	110.2	5.3	14.5	0.6
3. Certain Diseases of early infancy	102.3	39.4	13.4	4.3
4. Accidents—all	81.0	56.9	10.6	6.2
5. Tuberculosis—all forms	53.0	10.5	7.0	1.1
6. Heart Diseases	27.9	343.4	3.7	37.4
7. Malignant neoplasms	22.6	147.0	3.0	16.0
8. Nephritis and nephrosis	17.3	12.6	2.3	1.2
9. Congenital malformations	17.3	12.9	2.3	1.4
10. Vascular lesions affecting the central nervous system	14.6	103.6	1.9	11.3

[a] Prepared by Statistics and Analysis Section, USPHS, Albuquerque, New Mexico.

available to the Bureau of Indian Affairs and the United States Public Health Service?

Obviously, the accuracy of health statistics is a direct reflection of adequate coverage among any particular population group. Despite the fact that tremendous progress has been made in increasing medical service among the Navaho people during recent years, there is still a tremendous lag between medical needs and medical service rendered. There are still many Navahos who, either of their own accord or because of the problems of getting to hospitals and clinics, are unable to have proper medical care. There is every reason to believe that deaths are occurring which are not recorded, particularly among the infants. Even if the deaths are recorded, however, the notation may not be reliable in terms of the specific cause of the disease.

Another factor which affects the health statistics is that the Navahos are not a record-conscious people. One must bear in mind that many are nonliterate and do not feel a need for keeping records. They feel no urgency about reporting a birth or death to the health personnel.

In a study on the completeness of birth registration records which was carried out by the statistical office in the United States Public Health Service several years ago, it was found that approximately 60 per cent of the births had been recorded; thus, 40 per cent were not officially registered. Statisticians working with the Navahos also became aware of the fact that there may not even be an accurate base-line census for the reservation. Considering all these difficulties it is possible that the Navaho morbidity and mortality statistical tables reflect only the accessible data and are not too precise an indication of the incidence of particular diseases.

Be that as it may, it is clear that all medical teams which have made a survey on the Navaho reeservation, uniformly report that the Navahos have health standards far below those of the general United States population. It might be said that the health status of the Navahos is comparable with that of peoples in underdeveloped areas such as in the primitive regions of South America, Asia, or Africa. Certainly their life expectancy figures and infant mortality figures are comparable.

The striking differences in the leading causes of death among the Navahos as compared with the general United States population are indicated in the preceding table.

Health Status of Navahos and Other Americans

A popular method for comparing the health status of two population groups is the average life expectancy. The average life span of a Navaho is approximately 30 to 40 years, whereas the average United States citizen may expect to live 70 years.

The infant mortality rate (the number of infant deaths per 1,000 live births) is a more precise yardstick for measuring the health conditions of a population group. This figure also bears out the general view on Navaho health, for the infant mortality rate on the Navaho reservation is four times greater than the national rate. (The 1954 Navaho rate is 108.6, compared with the general United States rate of 26.6.)

J. Nixon Hadley, Statistician with the Division of Indian Health, United States Public Health Service, summarized the problem of evaluating the Navaho health situation in a recent report:[7]

> Measurement of health conditions among the Navahos is hampered by lack of complete data either on the base population involved or on deaths and illnesses. Even with this lack of specificity, however, it is obvious that mortality and morbidity rates for most of the major diseases are far in excess of the rates for the total United States population.

More than any other major disease, tuberculosis is the expression of the socio-economic conditions in a community. Indeed it has been authoritatively described as a disease of gross social mismanagement both on the individual and the community level.[8]

The extent of tuberculosis among the Navahos has never been fully determined for the total reservation population. However, reference to the vital statistics tables shows that the tuberculosis death rate among the Navahos is about five times that of the general population (53 as compared with 10.5 per 100,000). Mobile roentgenographic surveys that have been conducted in scattered communities on the reservation since the fall of 1952 have revealed active pulmonary tuberculosis ranging from 1 to 3 per cent of these population samples. On the basis of the sample mobile roentgenographic surveys, it would appear that there are probably two thousand or more cases of active pulmonary tuberculosis on the Navaho reservation.

The Navaho people have eagerly cooperated in accepting hospital treatment for tuberculosis even though they were required in most instances to go off the reservation for sanatorium care. (Approximately 500 of the 600 available beds for tuberculosis are situated 100 to 500 miles from the reservation.) With the advent, in 1952, of effective chemotherapy for tuberculosis and the inauguration of the expanded hospitalization program, the death rate from tuberculosis has fallen rapidly. It has been recognized that the Navaho tuberculosis patient will respond to appropriate medical and surgical management of his disease in the same fashion as the non-Navaho patient.

It can be expected that when effective antituberculosis treatment is fully developed, including ambulatory care, it may be possible to control the tuberculosis problem at a level now observed in non-Navaho United States society.

There are a host of factors which can influence the extent of tuberculosis among a group of people; the roles of hygiene, sanitation, housing, nutrition, and other factors are related to the severity of the tuberculosis problem.

Another major health problem among the Navaho has been

the high infant death rate from gastroenteritis and diarrhea. Diarrhea is ten times more frequent among the Navaho than in the general United States population. There is as yet no conclusive scientific study which has pointed up any common etiologic agent for all cases of the severe diarrhea of infants. However, most observers believe that the diarrheas are probably related to sanitation and hygiene. To date the most common bacterial agent found to account for the disease has been bacillary dysentery. It is often complicated by progressive dehydration which if not corrected may result in death. Because of the delay which frequently occurs in getting the patient to a medical facility, the infant arrives too late for the physician to initiate successful treatment.

With present-day medical technology, the diarrheas could easily be controlled. However, because of the factors determined by the environment and way of life of the people, diarrhea persists as a scourge among the Navahos and there is a predictable season of "summer complaint" as there was throughout all of our country many years ago.

Other major health problems which are seen on the Navaho reservation are respiratory illness, particularly pneumonias and influenza, conjunctivitis, trachoma, and chronic ear infections, and gall bladder disease.

There is yet too little known about diseases of the heart and blood vessels, cancer, hypersensitivity (that is, allergic diseases), high blood pressure, arthritic, metabolic, and mental diseases among the Navaho. Much more study is required before a statement can be made regarding the relative incidence of any of these disorders.

Improvement of Cross-Cultural Medical Service

What has been the approach of the United States Public Health Service during the approximately eighteen-month period since it became responsible for Indian health? At the outset, let it be emphasized that the career officers in the Public Health Service who have responsibility for the policy of the Indian health program are fully aware of the difficulties of attempting to introduce Western twentieth-century technology across a cultural barrier. Moreover, as individual officers, they had been sent to conduct the Indian Bureau's health program during the last year of its operations. Consequently, when the official interagency transfer of responsibility occurred, the men in charge of the new program were quite aware of the formidable nature of the task.

The basic approach followed consisted of: (1) expanding within budgetary limits the on-going program with special emphasis toward organizing an adequate field (that is, nonhospital) health program in the two largest areas, Alaska, and on the Navaho; (2) a general survey, principally by nongovernmental experts, of the health situation and needs of our Indian peoples with appropriate reference to their socioeconomic status; arrangement with university groups to conduct pilot research or demonstration programs on selected aspects of the total program.

On the Navaho reservation, the pre-existing hospital program has already been considerably expanded. At Tuba City, where an outmoded 35-bed hospital had been caring for most of the Western Navaho, a modern 125-bed hospital had just been completed by the Indian Bureau and was opened a few months before the actual transfer. It has been possible to staff this hospital with four physcans, one of whom is a fully accredited surgeon. The old hospital supposedly had two physicians but, more often than not, it had only one. In addition at this hospital, there are four Public Health Nurses where only one was available before and there is a full-time dentist.

For the reservation as a whole, in 1954, the government medical staff numbered 343 and by 1955 this was already increased to 436. In addition to the new hospital (constructed by the Bureau of Indian Affairs) at Tuba City, a new 200-bed general hospital is being constructed at Gallup, New Mexico, the business "capital" of the Navaho reservation.

The principal evidences of the organization of a proper

field health program to date are the increasing number of Public Health Nurses which totaled twenty-four by the end of 1955. Moreover, at all of the field hospitals there is now a physician whose major responsibility is with field health problems. Within the eighteen-month period it has not been possible to organize anything approaching a fully operating directed field program but a start has been made. Moreover, the construction of a number of strategically located Field Health Clinics are in various stages of development.

While the Public Health Service has been increasing the instrument for delivering more and better medical care to the Navahos, they have also enlisted the assistance of several university groups to perform both a research and to some extent a service program in health among the Navahos. The University of California Medical College is providing consultation, guidance, and personnel in a health education program. Cornell University Medical College has been chosen to conduct a pilot project in field health. This project has been centered at Manyfarms, Arizona, located in the geographic center of the reservation. It is the purpose of this field study to attempt to define the proper concerns of a health program among a people such as the Navahos and to attempt to develop, and determine the practicability by actual trial, of methods for the delivery of such health services as are found to be required. It is believed that the results of this study of the cross-cultural delivery of medical services will be a continuous source of information for the expanded Public Health Service program among the Navahos. It is also hoped that the observations made there will have generality for the health programs with the other Indian tribes and in so-called underdeveloped areas outside the United States.

To sum up this aspect of the discussion: It can be said that the increased health activities among the Navahos, which have been set up by the Public Health Service within the past eighteen months, represent a very considerable achievement. The problem is such a complex one, however, and has been neglected for so many decades that it will be some time before a reasonably acceptable program can be in full operation. Without question, one of the most immediate obstacles to a proper program is the necessity for constructing suitable housing for health personnel. For, in many of the areas in greatest need of medical services on the Navaho reservation, absolutely no housing exists for even one physician or nurse who might be recruited to deliver the badly needed services. Formidable difficulties exist in obtaining funds for the construction of such housing. This is particularly the case as the argument that "the Public Health Service should be able to do the job less expensively" was frequently voiced by well meaning non-governmental advocates seeking to persuade the Congress to legislate the transfer.

In the writers' opinion it seems clear that if a better cross-cultural medical service is to be rendered, it is necessary to discover the needs of the community and family, as well as that of the individual patient. To do this it is necessary to free ourselves from many ethnocentric and institution-bound ideas and practices and turn our attention to gaining knowledge of the way of life of the people we wish to treat.

What are some of the questions which must be answered before a reasonably adequate health program can be delivered to, and accepted by, the Navaho?

How does the patient feel about our medical service and how, from his point of view, could it be improved to meet his needs?

What are the causes of resistance to modern medicine when such resistance occurs?

How can a medical program that includes sanitation and health education learn to work effectively through community structure and leadership?

What are the basic factors which hinder effective medical interpretation and how can these be eliminated?

How can doctors and nurse's aides be recruited from among the Navahos and trained so that they can bridge the language barrier to the community and hogan?

We must seek answers to questions such as these on the level of the family and community.

The judicious borrowing from other cultures which typifies so much of Navaho behavior—as seen in time perspective—is also at work in his changing attitudes and responses to our Western medicine. New alternatives to the cures of the *singers* have been introduced; and when the medicine man has failed, the family of the patient seeks out the doctor to see what he can do. Or, as seen from the point of view of the medicine man:

> When I see that I am not getting anywhere with one of my patients I suggest that he go see the white doctor. But I always caution him first to come back and finish the ceremony that has been interrupted, or he will get sick again.

Two forces are at work here: First, there is the strong belief that once a ceremony has been started it must be finished; and second, the *singer* and the unacculturated Navaho generally speaking—as well as many highly acculturated ones—believes that even though the white doctor can rid the body of pain and "drive out the germs," still he cannot set the individual back in harmony with his environment. Anxiety is likely to be present upon discharge from the hospital—as it is with ourselves, but for different reasons—and this often persists until a *sing* has been held.

Changing attitudes of the *singers* are further documented by a speech that one of the tribal officers, himself a *singer*, made to an assembly of physicians at the Fort Defiance Hospital in 1955. He said:

> As I see it, all the diseases, which hurt the Navaho people may be divided into three kinds. There are those diseases that we medicine men have given up on. We know that you white doctors have better cures than we do. One of the diseases of that sort is tuberculosis. Then there is sickness which comes from getting too close to where lightning has struck. Right now there are probably some patients in this hospital

who are sick from that illness and you doctors have no way of even finding out what is wrong with them—but we medicine men can, and we are able to cure such cases. A third type of illness is snake bite. You can cure that, and we Navaho also have our own medicines for that.

These changing attitudes and beliefs are also shared by the diagnosticians, including the *listeners* and the *star gazers*. In 1957 at Manyfarms, Arizona, where a field clinic was recently inaugurated, four different *hand-tremblers* stated, upon questioning, that their hands "often shook towards the hospital," indicating that the patient's illness should be treated initially by the physician rather than the medicine man.

Effect of Antibiotics on Navahos

The Navaho's favorable outlook on our medicine has probably been accelerated in recent years by the "antibiotics" and other powerful drugs which have come into general use. Before these specific agents were developed, the physician was limited frequently to treating only the patients' symptoms and was unable to get at the underlying pathogenic causes. Treatment was often prolonged and not necessarily successful as in the case of tuberculosis and syphilis. Now the Navahos see positive cures in a shorter period of time for these and other diseases. They have been deeply impressed by the efficacy of this improved medical practice.

In 1940, when the Leightons wrote *The Navaho Door* they reported that many hospital beds were unused (although there was considerably more use of the hospital beds than as compared to the previous decade). Indeed, some hospitals were known as death traps—not unlike hospitals in our own culture less than a hundred years ago.

Hospitals became identified with death, and since death is contagious and the mere presence of a corpse in the same enclosure is contaminating in Navaho rationale, the hospitals were not utilized to the degree they are today.

These changes could be documented at greater length:

Whereas chest X-rays for tuberculosis case finding were resisted twenty years ago, today many Navaho patients ask for X rays to be taken if a pain of any sort is felt in the chest; vaccinations and "shots" have become routine in most community schools.

Relationship Between Medical People and Navahos

The physicians and nurses who are tolerant of Navaho belief and who recognize the psychologic dependence on the *sings* are likely to have a better relationship with the Navaho patients than those who are intolerant of their ways and attempt to force our beliefs and the scientific basis of our medicine on them.

There is good evidence that in the last thirty years doctors on the Navaho reservation, on the whole, have become more tolerant of the Navaho way of life, including their religion, than was formerly the case. They have found that permissive treatment is more effective than an uncompromising and authoritarian attitude.

Doctors at the Fort Defiance Sanatorium in recent years report that when they have suggested that patients have *sings* before and after sanatorium treatment, there has been less absence without medical advice once treatment in the ward is underway. This, of course, is preferable to allowing the patient to go home for a *sing* once chemotherapy has been started. But even that is better, in most instances, than denying such a request because the patient is likely to leave anyway and not return, but the patient who has been given such permission will come back.

Without waiting for further acculturation it is entirely possible for the practitioner of Western medicine to mould his scientific approach into the cultural frame of the Navaho people. In this way modern medical services might not only be made acceptable to the Navahos, but could be taken over as something of positive value and integrated into their own way of life.

References

1. *Navaho Year Book of Planning in Action,* Report no. 4 (Window Rock, Ariz.: Bureau of Indian Affairs, U.S. Department of the Interior, 1955).

2. In the fall of 1952, the Bureau of Indian Affairs was able to obtain the necessary funds to pay for the care of Navaho patients in tuberculosis sanatoriums located away from the reservation. Once this arrangement was set up, the lack of a case-finding program became the factors limiting adequate tuberculosis control.

3. Alexander and Dorothea Leighton, "Some Types of Uneasiness and Fear of a Navaho Community," *American Anthropologist* 44 (1942), pp. 199–209.

4. Clyde Kluckhohn, "Participation in Ceremonials in a Navaho Community," *American Anthropologist* 40 (1938), pp. 359–69.

5. Alexander and Dorothea Leighton, *The Navaho Door* (Cambridge, Mass.: Harvard University Press, 1944), p. 36.

6. Leland C. Wyman and Flora L. Bailey, "Two Examples of Navaho Physiotherapy," *American Anthropologist* 46, no. 3 (1944), pp. 329–37.

7. Nixon Hadley, "Health Conditions Among Navaho Indians," U.S. Public Health Reports, 70, no. 9 (Washington: U.S. Public Health Service, U.S. Department of Health, Education, and Welfare, September 1955), pp. 831–36.

8. R. J. Dubos and J. Dubos, *The White Plague: Tuberculosis, Man and Society* (Boston: Little, Brown and Company, 1952).

6

Introducing Modern Medicine
in a Navaho Community: 1
(The first of two parts.)

by Walsh McDermott, Kurt Deuschle, John Adair,
Hugh Fulmer, Bernice Loughlin

Walsh McDermott, M.D., is Livingston Farrand Professor, De-
partment of Public Health, New York Hospital at Cornell Univer-
sity Medical Center. Among the professional organizations with
which he is affiliated are the National Academy of Science, Ameri-
can Public Health Association, and the American Medical Associa-
tion. He has been the recipient of the Lasker Award and the first
recipient of the National Institutes of Health Lectureship Award
(1963). He is co-editor of Cecil-Loeb Textbook of Medicine *(12th*
ed.) Saunders, 1967.

Kurt W. Deuschle, M.D., is Chairman and Professor, Depart-
ment of Community Medicine, Mount Sinai School of Medicine,
New York. He was formerly affiliated with the Department of
Public Health and Preventive Medicine, New York Hospital at
Cornell University Medical Center, New York.

John Adair, Ph.D., is Professor of Anthropology, San Francisco
State College. Previously, he served at Cornell University and the
University of New Mexico. He has done extensive research and
writing on Indian life and culture. His publications include: First
Look at Strangers, *Rutgers University Press, 1959; co-author,* People
of the Middle Place: A Study of the Zuni Indians, *Human Relation*
Area Files, Inc., 1966; and co-author, Hastings to Culloden, *Dufour*
1964.

Hugh Fulmer, M.D., is Professor of Community Medicine, Uni-

111

versity of Massachusetts School of Medicine, Worcester, Massachu-setts.

Bernice W. Loughlin, M.P.H., is Director, Field Health Nursing Services, U.S. Public Health Service, Division of Indian Health, Field Health Station, Gallup, New Mexico. She served as a member of the Navajo-Cornell research group (sponsored by Cornell University in conjunction with United States Public Health Service) that was responsible for "Introducing Modern Medicine in a Navajo Community," Science (January 1960).

"Introducing Modern Medicine in a Navajo Community" (copyright 1960 by the American Association for the Advancement of Science) is reprinted with the permission of the authors and of the American Association for the Advancement of Science from Science, Vol. 131, 22 January 1960, pp. 197–205 and 29 January 1960, pp. 280–287.

Technologic development in the sense of the natural spread of a technique from one part of the world to another is presumably as old as man. Organized attempts to introduce technologies to a people either within or outside of the introducer's own country are likewise not new. Features today that are quite new, however, are the sheer size of the international technologic development movement, the changed sovereignty relationships of many of the recipient peoples, and the recently developed power to make rapid and truly significant changes in the status of their health. As health and agriculture (along with education) are the principal targets of most programs, the impact of technologic development today may be as much biologic as it is economic.

Of necessity, in such a hurriedly expanding international activity, the power to effect such widespread biologic and social changes must be wielded without much of the body of knowledge essential for its proper application. Thus, the activity carries with it the potential for harm as well as good.

The social scientists were quick to perceive this point, and there is now a rapidly expanding research effort being conducted by them on various aspects of the broad question of technologic development.[1] The social scientists can penetrate only so far, however, into the biologic aspects of the subject, and there has been relatively little research by medically trained investigators on what might be termed the "medical" aspects of technologic development. Indeed, some of the most important questions are of a nature that neither the social scientist nor the medical scientist is properly equipped to study alone. For example, with today's drugs it is possible to place in the hands of a barefoot, nonliterate villager more real power to affect the outcome of a child critically ill with, let us say, meningitis or pneumonia or tuberculosis than could have been exerted by the most highly trained urban physician of twenty-five years ago. This is a "technologic development" with truly great potential for either good or harm. Yet its full implications cannot be appropriately explored by either the social scientist or the medical scientist working alone. Moreover, in the usual course of events, even when the two are working together, as in the case of an operating program in the field, the requests for the physician to provide medical services to the people are usually so great that he is seldom able to participate in research.

In view of the importance of the basic issue, however, it seems wholly proper that attempts be made to subject some of the relevant questions to scientific scrutiny. Accordingly, in 1955 such an attempt was started, to utilize jointly the skills of the medical and the social scientists in a systematic investigation of the broad question of technologic development as it applies to medicine. The opportunity to initiate such a study was provided by the Navaho Tribal Government and the U.S. Public Health Service, which by congressional action had just been assigned responsibility for the health of Indians in the United States. The cultural, geographic, economic, and medical situations of the Navaho in 1955 closely resembled the corresponding factors in many economically underdeveloped areas of the world.[2] An opportunity was thus provided to do two things: to try to assist our government in its attempt to improve the situation of one of our own minority groups, and to study, from a vantage point not attainable in an operating government program, the wide variety of problems in this complex question of technologic aid to economically underdeveloped countries.

In this article, in the interest of brevity, we omit all discussion of such topics as the many steps involved in the choice of the project area; the negotiations with the Navaho tribal leaders and with the people of the area chosen; the organization of the project; and relationships of the project to the governmental activities in the larger Navaho area. These are all subjects of very considerable importance in the studies, but they will be presented elsewhere in detail. Suffice it to say (i) that the area chosen is representative in terms of both culture and terrain and consists of the 800-square-mile Manyfarms–Rough Rock area, with an estimated population of more than 2,000 people; and (ii) that the Navaho Tribal Council has annually appropriated $10,000 to $20,000 as its contribution to the research, in addition to the financial support provided by Cornell University, private foundations, industry, and the U.S. Public Health Service.[3]

In what follows, the research program is presented in brief outline, with the primary aim of describing the complex background, the goals, and the scope of the studies. In addition, the three-year results in a few of the projects are singled out for brief discussion. First, however, it is necessary to describe certain features of Navaho society, especially as they pertain to matters of health.[2, 4]

In May 1956 the study under discussion went into actual operation in the 800-square-mile Manyfarms–Rough Rock area in the approximate center of the Navaho territory. There were four avowed purposes: (i) to define the proper concerns of a health program among a people such as the Navaho; (ii) to find ways to adapt concepts of modern medicine for presentation in an acceptable form across formidable cultural and linguistic barriers without compromising essential medical standards in the process; (iii) to study, in so far as possible, the biologic and social consequences of this innovation in terms of the community (and the outside participants) ; and (iv) to see whether information of importance with respect to environment and disease in our present-day society can be obtained from study of a people who are emerging from a relatively primitive society and becoming part of the rural United States of today.

The total program may be considered in terms of three large general studies and a greater number of smaller and more sharply defined studies. To some extent this classification is arbitrary. In reality, the three general studies all tend to merge; conversely, the segmental or categorical studies have a way of developing subcategories once experience is gained in the study of a particular question.

The first of the three general studies consists of a socio-economic study of the community as a whole, with special reference to factors that might be relevant to a consideration of health and disease. The second study has to do with defining the pattern of disease in the community by performing complete physical examinations and appropriate laboratory studies on the individual members of the community. The third of the general studies is concerned with determining to what extent Navaho men and women with limited schooling can be trained to function as effective field auxiliaries of the public health nurses.

The use of the word *community* might be questioned when applied to 2,000 people scattered over an 800-square-mile area. The term seems justified, however, by the fact that the residents of Manyfarms and Rough Rock avowedly regard these two adjacent areas as "communities" to which they respectively belong, and the two areas together form an electoral district with a single seat on the 74-member Navaho Tribal Council. Representatives from the electoral district as a whole organized the exercises held at the inauguration of the project, at which time the medical facilities were "blessed" in appropriate religious ceremonies by Navaho medicine men. There is similar district-wide representation on the Chapter[6] health committee (several medicine men are members) , so that this committee, with which the research staff consults, nominally speaks for the residents of the entire 800-square-mile area.

Demographic Studies

The socioeconomic studies have revealed information about the Manyfarms–Rough Rock community of the same general sort as that presented above in the general description of Navaho society. The demographic data are of particular interest, however, because they are believed to represent the first reliable measurement of a Navaho birth rate. Formidable difficulties exist with respect to obtaining such information when an unknown proportion of births occur in remotely situated hogans. It was necessary, therefore, to expend a far greater effort in obtaining these data on births and deaths than would ordinarily be feasible except as a part of a research project.

The number of live births was 94 in 1956, 98 in 1957, and 94 in 1958 in a population that totalled 2,048 on 1 January 1959. Thus, the average annual birth rate over the three-year period was 48.7 per 1,000 persons. This extraordinarily high birth rate was associated with a high fertility rate—that is, the number of live births per 1,000 women aged 15 to 44. At the census point (1 January 1959) there were 436 women in this age group in the community. With a total of 286 live births (annual average, 95.3) during the preceding three years, the fertility rate was approximately 220.[7] Of this total of 286 live births, 48 percent occurred outside the hospital.

During the same three-year period (1956–1958) there were 47 deaths, or an average of 16 deaths per year in the community. This represents a death rate of 7.3 per 1,000 of the Navaho population. The infant mortality rate (deaths during the first year of life per 1,000 live births) was 73.1.

The information on deaths among the Navaho was even more difficult to validate than the data on births. In general, the major portion of a death rate is made up of deaths in the early years, especially in the early months, of life. It is this segment of the death rate that was so difficult to obtain. For in the Navaho country when a birth has occurred at home without medical or nursing supervision and the infant dies in the first few weeks of life, it is not at all unusual for the family to make no report of the event to the governmental authorities. There seems to be nothing particularly surreptitious about this. It is simply that members of the family appear to regard the death of their infant wholly in personal terms and hence as something of no conceivable interest to health authorities.

Accurate information on the rate of population increase is obviously of vital importance in technologic development programs, particularly in the planning for facilities in education and health. It is of considerable interest, therefore, that the concentrated study made on a continued basis in the 800-square-mile sample area revealed a birth rate so much higher than the official Navaho birth rate recorded for the tribe as a whole on the basis of routine reporting. For 1956, the official recorded birth rate for the tribe as a whole was 36.3 per 1,000,[5] in contrast to the rate of 49.6 for that same year in the sample area. Moreover, the annual rate of population increase during the three-year period in the sample area (4.0 percent) is almost twice the higher of the two rates (2.25 and 2.3) that form the present basis for government planning.[5] Both the Manyfarms data and the official data recorded for the Navaho area as a whole show a year-to-year consistency.

The question immediately arises as to whether this difference between 36.3 and 49.6 live births per 1,000 merely indicates that the 800-square-mile area at Manyfarms is not a representative sample of the much larger total Navaho area. In a sense, no arbitrarily selected region of a larger area can be truly representative of the area as a whole. What can be said about the Manyfarms area, however, is that in its chief socioeconomic characteristics it seems in no way atypical, and that in the opinion of long-time students of the Navaho scene it is not atypical. In this community of approximately 2,000 persons, the net gain in population (excess of births over deaths) in a three-year period was 239 persons. This represents a population expansion of "explosive" proportions.

Another finding in this general study of the community was that it was necessary to devise a wholly new system for such a mundane operation as medical record-keeping in order to fit the pattern of the society. It is not always realized that, as modern medicine was developed within the European culture, all medical record systems the world over are essentially the same. They are based on the "facts of life" of Western society and are simply "imposed" on everyone else. With the Navaho it was found that recording of kinship relationships was of considerable importance because two persons within the same immediate family may have different names. In order to recognize that two patients with a communicable disease seen at different times at the field clinic were in fact living together in the same hogan or camp, it was necessary to organize all of the individual charts of the patients by clan and by the composition of the extended and immediate (that is, nuclear) families. This was also of importance because, especially in the past, the Navahos, like many other peoples living in tribal societies throughout the world, have tended to pay little attention to the "Western" naming systems and have continued to depend on kin and clan designations. Consequently, an individual may be recorded by several completely different names in any set of records.

Defining the Pattern of Disease

The second general study merely represents the medical aspects of the first study and has to do with defining the pattern of disease in the community. A systematic attempt was made to obtain detailed and complete physical examinations and appropriate laboratory studies on every member of the community with whom the staff had any medical relationships.

The disease pattern found in the first 1,600 persons examined was exactly what one would have expected from the nature of the society. Approximately three-quarters of the disease (76 percent) was either microbial disease or the preventable consequences of microbial disease (Table I). An example of the latter is the permanent impairment of hearing that may result from an untreated streptococcal infection of the inner ear. Only two components of the disease pattern would seem exotic to a physician trained in the United States: the presence of trachoma and the extraordinarily high prevalence of "congenital" dislocation of the hip. Both of these diseases have long been recognized as prevalent among the Navaho.[8]

The prevalence of tuberculosis was found to be high, but the incidence (the number of new infections per unit of time) has fallen substantially during the three-year period. In 1957 an intensive roentgenographic and tuberculin survey was made of one half of the population in the project area (in Manyfarms but not in Rough Rock). The prevalence of tuberculosis of all forms was 9.0 percent. Pulmonary tuberculosis, not including primary tuberculosis, was present in 7.0 percent of the approximately one thousand people. In 2.1 percent of the group, the pulmonary lesions were active or presumably active. Evidence that the incidence of tuberculous infection is falling was obtained from the steady fall in positive cutaneous reactions to tuberculin among the school children, almost all of whom were between five and ten years of age. In May 1956 the prevalence of individuals who reacted positively to tuberculin was 33.3 percent among 168 children.[9] In October 1956 it was 29.4 percent, and in October 1957 the figure was 26.4 percent. A much more dramatic indication of what is going on is provided by the prevalence of positive tuberculin reactors among the 49 five-year-olds who formed the "beginners" class in the fall of 1958. Of the 49, only eight (16.3 percent) reacted positively to tuberculin, and in all but two instances the fact that the child did react positively was already known.

It is believed that this impressive fall may be in part a consequence of the Manyfarms–Rough Rock chemotherapy and chemoprophylaxis program but that it is in greater part the result of two innovations made in 1952. These were the Navaho-Cornell studies in tuberculosis chemotherapy at Tuba City and Fort Defiance and the off-reservation sanatorium program organized through the Fort Defiance facility by the Bureau of Indian Affairs.[10] Certain of the problems involved in the ambulatory chemotherapy program are considered below, in the presentation of the segmental programs.

Respiratory disease caused by microbes other than *Mycobacterium tuberculosis* was also found to be common. Most of these respiratory infections are either definitely or presumably viral in origin. They consist of the familiar influenza-like illnesses, the respiratory complications of measles and chicken pox, and the numerous forms of "colds and bronchitis" that may afflict adults but are especially prevalent among young children. As for the *occurrence* of these illnesses, the situation among the Navaho is not particularly different from that elsewhere in the United States. Wherever infants and children are raised, families go through periods in which there seems to be simply one respiratory infection after another. The difference in the situation in an economically underdeveloped area such as the Navaho reservation lies not in the occurrence of these illnesses but in the fact that preventable serious secondary complications are much more likely to occur.

Secondary Complications Are Serious

For example, it is well recognized that measles is generally not too serious an illness in early life, in contrast to the serious nature of the disease among adults. Yet in the late winter of 1957-1958, measles was widely prevalent in the Manyfarms–Rough Rock area, and 130 children of preschool age were seen. In approximately one-half of these children a pneumonia developed, and the pneumonia was of a type not readily controllable by present-day antimicrobial drugs. Although precise data on this point from elsewhere in the United States are now difficult to obtain, consultation with a number of eminent pediatricians revealed agreement that this was a considerably higher incidence of postmeasles pneumonia than they ordinarily found in the cities of the United States. The

TABLE 1. PATTERN OF DISEASE IN THE FIRST 1,600 PERSONS EXAMINED IN THREE YEARS AT MANYFARMS.

Diagnosis	Percentage of total disease
Almost entirely microbial (76.3%)	
Respiratory diseases (pneumonia, influenza, and tuberculosis)	26.8
Other microbial diseases (exclusive of tuberculosis and infant diarrhea)	19.0
Sensory organs and nervous system (principally meningitis, deafness, and eye diseases, all resulting from infection)	15.5
Diseases of digestive system (principally infant diarrhea and gallbladder disease)	8.6
Disease of skin (principally infection)	6.4
Anemia, congenital hip disease, accidents (11.3%)	
Accidents	5.1
Anemia and other blood disorders	3.4
Diseases of bone (includes congenital disease of hip)	2.8
Diseases common in U.S. society (4.0%)	
Diseases of circulatory system (includes diseases of heart and vessels, principally rheumatic fever)	2.2
Allergic and endocrine and metabolic diseases (includes asthma and hyperthyroidism)	1.1
Cancer	0.2
Mental diseases	0.5
Miscellaneous (8.4%)	
Pregnancy, genitourinary diseases, congenital malformations, and so on	8.4
Total	100.0

point was made, however, that in the first quarter of this century it was part of the medical folklore that whereas measles was generally mild, with a low incidence of pneumonia in "middle class" urban dwellers, the disease was considerably more severe, with a higher incidence of pneumonia, in slum dwellers. In effect, therefore, a viral disease widely prevalent in our society and virtually inescapable in youth is not too serious under present-day general living conditions of the United States but becomes a considerably more serious medical problem in young children living in the hogans. It should be noted that there is no evidence at all that the measles per se is any more virulent among the Indian than among the non-Indian population. Indeed, despite the high incidence of pneumonia in this 1958 epidemic, no deaths occurred among the 130 children.

Another example of disease common in non-Indian society that is more serious when it occurs among the Navaho is streptococcal infections. These are the infections that produce sore throats and that, in children, sometimes involve the ear. With modern medical care in the non-Indian United States, serious ear complications of this common infection have been reduced to a negligible level. With the Navaho, however, inflammation of the middle ear of infants and children is commonplace and, indeed, is an important cause of deafness.

As a part of the Manyfarms study, an examination of hearing loss in some 270 school children aged six to ten in the project area was made. It was found that 16 percent of this group of children showed some significant loss in hearing. When a partial loss of hearing is added to the problem of attempting to receive an education in an alien language, the implications of these streptococcal infections are very great.

The same viral respiratory infections that attack the Navaho children in some cases attack the adults, and here, too, serious complication may result. For example, various potentially serious forms of nonviral pneumonia and meningitis may develop, and to a considerable extent the occurrence of these illnesses is facilitated by a preceding viral respiratory infection. In the case of the adults, however, the relatively few serious complications that arise could be readily managed in the hospitals, as they are in the United States in general, provided it is possible to get the Navaho patient to the hospital in proper time.

Infant Diarrhea

Diarrheal disease, likewise, is not really a problem among the Navaho adults or school children, despite the fact that the home sanitary practices with respect to drinking water, food preparation, and the disposal of feces are relatively unsatisfactory. Yet diarrheal disease is an exceedingly important problem among the infants and preschool children.

A total of 506 diarrheal episodes were observed in the clinic in a 27-month period at Manyfarms. Of the 506 episodes, 484 were observed by a physician, and 22 were not. In 23 cases it was necessary to send the patient to the hospital. The age distribution of these 506 diarrheal episodes was quite sharp, with 75 percent of the illnesses occurring in infants or in preschool children. From the epidemiologic pattern of this illness in the Manyfarms studies, and from recent studies in virology, the suspicion is growing that the major portion of this diarrheal illness represents a viral or a combined viral-bacterial infection.

The pattern of illness fits this concept extremely well, and it appears that the infection is something that first occurs soon after the early months of life, at a time when (i) breast feedings are first supplemented with other food; (ii) the child starts crawling around on its own; and (iii) the effects of any immunity that might have been transmitted by the mother at birth would have begun to wear off. This suggests that when sanitary conditions are poor the infection is probably universal, and that a significant immunity to it develops from infection in infancy or early childhood. In most circumstances the disease is not particularly severe, but if the child remains untreated the disease may progress, and it is not infrequently fatal. The emphasis on this entity of infant diarrhea does not mean that isolated outbreaks of other forms of diarrhea in all age groups do not occur as a result of lapses in sanitation. In general, however, such outbreaks are clearly bacterial in origin, are confined to only one or two persons in a single camp, and do not represent numerically the serious health problem presented by the diarrheal disease of infants and young children.

Trachoma

Trachoma in an active stage was found to be present in 2.9 percent of the Manyfarms-Rough Rock school children less than ten years of age. This prevalence of active disease among the children was considerably less than was found at about the same time among adolescents (14 to 16 years of age) assembled from various parts of the reservation at a school for special training in Utah. In 1957 and 1958, at the fall opening of this school, the prevalence of active trachoma was 15.8 and 19.6 percent, respectively. It is evident that these considerable differences in prevalence are not explainable by differences in diagnostic criteria, for an appropriately chosen sample of the Manyfarms–Rough Rock community was reexamined in early 1959 by the same consultants[11] who had made the examinations in Utah, and the 2.9 percent prevalence of active trachoma among the young school children at Manyfarms was confirmed. The possibility that Manyfarms was in some way atypical with respect to trachoma seems unlikely in view of the fact that the prevalence of *inactive* trachoma found there was 16.8 percent, whereas more than 40 percent of persons more than 25 years of age showed evidences of previous disease.

It is generally accepted that the "natural" pathway for the spread of trachoma is from mother to infant. In the present situation, however, it appears that some additional factor is operating and that it favors a considerable spreading of the disease among children more than ten years of age. A factor that could operate in this way would be a lapse in accepted practices of sanitation in the reservation boarding schools.

In actuality, such lapses are known to have occurred due to water shortages or the use of communal towels, and at least two localized epidemics of trachoma have recently been observed soon after the children started living together, at the beginning of the school year. It is believed, therefore, that the situation described for trachoma represents merely one more example of the phenomenon familiar in social development, wherein a particular step from Arcadia to urban-type living may upset the balance between a people and its diseases.

Nonmicrobial Diseases

Of the nonmicrobial diseases, cholelithiasis was relatively common, with 45 instances among the 1,600 persons of all ages who were examined. Neoplastic disease was quite rare, presumably not because of ethnic factors but because of the predominant youth of the population and its relative lack of exposure to such environmental factors as cigarette smoking and atmospheric pollution. Certain diseases relatively prominent in non-Indian society in the United States, such as Graves' disease (hyperthyroidism), paralytic poliomyelitis, asthma, peptic ulcer, and hypertension, were either quite rare or were not encountered at all.

References

1. B. Paul, *Health, Culture, and Community* (Russell Sage Foundation, New York, 1955); G. Foster, *Problems in Intercultural Health Programs* (Social Science Research Council, New York, 1958).

2. J. Adair, K. Deuschle, W. McDermott, *Ann. Am. Acad. Polit. Social Sci.* 311, 80 (1957).

3. The project has received substantial support from the Division of Indian Health and, by research grant (RG–5209), from the Division of General Medical Sciences, National Institutes of Health, U.S. Public Health Service. The project is also supported in part by grants from the Russell Sage Foundation and the Max C. Fleischmann Foundation. Generous gifts of valuable commodities or equipment have been made by firms in private industry, including the

Hyland Laboratories (Los Angeles), Chas. Pfizer and Company (Brooklyn), the E. R. Squibb Division of Olin-Mathieson (New York), and the Santa Fe Railroad.

4. A. Leighton and D. Leighton, *The Navajo Door* (Harvard Univ. Press, Cambridge, 1944).

5. R. W. Young, Ed., "The Navajo Yearbook," *Rept. No. 6 of Navajo Agency, Window Rock, Arizona* (1957).

6. The "Chapter" is a loosely defined rudimentary form of "local" tribal government.

7. In 1957 the highest fertility rate in New York City was among non-whites and was 117.3.

8. L. Merriam, *The Problem of Indian Administration* (Johns Hopkins Press, Baltimore, 1928).

9. In 1954, the prevalence, among U.S. Navy Recruits (whites and non-whites), of individuals who reacted positively to tuberculin was 4.6 percent. See G. J. Drolet and A. M. Lowell, *Am. Rev. Tuberc. Pulmonary Diseases* 72, 419 (1955).

10. K. Deuschle, *Am. Rev. Respirat. Diseases* 80, 200 (1959).

11. The consultants were C. Dawson, senior investigator of the Epidemic Intelligence Service, U.S. Public Health Service, and representatives of the Hooper Foundation, University of California Medical School, San Francisco.

Introducing Modern Medicine
in a Navaho Community: 2
(The second of two parts.)

by Walsh McDermott, Kurt Deuschle, John Adair,
Hugh Fulmer, Bernice Loughlin

In part I of this article were presented the background, the goals, and certain of the preliminary findings of a joint medical-anthropologic research program on cross-cultural technologic development in the field of health. The studies are being conducted with the cooperation of the Navaho Tribe and the U.S. Public Health Service in an 800-square-mile area situated in the approximate center of the Navaho land in the southwestern United States.

Few better illustrations of the significance of cross-cultural matters in medicine can be cited from the present study than the situation observed with respect to congenital dislocation of the hip. Indeed the experience has been an excellent lesson in the basic principle that what constitutes a "disease" in one culture does not necessarily constitute a "disease" in another culture.

"Congenital" Hip

As had been expected, the prevalence of congenital dislocation of the hip at Manyfarms–Rough Rock was found to be quite high. Indeed the number of cases found represents a prevalence rate of 1,090 persons afflicted per 100,000 population, in contrast to a rate of 3.8 persons per 100,000 in New York City. To what extent this disease is truly hereditary has never been precisely established, although it is generally designated as a congenital disorder. It has also been strongly suspected that cultural factors, notably the use of cradleboards, contribute substantially either to the condition itself or to the degree of permanent disability resulting from it. For, on the cradleboard, the infant is securely laced with the outstretched legs bound together in a position that does not favor continued insertion of the head of the femur in the pelvic joint.

Irrespective of the relative roles of genes and culture in causation, there is an increasing body of evidence that the major portion of the disability in congenital hip disease can be prevented if the condition is discovered and appropriate nonsurgical treatment is started during the first year, or at most the first two years, of life. During the next two years (ages three and four), the only satisfactory treatment is surgical and consists of exposing the joint and inserting the femur in its proper location. Once the child has attained the age of five or six years (school age), the only treatments available are the more elaborate surgical procedures of attempting to create a "shelf" of bone, or, if this fails, fusing the hip joint. The latter operation is seldom employed as the initial treatment unless the child has reached the age of twelve or thirteen years, and the operation results in a completely stiff and "frozen" hip joint. The reason for purposely producing the obvious physical handicap of a completely fused hip joint is that unless this is done, the patient runs a considerable risk of having a chronically painful traumatic arthritis of the hip when he or she attains the age of forty or forty-five.

When in the course of the research program the time seemed appropriate to begin a special study of congenital hip disease, it became abundantly clear from the reactions of the Navaho staff that a highly "tender" area was being approached. Contrary to the immediate assumption, moreover, it speedily became clear that the delicate nature of the matter was quite unrelated to its obvious familial connotations. Something quite different was at issue—namely, that in Navaho culture congenital dislocation of the hip, even when bilateral, is not viewed as a disease or even as a particularly important disability. Boys with this condition are not generally mocked, and girls who have it have no difficulty in obtaining husbands and raising families. Indeed, the fact that one child in a family has congenital hip disease appears to be regarded, not quite as a positive blessing, but as a sort of continuously visible relative blessing. By this is meant a blessing in the sense that when evil struck the family, this was the worst it could do, and evil is not apt to strike one family on too many occasions.

What made the issue such a delicate one was the fact that a number of years previously the members of our Navaho staff had happened to witness the consequences of the surgical treatment of congenital hip in older children in their own homes. As explained above, when congenital hip disease is not discovered until the child has passed a certain age, surgical fusion may be all that can be done. Moreover, this procedure is a perfectly sensible one for an older child or adolescent in the non-Indian culture of the United States. The stiff hip does not prevent the child from getting around, and the risk of a more serious handicap in mid-adult life is prevented. With a Navaho child whose hip joint is fused, however, the situation is completely different. Life around a hogan is enormously complicated for one with a stiff hip. For example, such a person cannot join the family for meals because the whole family usually sits on the ground or on sheepskins at mealtime. Moreover, such a child is unable to ride horseback. In Navaho eyes, these are present realities that cannot be effectively offset by the thought that some other disability, not too well understood, will not be present twenty or thirty years hence.

From the viewpoint of the Navaho staff, therefore, the sole contribution of modern medicine to the question of congenital hip disease was to transform something that was no real handicap, and was almost a blessing, into something that represented a very serious handicap indeed. Once it became clear what was bothering the staff, it was possible to design a study with the initial object of developing ways to identify congenital hip disease sufficiently early in life so that nonsurgical treatment might be applied. A genealogic study of the occurrence of congenital hip disease has been started, with the thought that, if it could be established that the condition is genetically determined, the use of diagnostic X ray could be limited to infants in families that had a history of hip disease. Although this study is only in its early stages, there appears to be no cultural problem at all with respect to asking questions about antecedents, because kinship relations are matters of considerable interest in Navaho society.

This episode is cited because it illustrates the danger in attempting to build a health program on the illusory concept that health is the absence of disease. In reality, "health" is a relative matter and signifies the degree to which a person can operate effectively within the particular circumstances of his heredity *and environment.* The wisdom of our Navaho staff on this point undoubtedly saved us from considerable difficulty.

From this study of the disease pattern of the community certain general findings appear significant. First, the virtual absence of most of the diseases that are fatal in non-Indian society in the United States serves to emphasize the fact that in reality all societies are disease-ridden; it is only in the disease pattern that the great differences lie.[1] In economically underdeveloped areas such as the Navaho country, the disease pattern is one of high infant mortality, juvenile invalidism, and premature death, in contrast to the disease pattern in the non-Indian part of the United States, which permits many decades of productive life. Second, in the Manyfarms–Rough Rock community, microbial diseases or their consequences constituted more than three-quarters of the disease found. For most of the diseases, and for virtually all of the fatal ones, effective and practicable measures for treatment or prevention exist. Third, more than 97 percent of the illness encountered could be quite properly and effectively treated in the field clinic facility. Fourth, in such a society, a health program based on the school children is largely a "repair the damage" program.

By the time the child arrives at school at five or six years of age, much of what is going to happen has already happened, and he is a "veteran" of human disease. He may be infected with tubercle bacilli, may be deaf from streptococcal infections of the ear, may have some visual difficulties because of trachoma, and may have been walking since infancy with a congenitally dislocated hip. Obviously, therefore, a program in *preventive* medicine, to be fully effective, must be inaugurated with the preschool children. In a society in which the people live in compact villages, the preschool children are relatively accessible. In a society such as the Navaho, with its vast distances between homes, a considerably greater effort is required, in terms of staff and facilities, to organize a health program for preschool children than to organize such a program for any other age group.

"Health Visitors"

The third of the three general studies undertaken by the medical-anthropologic research group has to do with determining to what extent only partially educated Navaho men and women can be trained to function as effective field auxiliaries of the public health nurses. This program is designated the "Health Visitor" program. In a very real sense this program in medical and nursing research represents an attempt to study certain of the implications of the technologic revolution represented by the development of powerful and simply administered antimicrobial drugs.

In conditions such as those that obtain in the Navaho country, where the population is thinly dispersed over the rugged terrain, it is quite difficult for a trained public health nurse to make more than one or two home visits per day. Moreover, she must be accompanied by a driver-interpreter. Obviously no proper field program could be set up until some way could be found to multiply the effectiveness of the highly trained public health nurse. An essential feature of the study under discussion is the concept of a *single* all-purpose subprofessional worker—that is, an auxiliary to the field nurse, a driver-interpreter, a sanitarian, and a community worker all in one.

It must be emphasized that the Health Visitor program is not one of training "feldshers," or "half-baked" physicians, but rather a study of the use of subprofessional workers who are constantly under the direction of the public health nurse. Each Health Visitor has an assigned group of patients all residing in a particular area, and when out in the field, the Health Visitor regularly communicates with and receives instructions from either the nurse or the physician by radiotelephone installed in the automobile. At the present time a single public health nurse can manage the activities of three or four Health Visitors. The latter can perform all immunization procedures, can administer penicillin and other medication that must be injected, can obtain the patient's basic history, can assist in obtaining the history of the current complaint, and can perform many of the tasks that so frequently consume the time of more highly trained personnel. The types of relationships that are developing between the Navaho Health Visitors and the community on the one hand, and between Health Visitors and the professional staff on the other hand, are being studied in detail by the social scientists.

Segmental Studies

The term *segmental* is used to describe studies in areas that are more sharply defined than the three areas of the general investigations. The range of subject matter in the segmental studies is understandably broad. As a consequence, the research necessarily involves the use of both "field" techniques, in the epidemiologic, genetic, and social-anthropologic studies, and laboratory techniques, for such studies as those on viral disease, anemias, and coronary arterial disease. Segmental studies are in progress for each of the problem disease areas included in the community disease-pattern investigation, and such studies are also in progress in a number of other areas. No attempt will be made to present a complete listing of the studies, but four are briefly outlined to illustrate the varied techniques involved, the type of problem encountered, and the fact that the particular questions chosen could not really be profitably studied by either the medical or the anthropologic investigators working alone.

Self-Administration of Drugs

The first is a study of the extent to which an uneducated, nonliterate people (with partially educated children) can assume personal responsibility in a tuberculosis therapy or prophylaxis program based on the long-continued daily self-administration of isoniazid tablets. Although this question is being studied in terms of drug therapy in tuberculosis, in reality the point at issue has far wider implications. For one of the major trends in medicine today is the unprecedented extent to which successful control of disease has come to depend on long-continued daily self-administration of a variety of powerful drugs by completely asymptomatic patients. To be faithful in the daily ingestion of a pill appears to be strangely difficult in any society. As the act is usually closely related to such personal habits as morning ablutions, the circumstances that surround it may be quite different in different cultures. The first step chosen in the study under discussion was simply to prescribe daily isoniazid tablets for an 18-month period for a group of 150 persons, two-thirds of whom were children. The degree of effectiveness of this practice was evaluated by the only means then available—namely, analysis of the patients' requests for additional supplies of the drug, supplemented by random visits for "pill inventory" in the hogans. By this admittedly crude method it was estimated that approximately 75 percent of the people managed their chemotherapy satisfactorily; an additional 10 percent did so if they were regularly prodded and supervised; and approximately 15 per cent of the group, for one reason or another, could not be relied upon to do their part. The obvious next step was to define these three crudely differentiated groups more precisely, so that the relevant individual factors might be identified. Before this could be done, however, it was first necessary to develop a laboratory technique, suitable for field conditions, whereby the fact that the drug had been recently ingested could be established. Several procedures for chemical analysis of the urine were available but were not satisfactory for conditions as they existed in the field.[2] For it was essential that the procedure should not involve the administration of any new chemical compound of undefined toxicity; the discoloration of the urine or a marked change in its odor; or any chemical extraction process or technique of similar complexity, beyond the capacity of the subprofessional Navaho laboratory workers to carry out. In association with Gladys Hobby, a technique was developed that met these criteria.[3] The vitamin riboflavin is incorporated in the isoniazid tablet, and the presence of the riboflavin in the urine is easily detected by its capacity to fluoresce. It has thus become technologically possible to return to the field studies, but because of certain social problems it is essential to proceed with caution. For in order for the technique to be useful, it will be necessary at some time to reveal the information it discloses. Once this is done, there will occur a change in the relationship of family and physician from one of trust to one of resentment of a mysterious form of "inspection." This problem in itself can presumably be managed through careful conduct, but there is a further problem that is even more delicate. This has to do with the fact that certain Navaho are members of a cult that use the alkaloid peyote in a religious ceremony. This practice has been outlawed by the Tribal Council, and if the practice of peyotism can be proved, the user is subject to a sentence in jail. In the course of the tuberculosis studies at Manyfarms, but before the particular riboflavin technique had been developed, it was discovered that families from certain camps were reluctant to participate. On discreet inquiry it developed that they had heard a rumor that a test was available for the identification of peyotists by detection of the material in the urine. By treading a difficult course between the obvious wishes of the Tribal Council to stamp out peyotism on the one hand and the desire to obtain the cooperation of patients on the other, it was possible to "get the word around" that no such test was known to the staff. This process now has to be repeated, and whether this can be done successfully remains to be seen.

Thus it is that a "drug self-administration" study that has proceeded "logically" from the investigator's standpoint has developed its own set of complications. The experience represents one more example of a principle familiar in cross-cultural work in any field—namely, that a technique which produces information is looked upon as something quite mysterious, and hence may be accorded a completely unpredictable role in terms of the prevailing fears of the culture.

Translation of Medical Concepts

The second of the segmental studies that deserves mention is that on the subject of "conceptual transfer." This study is being conducted by both the social and the medical scientists in association with a noted student of the Navaho language, Robert Young. The basic techniques involve the paraphrasing of passages from a selected medical textbook into two English versions—a version readily intelligible to a person of average education in the United States, and a version thought to fit Navaho concepts. The two versions are then translated orally into Navaho by a number of persons who bear a greater or lesser responsibility as interpreters at medical facilities in the Navaho country. The translations are recorded and are analyzed as they are retranslated into English. The disease descriptions include diseases familiar to the Navaho and diseases concerning which they have no knowledge.

Certain of the points established thus far are general ones that are presumably valid in fields other than health. For example, it was discovered that the common practice of defining with synonyms gave rise to considerable difficulty. Some interpreters presented with the statement "the disease known as arthritis or rheumatism" would proceed to attempt to describe two separate diseases from that point on. A more important specific finding, however, has been that the problem of physician-patient communication with Navaho people is a formidable one, not so much because there are wide differences between the Navaho and the English language as because there are wide differences between the two cultures with respect to concepts of bodily disease. If both cultures had essentially the same concepts of disease and its treatment, any person reasonably fluent in both languages could serve as a satisfactory "bridge" between the patient and his physician. As it stands, however, with the wide difference in medical concepts that exist, an interpreter may be completely bilingual in discussing the ordinary affairs of life yet wholly unreliable in discussing medical matters unless he is quite generally familiar with the medical concepts of both cultures.

To be sure, this same principle applies in some degree to technologies other than medicine. But in most other technologies—for example, animal husbandry or agriculture—the two people involved in the attempt at communication are both usually concerned with the visible world around them and not with the inner feelings of one of the two persons. By contrast, for the proper application of modern medicine the physician depends to a very considerable extent (exclusively, for some diseases) on the subtleties and minor gradations in the patient's own account of how he feels as compared with his usual state.

Thus, in the case of the Navaho, the patient's own standards, by which he judges his degree of well-being, are not only not known to the physician but they derive from concepts of whose very existence the physician may be unaware. It is possible to learn about the concepts from the person serving as interpreter, but this is a lengthy process and the sessions must be conducted in private. For to establish effective interchange with the patient it is essential that the interpreter should not be placed in a position of embarrassment with one of his own people because of a particular approach used in questioning. Ideally, the physician should learn both the concepts of health and the language of the community in which he is working. But for him to acquire the language, particularly to a degree that would permit him to make fine distinctions among symptoms, is frequently not practicable.

An approach that is practicable is to train the physician and the technicians to work effectively through interpreters. The principal lesson already learned, however, is that for effective interchange it is necessary for both the physician and the interpreter to acquire a very considerable body of information concerning the disease concepts in the two cultures. And the educational effort necessary to train the interpreter in "Western" medical concepts is very little less than that necessary to train him as an effective subprofessional technician. Consequently, at least in the specific case of cross-cultural work in medicine and health, there is no real place for a special training school for interpreters. It is more realistic to go the whole way and train the subprofessional auxiliaries of the physicians and nurses.

Ischemic Heart Disease

The third study for mention is one concerned with ischemic heart disease—that is, the myocardial damage that results from coronary arterial disease. Impressive evidence has been accumulated in recent years that this disease is culture-linked. The factor in various cultures that is most often singled out as perhaps the most significant in this disease is the amount of fat, specifically the amount of hydrogenated fat, in the diet. It has been thought that the Navaho, like many peoples who live in relatively primitive surroundings, have a low prevalence of ischemic heart disease, but that, unlike most such peoples, the Navaho consume a diet high in animal fat. It seemed of importance, therefore, to test the long-held clinical impressions that ischemic heart disease was rare among the Navaho by making detailed clinical, electrocardiographic, and other laboratory studies on all members of the Manyfarms–Rough Rock population who were thirty years of age or older. If the suspected low prevalence were to be confirmed, the impression that the people consume relatively large quantities of animal fat could then be tested, and indeed any other culturally linked factors that might reasonably be thought to have significance could be studied.

The suspicion that the prevalence of ischemic heart disease was low was definitely confirmed, and the other studies were started. The observations made thus far have included complete histories and physical examinations on approximately 500 of the 600 persons thirty years of age or older; electrocardiograms with standard and unipolar leads; measurement of the serum cholesterol; determinations (in selected groups) of the pattern of urinary excretion of 17-ketosteroids and ketogenic steroids;[4] characterization of the daily diet by investigators who arranged either to live with a number of the families or who made systematic visits to a larger sample at mealtime; determination (by the same observers) of sleeping habits; measurements of cigarette consumption; and crude estimates, based merely on observation, of the amount of physical exercise generally involved in hogan living. In addition, studies of the fatty-acid composition of samples of fat obtained by biopsy of appropriately selected subjects are in progress; actual measurement of physical exercise has been made; and an attempt is being made to measure crudely what might be termed "relative peace of mind" by ascertaining the number and the effectiveness of religious ceremonials held for this purpose among an appropriately selected population sample. (Navaho religious ceremonies are not held on a regularly scheduled basis but are organized on an *ad hoc* basis, according to the particular needs of an individual.)

As indicated above, virtually all of these data have been obtained, except in the last three areas, and the data are now undergoing analysis. Consequently, only very tentative statements can be made at this time. When due allowance has been made for this fact, however, it appears that the prevalence of ischemic heart disease is indeed low [three cases in a three-year period among the approximately 600 (actually 607) people thirty years or older]; that the apparent absence of angina pectoris is not a reflection of failure of "conceptual transfer" on the part of the interpreters; that the range of values for serum cholesterol is the same as for urban dwellers in the United States; and that consumption of cigarettes is rare and, when found, is low (maximal consumption being forty cigarettes weekly). It further appears (although the analyses are less complete) that the usual diet will be found to approach the United States average in terms of content of fat; that the obvious differences between Navaho and non-Navaho in terms of hair distribution are not accompanied by significant changes in the pattern of hormone excretion in the urine; and that aortic calcification occurs at a later age in the fifty- to sixty-nine-year age group among Navaho than among non-Navaho. It is believed, therefore, but it cannot as yet be stated as definite, that of the factors studied, the principal differences between the Manyfarms–Rough Rock Navaho and residents of urban communities in the United States may be found in such factors as amount of physical exercise, duration of sleep, consumption of cigarettes, and perhaps relative "peace of mind."

Medicine Man and Physician

The fourth segmental study to be mentioned has to do with relationships between the Navaho medicine man and the "Western" physician, and the effects of these relationships on community life. This study has two components. The first is an investigation of what might be termed "the healing process" in a selected sample of nine families. An attempt is being made to determine what is considered to be a health problem in the home and what factors appear to determine whether help is first sought from the Navaho medicine man or from the physician. The other component of the study has to do with the reactions of the medicine men themselves and with whether, as a consequence of the availability of "Western" medicine, young men are no longer willing to expend the not inconsiderable effort necessary to acquire status as medicine men. Thus far the relationships between the medicine men in the community and members of the project staff have been excellent. Every effort is made to accord the medicine men the respect they deserve as the spiritual leaders of the community. Many of the medicine men themselves consult the physicians as patients, and they have raised no objections to the use of "Western" medical methods for patients they are caring for by Navaho methods. Nevertheless, an obvious potential problem exists in any attempt to preserve the spiritual influence of the medicine man while removing from him responsibility for the management of "somatic" disease. The medicine men believe they can distinguish between the type of "illness" most likely to be benefited by their procedures and the type that is better managed by the project staff. Moreover, they are quick to recommend the employment of both sets of "healers" in situations that appear to have any urgency. The danger obviously exists, however, that an acute illness that could be easily treated by modern medical methods might be allowed to progress significantly while Navaho medicine men were being employed. Thus far this has happened only rarely. It is to be hoped that the issue may not become serious and that the present good relations can lead both parties to make adaptations in their practice that will make it possible to preserve the essentials of both "ways."

Significance of the Study

It seems appropriate to comment on the problems involved in the evaluation of studies such as those under discussion and on the possible applicability of any findings to cross-cultural medical technologic development in general.

One of the obvious problems that has to be faced in mixing medical and social-science studies in a single whole is that methods suitable for evaluation in one field cannot always be adapted to another. In the Manyfarms project, the drawing of inferences from the data consists of evaluating a variety of observations, of widely different nature, on the influence of the technology on the community. Some of these observations can be expressed numerically, but many cannot. Thus we have to find ways of arriving at conclusions based on a mixture of various types of evidence.

It would be foolish to defer facing the fact that in many of the issues of greatest importance, the major inferences, in the last analysis, are in the form of subjective judgments. Every effort has been made, therefore, to ensure that the observations and the subjective judgments are made in as systematic and organized a way as possible, and that the conclusions represent the consensus of the greatest number of people in a position to make an informed judgment. It appears that the strictly medical findings should have generality. What cannot be decided at present, however, is whether the particular observations that have to do with working with a people represent research findings that have generality, or whether they merely represent experience, and a certain wisdom presumably acquired thereby, that must remain an essentially individual affair.

Many problems remain that are not being studied. Certain of these are beyond the scope of the project or the competence of the present investigators; others represent wholly proper research subjects for which no approach has as yet been imagined. Nevertheless, they deserve brief mention.

There is the fascinating question of the character of the period during which a community might have the "best of both worlds," when its "primitive" pattern of disease has been suddenly suppressed artificially, rather than by the century and a half of socio-economic development that produced the same result in our society. Is it not possible that we achieved this result at too high a price, as reflected by the particular diseases that are plaguing us today? Will the artificially altered communities necessarily follow directly in our footsteps, as seems to be tacitly assumed. Might it not be that a people who will necessarily continue to live for some time in a rustic environment will develop wholly new disease patterns, quite unlike our own, as they adapt to this relatively isolated but drastic change in their environment. This whole subject is obviously no mere philosophic speculation, for even the preliminary data on births and deaths at Manyfarms strongly suggest the emergence there of just such a phrase as "the best of both worlds."

Another major area has to do with the markedly changed sovereignty relationships of recent years, whereby technologic development activities are now almost invariably conducted with recipient governments and peoples who are politically independent of the nations supplying the bulk of the technicians. Even a nation's own trained people are frequently quite alien to its rural peoples and exert only nominal political authority over them. This general phenomenon has many implications, but a major one is that to all intents and purposes public health programs today are obliged to proceed solely by persuasion. But "persuasion" in a cross-cultural situation is a highly deceptive word, for it really means the use of an enormous body of information and skills that have nothing to do with technological knowledge. Moreover, in most economically underdeveloped areas, persuasion in the area of health must proceed without the powerful support of an immediate prospect of rapid change in social and economic status. Such a hope for improvement of social status has undoubtedly been a very powerful force in determining our own hygienic practices as individuals.

It must also be noted, as was recently emphasized by the Banfields,[5] that the degree of community organization necessary for the exploitation of a technology does not necessarily arise automatically just because the technology is made easily available, and that in some cultures the necessary organization may not arise at all. With the Navaho, the problem of organization should not prove too difficult because the tribal organization is rapidly assuming a well-directed responsibility for the management of its affairs. Inevitably there will be some lag between effective organization at the general tribal level and effective participation by the individual communities in their own affairs. The latter is something that differs widely in degree at present among the many "communities" of the large tribal area.

How Rapid the Change?

It would not seem proper to close this consideration of certain aspects of research in technologic development without mention of the pace or rate of the introduction of a technology. Certainly it is not clear whether this is something that is controllable or even susceptible to study or whether, once a significant innovation is made, others inevitably follow in an essentially uncontrollable fashion. In large measure, any attempt to control the pace of introduction of a technology involves ethical considerations, and these become of primary importance when the technology is medical. With the Manyfarms project we have not really had to face up to this formidable question. For many delays, of a type to be expected in any field program, resulted in a situation in which we could not have simultaneously introduced the many individual elements of a total program even if we had wanted to do so. Consequently, we have tended to introduce one thing at a time. Moreover, in making our choices we derived considerable freedom from the fact that the governmental and tribal programs are both expanding at such a rate that by the time our long-term studies are completed, any appropriate services from our program can be maintained.

In most development programs in health, however, this question of pace looms importantly, especially in the case of programs devoted to the control of a single disease, such as tuberculosis. Unless we can acquire wisdom in this matter, the possibility of actually doing harm through technologic development programs in health is very real. At the present time, however, we cannot pretend that we have found a way to investigate this question of "rate of introduction" in the Manyfarms studies and can only state that we are devoting considerable attention to attempts to find such a way. In the meantime, in our thinking we try to be guided by the thought expressed several years ago by the distinguished former United States diplomat George Kennan:[6] "Wherever the authority of the past is too suddenly and too drastically undermined— wherever the past ceases to be the great and reliable reference book of human problems—wherever, above all, the experience of the father becomes irrelevant to the trials and searchings of the son—there the foundations of man's inner health and stability begin to crumble. Insecurity and panic begin to take over, conduct becomes erratic and aggressive. These, unfortunately, are the marks of an era of rapid technological or social change. A great portion of our globe is today thus affected. And if the price of adjustment to rapid population growth is to cut man's ties to the past and to catapult him violently across centuries of adjustment into some new and unfamiliar technological stratosphere, then I am not sure that the achievement is worth the price."

References

1. R. J. Dubos, *Mirage of Health: Utopias, Progress and Biological Change* (Harper, New York, 1959).

2. W. Fox, *Tubercle* 39, 269 (1958); R. Roberts and K. Deuschle, *Am. Rev. Respiratory Diseases* 80 (1959).

3. G. Hobby and K. Deuschle, *Am. Rev. Respiratory Diseases* 80, 415 (1959).

4. The determinations of the patterns of urinary excretion of ketosteroids are being performed by Thomas F. Gallagher and his co-workers at the Sloan-Kettering Division of Cornell University Graduate School.

5. E. C. Banfield, *The Moral Basis of a Backward Society* (Free Press, Glencoe, Ill., 1958).

6. G. Kennan, *Realities of American Foreign Policy* (Princeton Univ. Press, Princeton, N.J., 1954).

7

Pregnancy in the Navaho Culture

Bernice W. Loughlin

Bernice W. Loughlin, M.P.H., is Director, Field Health Nursing Services, U.S. Public Health Service, Division of Indian Health, Field Health Station, Gallup, New Mexico. She served as a member of the Navajo-Cornell research group (sponsored by Cornell University in conjunction with United States Public Health Service), which was responsible for "Introducing Modern Medicine in a Navajo Community," Science, (January 1960). "Pregnancy in the Navajo Culture" is reproduced with the permission of the author and of the American Journal of Nursing Company from Nursing Outlook, *March, 1965, pp. 55–58.*

As a participant in the Navaho-Cornell Health Research Project to determine the health needs of the Navaho people, I was particularly fascinated by one of the findings: Although only an average of 58.6 percent of the babies were delivered by physicians, there had been no maternal deaths in nineteen years, and only a very small percentage of the infant deaths (0.99) occurred in the perinatal period.[1]

This information prompted me to undertake another study to explore the needs of a selected group of pregnant Navaho women, with the hope that my study might contribute to future planning for maternal and child health programs.

The data presented in this study were gathered through careful examination of the medical records of 230 women who had delivered 428 live children between October 31, 1956, and December 31, 1960. All data which might prove significant in planning future programs and in defining the needs of this group of women were tabulated. As far as possible, all data were verified by the use of documented records. Interviews were conducted with the women to determine their attitudes toward scientific medicine, reasons for seeking care, and the kinds of care which were most acceptable.

Life on the Reservation

The Navaho Reservation comprises 25,000 square miles in Arizona, New Mexico, Utah, and Colorado, called the "Four-Corners" area. The land is at once harsh, desolate desert, beautiful vistas and blue hazy mountains, all covered by a deep blue sky. There are areas of severe erosion, as well as lush ponderosa forests. The reservation cannot begin to support the 85,000 Navahos living there.

The Navaho people, until recently, averaged no more than a third-grade education. The majority continue to use the Navaho language and many speak no English at all. They work off the reservation as itinerant, part-time workers in agriculture, on railroads, and in a variety of unskilled and semiskilled jobs. Those who remain on the reservation subsist largely on a sheep economy. The annual per capita income in 1960 was estimated at about $520.

There are but a few all weather roads, so the people remain isolated. The majority still live in the traditional one-room, log-and-mud octagonal structures, called hogans. A hole in the roof allows smoke to escape from the single potbellied stove used for heating and cooking, and also provides ventilation. Water for personal and household use is hauled, occasionally as far as ten miles, by horse and wagon or by pickup truck.

The Navahos are straddling two cultures, the traditional culture of the "ancient ones" and the tradition-shattering culture of the twentieth century. The traditional family is matrilocal and matrilineal. The matriarch is the leader of her family, although not necessarily its spokesman, and her daughters and their families live close to her. Few major decisions are made without consulting her.

The Navaho concepts of health and disease are interwoven with their concepts of the supernatural. Good health is an indication of a balanced relationship between man and the supernatural forces. If that balance is disturbed, illness is one result.

The Navaho regard for individual autonomy is extremely high. Birth is a personal matter and thus cannot possibly be of interest to anyone else. Modesty creates problems in the examining room except in the very young. Fear of witchcraft often makes it difficult to obtain specimens, such as urine for analysis. Culture values decree that the people endure pain and discomfort without external evidence. Many Navahos still adhere to the traditional *sing,* a curing ceremony in which the medicine man uses a complex interweaving of prayer, chants, and herbal infusions. The very words used to describe illnesses are associated with tradition and cannot easily be used to interpret scientific knowledge.

Poor roads, low level of English literacy, inability to understand scientific concepts of disease, lack of transportation (about one-third of the families have no vehicle), and the widely dispersed hospital facilities all combine to hinder early and adequate care.

Childbearing

Among the Navahos, childbearing is a natural life experience. It is the ultimate goal of the women to bear children, and it is never considered an illness to be endured for nine months. There are many taboos and rituals to be observed during the pregnancy, not only by the prospective parents but by the entire family. The new arrival is truly anticipated and much to be desired, whether he be the first or the fifteenth. Very little preparation can be made, however, because of a taboo that this might cause illness, injury, or even death to the unborn baby.

The expectant mother continues with her usual chores, including wood chopping. She goes horseback riding and takes long walks. She makes no changes in her dietary habits. This simple way of life, the continuance of normal activities, the expectant happiness, the traditional nonbinding clothes, and the customary diet probably all contribute to slow acceptance of medical supervision which might impose adjustments or changes during pregnancy and the puerperium.

The antepartal period is a time of new activity for the Navaho woman as well as happiness for every member of the family. The expectant mother may be concentrating on weaning her soon-to-be-displaced baby; an older child may be planning for his responsibility to administer the cold bath which traditionally takes the present baby out of babyhood and into childhood; father may be selecting a tall, straight pine tree which will make a cradleboard for the baby after it arrives; even the toddler may have been made responsible for carrying kindling.

The extended, closely knit family provides a great deal of mental and emotional support as well as physical help. Although a basic tenet of the Navaho is their belief in individual autonomy, it is still the prerogative of the matriarch to advise and help when asked. The grandmother of the expectant mother is close to her during this time as are the grandmother's sisters (also called grandmother). The designation of all the maternal aunts as "mother" is an indication of their deep-seated family cohesiveness.

Since the clinic population in this study was young (78 percent under age thirty-four with 54 percent of these under age twenty) there was a real need for the support and advice of the matriarchs. Further, the expectant woman who had so many mothers, all of whom lived nearby, did not suffer from baby sitter problems.

The Navahos, as many ethnic groups, have a reverence for

the aged. They ask, "Who could know [about childbirth] better than my grandmother who has had many, many children? What can a man [doctor] or a young woman [nurse] know of the feelings of a pregnant woman? Have they ever had one baby?" Many still prefer to deliver at home, surrounded by family and warmth, in a squatting position, rather than on a hard table in an uncomfortable position, with the glare of surgical lights, and not one person from the family there to help.

Gradually, the younger, better educated women are going to the hospital to deliver, often not because it is safer, but because it removes the necessity for observing the taboos which many now find tedious. Often, too, the young woman lives in town, and the hospital is closer than the family hogan. Conversely, there may be no transportation at the hogan when labor starts, and mother may have to be content with the traditional ministrations.

There is an almost complete lack of any obvious censure for the unmarried pregnant woman. Because the people feel so strongly that procreation is woman's function, they realize that an extended period of education discourages early marriages, thereby creating sexual problems which may lead to extramarital intercourse. Often the girl's mother has no "creeping" baby and she welcomes the newcomer as her own, while the unwed mother returns to school to complete her studies.

Whereas pregnancy is a natural and normal physiological experience, not all women of childbearing age are physiologically normal. Since the Navaho woman never considers herself to be ill because of a pregnancy and since health is a state of balance between the individual and the supernatural, there is no felt need for a medical examination.

Some Project Findings

The 230 women in the sample study group ranged in age from thirteen to forty-eight, and in gravidity from one to seventeen. During the study period, they had a total of 428 live births. There were four sets of twins, no stillbirths, but 22 abortions of 26 weeks gestation or less. The women in this study had an average of six children each; their average age at first delivery was slightly over twenty.

The fertility rate for this study group was 236.9 per 1,000 women aged fifteen to forty-four years as compared to the United States rate of 120 per 1,000; 68.3 percent of these deliveries occurred at intervals of two years or less. In the total group which was separated into five-year age intervals, beginning with ages fifteen to nineteen, twenty to twenty-four, and so on, every age group included from one to four women who conceived out of wedlock. Under age twenty-nine, these were primarily women who stated they were single; over thirty, they were primarily widows. One significant factor was apparent. Of the women in these groups, only one had any antepartal care. Could this have been because of the known censure in the Anglo culture?

Only 13 percent of the women were seen for the first time in the antepartal period in the first trimester, 17 percent in the second trimester, 23 percent in the third trimester, and 47 percent received no antepartal care from the clinic. While medical care in the first trimester does not of itself insure adequate care, the possibility of adequate care is less likely if it does start in the first trimester. (Adequate care is defined here as one visit in the first trimester, one in the second, one early and one late in the third trimester.)

Of the 230 women in the study, 36 had complications, including anemia, mild toxemias, hemorrhage, malformed infants, and abortions. It was further found that the probability of complications increased with gravidity; the risk increased with succeeding pregnancies.

Mortality statistics point out that the greatest number of child health failures occur among postneonatal infants, 58 percent of the deaths occurring from age twenty-eight days through age one year. The causes of these deaths are, most often, infections. About one-third of these deaths are due to influenza and pneumonia, including pneumonia of the newborn; another third was due to the diarrheas and dysenteries, including the newborn.

In the course of the Navaho-Cornell project, almost every family was visited every three to six months by the nursing team, regardless of morbidities or priorities. In this way, most antepartal patients were found, and every effort was made to give them information about antepartal care.

The project elicited the fact that there was a close correlation between home visitation and the frequency of visits made to the clinic for medical supervision. Nineteen women who were not visited (or visited too early to detect obvious pregnancy) sought no medical care, while most of those who were visited in their hogans three or more times received adequate care during the pregnancy. Within the study period these same women sought earlier and more care with each succeeding pregnancy.

Acceptance of preventive care has been slow to accomplish, but immunizations are already well accepted, and other preventive measures are being adopted as the people observe their effectiveness.

Implications for the Nurse

Anthropologists have long advocated a close scrutiny of the cultural values (often with emotional overtones) that people place on both traditional and scientific care programs. It seems rather unnecessary to suggest that we, as nurses, should learn about existing cultural patterns before we suggest new methods. What are the maternal health needs of these people? Is the traditional care adequate? Why do they participate in some health programs and not in others? To what extent can mortality rates be relied on to give the foundation of a program? How much can be accomplished, and what is the irreducible minimum?

In the small group studied the question arises as to whether we have a sound basis for insisting that patients be delivered in the hospital. Should women be encouraged to make their own choice as to place of delivery? Should they be offered support in whatever choice they make and recognition be given to tribal customs and taboos? Despite the lack of proved mortality, it is a fact that most of the morbidities of pregnancy are preventable and at least the small, high-risk group should seek medical care. In this study, this group included the 5 percent of primiparas, under twenty and over thirty; the 15.7 percent with significant histories of previous maternity complications or chronic illnesses; and the 5.3 percent of babies weighing less than 2,500 and over 4,500 grams at birth.

The study has shown that casefinding can best be done as a part of an integrated family public health nursing team service. The best rapport was obtained when the support of the pregnant woman was only one facet of the family visit. Typically, these prospective mothers were more concerned about a sick son or daughter than about care for themselves. As the nurse became known to the people they responded more readily to her suggestions, and with each succeeding pregnancy, they sought earlier and more medical care. As home visits by the nursing team increased, the number of patients who sought medical care increased in direct proportion to the increased number of visits. This implies that the nurse was able to allay fears by advising them of what to expect and by explaining some of the problems which medical care could alleviate.

Over half of the antepartal visits to the medical care center were primarily because of a morbidity. This may point to a need for general rather than specialized clinic programs. It would also seem to indicate that there is a need for more well-qualified public health nurses to serve small districts than is now possible, so that they could become known and respected. (The "average" nurse on the Navaho reservation covers 1,500 square miles and has 6,000 patients.)

There were indications that as families moved into urban and away from rural living, the size of the family presented a problem. A program of family planning could well fill an emotional as well as economic need and should be available to those who wish to limit the size of their family.

Since it seemed apparent from this study that the extended, traditional family offered many strengths, it would be interesting to study a group of women who have moved out of the "family nucleus" setting, to learn about their feelings and problems. As is true of any group in transition, the Navaho tribe today includes the gamut of personality types—from those completely Anglicized and in top-level jobs to those still completely traditional and resistive of all scientific methods.

The high fertility rate and the close spacing of the children, together with the high postneonatal death rates, could well indicate that the period of weaning is the most critical time. A coordinated and comprehensive program of personal and environmental hygiene, utilizing all health disciplines and including some means of implementing improvements, is most important to the people.

Any program of action designed to change attitudes must take into consideration the values and pressures involved in old attitudes and resistance to change, especially those attitudes laid down by cultures which have prospered over centuries of time. It would seem here, as elsewhere in the world, that the health of the individual cannot be sustained or improved without the coordination of all forces which influence daily living—environmental, socio-economic, emotional, and cultural—nor can the health of the individual be markedly improved without some change in the total group. Further studies involving other segments of the Navaho people are needed to substantiate or refute the findings of this study, but some conclusions have been drawn which might point the way to further studies and to future planning in maternal and child health services.

Note

1. The Navaho-Cornell Field Health Research Project was conducted under the direction of Cornell University Medical College Department of Public Health, in cooperation with the U.S. Public Health Service Division of Indian Health and the Navaho Tribal Council. It was located in the middle of the vast reservation in the Manyfarms–Rough Rock area on which 2,237 persons lived, as of January 1, 1961. The author was on loan from USPHS when she participated in the project.

Bibliography

McDermott, Walsh, and others. Introducing modern medicine in a Navajo community. *Science* 131:197–205; 280–287, Jan. 22 and 29, 1960.
The Navajo Yearbook; a Decade of Progress. (Report no. 8) Window Rock, Ariz., Navajo Agency, 1961.

8

Suggested Techniques for Inducing Navaho Women to Accept Hospitalization During Childbirth and for Implementing Health Education[1]

Flora L. Bailey

Flora L. Bailey, Ph.D., is Supervisor of Physical Education, K-VI Schools, School District of South Orange and Maplewood, New Jersey. She formerly served in a similar capacity at the Tuscan School, Maplewood. Her interest and life work have been in health education and physical development of children. Her "Suggested Techniques for Inducing Navaho Women to Accept Hospitalization during Childbirth and for Implementing Health Education" is reprinted with the permission of the author and The American Public Health Association, Inc., from American Journal of Public Health, *Vol. 38, No. 10 (Oct. 1948), pp. 1418–1423.*

Some interesting and valuable suggestions on the implementation of health education and medical procedures among the Navahos have been made by Alexander and Dorothea Leighton.[2] Since I agree with them that a sympathetic approach to this important problem is necessary, I should like to offer a number of additional suggestions based on my investigation of the beliefs and practices of the Navaho Indians pertaining to the reproductive cycle.[3] This material was gathered from three areas in New Mexico, namely, the Ramah, Pinedale, and Chaco Canyon regions. Sixty-six informants, both men and women, furnished the data. The investigation was made with a view to laying the background for a better understanding of Navaho attitudes toward health and particularly toward the problems of childbirth. Hospitals which serve the Navahos, both government and private, have made efforts to inculcate certain health principles into the minds of those whom they contact but the extent to which they have been successful is undetermined. Recent figures estimate that perhaps 25 percent of the women seek medical assistance during childbirth.

In analyzing the data, a considerable degree of homogeneity of belief was found to exist, with certain deviations of opinion surrounding the central pattern. Definite patterns of thought, however, could be distinguished throughout all the material. For example, Navaho beliefs and practices pertaining to the reproductive cycle are dependent upon mythological and religious sanctions. Pregnancy restrictions and behavior patterns for facilitating delivery are based on the premise that *like produces like,* or that an effect resembles its cause, and various forms of sympathetic magic are indulged in so that nature will be forced into the path which is desired. It was also discovered that there is a strong emotional response in relation to hospitalization and medical aid. Although many informants did not refer to hospitals, others expressed a violent feeling either for or against these institutions and even mentioned individual doctors by name, discussing them with strong feeling.

Because certain Navaho practices are sanctioned by mythology and reinforced by ritual, they offer great resistance to change unless such changes can be made to fit the pattern of Navaho logic rather than that used by administrators of educational and medical programs. It is suggested, therefore, that medical workers and health educators accept without adverse comment the pregnancy restrictions and rules of conduct which are traditional with the Navaho. Then, using a pattern of logic which parallels that expressed in Navaho thought, they could present new restrictions and rituals based on modern medical knowledge which would assist the woman to achieve the desired result, namely, the safe and easy delivery of a healthy child.

Specific recommendations, based on these conclusions, have been proposed and will be presented here in conjunction with the native practices which can be used to reinforce or redirect the pattern.

It is of primary importance to gain the support and confidence of influential members in each family group if a program of health education is to be successfully implemented. Group decisions in matters of health are a common practice when a healing ceremonial is involved. There is considerable carry-over, it is safe to venture, in decisions regarding hospitalization. There is little doubt that many women would welcome medical advice and assistance during pregnancy and childbirth if they had the support of older members in the family and heard favorable reports from those of their friends who had experienced hospital care.

One *singer* reported, "For a while, after one woman around here had gone to the hospital and come back with the news that they gave her something to put her to sleep and she had no pain with the baby, many women thought it was better to go to the hospital than to stay home." If, as a result of one woman's confidence and satisfaction, "many" women wish to make use of medical assistance, it should be a matter of principle for each woman receiving help to be sent away feeling secure and happy so that her enthusiasm would create support and confidence among her neighbors.

In explaining why women hesitate to make use of medical facilities the statement was made, "Women know what to do at home, and they don't know about hospitals, so they don't go to hospitals." This, according to Dr. Clyde Kluckhohn's analysis of Navaho thought patterns,[4] is a basic reaction closely linked with others by which they win security. Regarding unfamiliar human beings as threats the women withdraw and do nothing when confronted with a new and potentially dangerous situation. Facing such a situation, with which she feels unable to cope, the woman solves her problem by refusing to have anything to do with doctors. The medical staff, by anticipating this reaction, could prepare the way for a more constructive solution of her problem through field clinics, individual conferences, and educational procedures designed to reassure the patient through an explanation of hospital routine.

Even a white patient, entering a hospital for the first time, is confused and apprehensive if the routine has not been explained. How much greater must this apprehension be for a woman who enters an alien world where the language is strange, where nothing fulfills her expectations of how things should be done, and where she is liable to "ghost infection" (as the Navahos term the disease) if she comes in contact with articles previously used by those who have died there.

After orientation and reassurance have been given her, the staff of the hospital, or the visiting field worker, should continue to seek ways of reinforcing the woman's emotional security and peace of mind. The fear and anxiety of pregnant women in connection with hospitalization could doubtless be reduced by encouraging early admittance, thereby lowering the mortality rate. Reports show that the majority of maternal deaths in the hospital are caused by a retained placenta since the women are so afraid to face an unknown situation that they arrive at the hospital only in time to die there. One young woman remarked, "If a baby doesn't come for two or three days they get scared and go to the hospital." This tendency to seek hospitalization only in an emergency, or if death is imminent, is not unusual. As a result, one hears such bitter reports as that which came from an older woman who had lost two daughters in childbirth at the hospital after each had successfully delivered other children at home. Obviously, in her opinion, there was only one deduction—the white doctors had killed her daughters!

Any effort made by health educators, therefore, to persuade

women to seek hospitalization at the proper time would be valuable in that rumors of death due to the fault of the hospital would be minimized, and the fear which serves as an emotional block for some women could thereby be counteracted.

One anxiety, however, which might be exploited in persuading women to accept aid is the extreme fear of contact with the birth discharge. It is linked with the even greater fear of contact with menstrual blood. One man reported, "This blood is not as bad as menstrual blood but it will break the back or the breast." The "breaking" thus referred to is *arthritis deformans,* for it is believed that deformation will result from contact with the birth discharge. Other ill effects were detailed by a young woman as follows: "If a ghost-bird, or a bluebird, or a coyote eats it, the woman won't get well for a long time; she stops having babies; it gives the woman more pain; it kills the mother; the baby won't have any sense; it will cripple animals; and witches will get it." In the face of such formidable dangers which follow the improper disposal of the birth discharge, medical authorities might offer to relieve the woman of this responsibility, assuring her that if she comes to the hospital the nurses would take care of the disposal, thereby avoiding the possibility of exposing any of her family to contact with the blood and the resulting infection.

In dealing with patients during pregnancy, as well as after their admission to the hospital, it is important to phrase medical suggestions in terms of Navaho logic. For example: Navaho methods of keeping the fetus small, to insure an easy delivery, include hard work, exercise, and not sleeping in the daytime, as well as the magical application of certain medicines which work on the *like produces like* formula such as sucking honey from the pentstemon (called hummingbird's food) or eating a hummingbird's egg, shell and all, because this bird is so tiny. If the medical worker suggests other methods such as moderate exercise, the use of vitamins, or an increased calcium intake, he might explain them by using the Navaho phraseology, "It will make the baby strong, even though he remains small, so he will be born easily." It might also be pointed out that exercise keeps a person lean and in good condition, therefore it would, as they say, "keep the baby small."

There are certain parallels between Navaho and white medical practice which might be capitalized on by the hospital staff to expedite the delivery in a manner satisfactory to all concerned. Since the woman is accustomed to the native pattern of male assistants in the hogan, the presence of a male physician should be acceptable to her, and the Navaho practice of manipulating the abdominal walls in order to secure a favorable presentation could be related to any similar manipulation which might be undertaken by the doctor. Both these patterns have mythological sanction, for Washington Matthews notes that abdominal manipulation to secure a favorable presentation was used by the two male gods, Talking God and Water Sprinkler, when they assisted at the delivery of Changing Woman and White Shell Woman.[5]

Native forms of modesty should be respected for a Navaho woman expresses her modesty in a slightly different manner from a white woman. That is, she does not consider exposure of the breasts an immodest act but places great emphasis on being adequately covered from waist to ankle. In their ceremonials women strip to one or two skirts and are very skillful in participating in events, even in the ceremonial bath, without exposing the lower part of the body. It is not strange, therefore, that hospital procedures involving a short bedgown and exposure during nursing care should be disliked. Manual examination should be undertaken with as little exposure as possible. However, since women are accustomed to a *singer* pressing and manipulating the body for ceremonial purposes, the doctor might minimize his problem by relating his examination to some such act with which she is familiar.

If internal version is indicated there is precedent in native practice for this also. Cactus salve is rubbed on the hands to make them slippery and the midwife then reaches into the orifice, using her hands as forceps, to deliver the child. However, one woman said, "It is a bad thing to reach in for the baby. I saw it done and it killed the woman." It should be explained to the patient, therefore, that under sterile conditions such emergency measures involve less danger than she anticipates in the hogan.

Navaho medical practices include the application of medicines externally and drinking of draughts during the period of pregnancy as well as at the onset of labor. Thus, any medicine which needs to be administered could be given with the explanation that it will, as the Navahos say, "help bring the baby easier," or "bring the placenta right away," or "stop the pain and clean out the blood." These are the results toward which their native medications are oriented and will, therefore, have meaning for them. No more than the exact amount, however, should be left where the patient has access to it, unless drinking a large quantity will make no difference, for the usual dose of native medicine is prescribed as "drink lots of it, drink one or two cups of that medicine."

If there is need for the use of diathermy, X ray, or similar treatments these might be related to the healing properties of the sun prominent in Navaho ceremonial lore.

Since women are used to hot applications (made by heating the branches of juniper and packing them around the body) a parallel will be easily grasped, if heat needs to be applied, by using the Navaho cliché, "it will stop the pain."

If lacerations occur it is customary to use lotions, salves, or dusting powders. Steam baths, produced with water and herbs called Life Medicine, are also recommended. If similar treatments, ordered in the hospital, are tactfully introduced, objections might be avoided. Surgery, however, is not a native practice and this would have to be presented as a special technique used by white doctors.

A few days after delivery the woman takes a bath in certain

herbs, including those called Life Medicine, to counteract the danger from contact with the birth discharge. It would be easy for a nurse to mention that the daily bath water contained a kind of Life Medicine possessing purifying qualities, thereby easing the patient's mind.

If a woman does not have sufficient milk to nurse her child she may resort to artificial means of increasing lactation. This follows the familiar pattern of *like causes like* since liquids (particularly soups) are taken internally, and milkweed plants are applied to the breasts. On the basis of Navaho logic, therefore, the staff could introduce milk into the diet or, if desirable, force liquids. Certain other practices which have mythological sanction and therefore deep emotional significance for the parturient might be permitted, or even suggested, by the medical staff. If the doctor, for example, would advise the woman to have a Blessingway ceremonial sung for her, prior to entering the hospital, it would fall into a pattern which is familiar to her and make her feel that there was sympathetic cooperation between the white doctor and the native *singer*.

The kneeling position, which the woman by tradition assumes for her delivery, has mythological sanction and is more in keeping with her sense of modesty than the modern obstetrical position. If the hospital could adapt its methods to allow delivery in the native position it might reduce emotional tension and prove valuable psychologically. Perhaps the dragrope, which in the legend was either a rainbow or a sunbeam, could be adapted for the woman's support, and certainly such small rituals as placing pollen ceremonially on the objects to be used, or applying pregnancy charms to her body, could do no harm. Corn pollen, sprinkled on a living horned toad at the moment it is born and then gathered, is always carried by a pregnant woman for use in this emergency. They say, "Take live pollen from the horned toad's babies and when the pains begin the woman takes a pinch and drops it inside her blouse because when the little toads are first dropped they can run away fast. They are strong." Mythologically the horned toad is protected against danger. For a nurse to suggest that the woman make use of such ritual assistance might easily serve to strengthen her feeling of security so that the subsequent ordeal would be eased.

Since the ritual act of *untying* plays an important part in native precautions at birth, if the woman were allowed to unbind her hair and remove her jewelry, and in cases of unusual emotional tension if the nurses would also make some gesture toward untying or unbinding their own persons, this would reinforce her morale.

The Navahos say, "No one should be around who gave any trouble to his mother at birth." Perhaps the hospital assistants could let it be known that they themselves had been born with great dispatch and little trouble. Anything that can be related to the *like causes like* formula would serve to bring reassurance.

That Navaho women find the smell of blood objectionable is evidenced by the fact that they use pungent herbs as an inhalant with the explanation that this will prevent fainting from smelling the blood. This may be partly psychological, related to the fear of contact with the birth discharge, but it would be easy to present the woman with a small bunch of sagebrush or a twig of wet juniper and might help her through a trying time. Familiar odors are known to be powerful stimulants to the emotions and would be gratefully welcomed in an atmosphere of strong, unfamiliar, and doubtless unpleasant odors.

One of the reasons women dislike hospitalization is that the food is unfamiliar and sometimes, to them, unpalatable. The food which the post-parturient expects to receive immediately after delivery is a ceremonial food sanctioned by mythology. It is a special type of blue cornmeal mush without the juniper ashes usually added to cornmeal breads. Any woman who has eaten mush ceremonially must eat it following childbirth. Where Navaho women assist in the hospital kitchens it should be possible to serve this specialty and thereby add to the patient's mental and physical comfort.

Since the woman is used to having the newborn baby close to her side it might be advantageous to let the infant remain near its mother in the hospital rather than to exile it to the nursery. This practice is not without precedent in certain modern hospitals where the philosophy of purely objective routine and seclusion for the infant has been replaced by one advocating closer physical contacts.

Molding or pressing the body of the newborn baby is believed to produce strength and beauty. This manipulation is based on mythology, being related to the pressing in the "Girl's Puberty Rite." Women who have had children born in hospitals say that the children did not develop normally due to lack of this ritual. One young mother said, "You press his forehead and nose, and body to make him beautiful. My oldest girl was born in the hospital and they didn't do that to her, and her nose is little and her forehead sticks out." Certainly it would do no harm to suggest this ritual pressing and would satisfy a need.

Legend tells us, "It is thought the sun fed the infant on pollen, for there was no one to nurse it." This statement gives the sanction for the first food given to the child. Allowing the mother to offer a pinch of corn pollen to her baby would do him no harm and might do the mother considerable good. It might be practical, also, if the mother has enough milk, to allow her to nurse the child whenever it cries. This would follow a familiar native pattern yet would not be out of line with the newest practices in child care.

If the mother remains in the hospital until after the navel of the infant has healed it is important that the cord be given her to take home rather than discarded. The strong emotional tone in which the magical properties of the cord are discussed would indicate that cooperation in its proper ritual disposal would be appreciated.

When the mother and child are discharged from the hospital it is to be hoped that confidence will have been established between the medical adviser and the Navaho patient. Toward that end the preceding recommendations have been offered with the hope that they may point out specific ways of adjusting one culture to another and of lessening the tensions which are inevitable from such contacts.

References

1. This paper was presented before the Section on Anthropology of the American Association for the Advancement of Science at the One Hundred and Fourteenth Meeting in Chicago, Ill., December 26, 1947.

2. Leighton, Alexander H., and Leighton, Dorothea C. *The Navaho Door*. Cambridge, Mass.: Harvard University Press, 1944.

3. The writer is indebted to Dr. Clyde Kluckhohn of Harvard University and Dr. Leland C. Wyman of Boston University for their encouragement and advice in the conduct of this study.

4. Kluckhohn, Clyde, and Leighton, Dorothea. *The Navaho*. Cambridge, Mass.: Harvard University Press, 1946.

5. Matthews, Washington. "Navaho Legends," *Memoirs*. American Folklore Society, 5, 1897, p. 231.

9

Helping A People To Understand

Annie D. Wauneka

Mrs. Annie D. Wauneka is the only woman member of the Navajo Tribal Council and is chairman of the council's Committee on Health and Welfare. She has received many honors for her work in this area. In 1959, she was cited by the Arizona Public Health Association as the state's outstanding worker in public health. Also in 1959, she was presented the Indian Council Achievement Award. "Helping a People to Understand" is reprinted with permission of the author and of the American Journal of Nursing from the American Journal of Nursing, *Vol. 62, July, 1962, pp. 88–90.*

In 1951, my first year on the Navaho Tribal Council, one of the doctors reported on the difficulties of helping Navaho patients with tuberculosis. At that time, although Navaho patients were flown to sanatoriums, some of which were located out of the state, once there, they often refused treatment. Some even walked out in their pajamas and went home by whatever transportation was available. Sometimes, when visiting, parents took their children home with them. This caused quite a disturbance among the health workers and, of course, members of the Tribal Council were concerned that their own sick people were refusing services.

I was appointed by the council to look into this problem and see if I could find a way to convince Navaho patients to remain in the sanatoriums for treatment. It was thought that a woman and mother could better understand their problems.

The doctors had told patients that tuberculosis was caused by a germ that could be transferred from one individual to another through contact. But this idea was not understood by many Navaho, especially those who were uneducated. Even today, out of 100 Navaho people, 85 are illiterate.

It was difficult for me to realize that I would be working among my people on the prevention and treatment of tuberculosis, because I was just as unknowing about the disease as any Navaho on the reservation. I admit that I was definitely afraid to tackle the problem. I told my husband of the appointment and explained what I was supposed to do. He immediately objected saying that I would contract the disease and the rest of the family would get it. We were all afraid of tuberculosis.

I thought about the problem for a long time. I did not know anything about tuberculosis, how to talk about it, whether it really was caused by a germ, or whether the doctors had made up the whole story about "bugs." To explain to other Navaho about tuberculosis, to know what I was talking about, to convince sick Navaho to return to the sanatoriums, I had to find out all about it—what it could do to a human being, where it came from.

I spent a lot of time talking to doctors about it and, over a period of several months, visited the laboratory. I wanted to see with my own eyes what kind of bugs the doctors were talking about. I had to know that there actually were germs.

When I understood enough about tuberculosis, when I learned that tuberculosis could affect not only the lungs but many parts of the body, when I knew I could answer questions, then I was prepared to tell my people that only "white man's medicine" could cure tuberculosis.

But first I spoke to the medicine men on the reservation about what I had learned. In turn, the medicine men explained to me the old Navaho beliefs about what causes illness. It was hard for me, but I had to learn both the old and the new to be able to interpret to the Navaho.

Beliefs and Customs

Today, when a Navaho becomes ill, he must choose between the white man's doctor and his own medicine man. He has to decide which one will cure him. In the past, the Navaho people did not believe in the spread of disease, and this is still true today with a majority of them.

There is no word for "germ" in our language. This makes it hard for the Navaho people to understand sickness, particularly tuberculosis.

I asked the medicine men what they thought caused the lungs to be destroyed; what caused the coughing and the spitting up of blood. According to the stories learned from their ancestors, tuberculosis is caused by lightning. If lightning struck a tree and a person used that tree for firewood or anything, it would make him sick, cause blisters to develop in his throat and abscesses in his lungs. There are other beliefs besides this.

It is difficult for the Navaho people to believe that tuberculosis is not caused by lightning but by a germ that multiplies.

To talk about tuberculosis or health care to a Navaho, one must approach him with courtesy and respect. When we enter a hogan or visit with patients in the sanatoriums, we first talk about each other's relations. This is particularly necessary with the elderly Navaho people. By beginning in this way, we show that we are friendly and interested in the person and have respect for him and that we are, in a fashion, related.

Next we talk about everyday chores, how the family is getting along, whom they visit, how they are making out with the livestock or other sources of income. We ask if they are getting any kind of help. This leads to talk about welfare, sanitation, and, finally, about tuberculosis.

We explain to the whole family how tuberculosis is spread and how the bugs can actually be seen through a microscope. We describe how the sick person starts to lose weight, how he coughs, then starts spitting up blood. We tell about X rays, that taking them is just like taking a picture of anyone. They usually listen eagerly.

It takes them a long time to answer, because they are thinking about what we have said. They tell us about their family problems and ask who will take care of their loved ones at home, who will look after the sheep and horses if they go to the sanatorium. We discuss these problems and tell them that their families will be taken care of when they go to the sanatorium.

In most cases, it is not necessary to look for help outside the family group, because Navaho families are closely united, and not only in blood lines. They live close to one another. Married daughters, aunts and uncles, and in-laws usually are available to help.

This encouragement we give makes patients less reluctant to go back to the hospital for treatment and cure. It is very hard for the Navaho, especially the older ones who have tuberculosis, to go far from home, because they have never been off the reservation or far from their loved ones.

Adjusting to Hospitals

A hospital is totally strange to them—strange people, strange food, strange ways of treating the sick. Bathing facilities, running water, electric lights, and thermometers are all strange.

Among other things, the Navaho do not like to have their persons touched. They do not like someone looking at their bodies without their consent. The Navaho do not like to expose their bodies. Bed rest is also strange to them, particularly if they are at home. They know that they must make a living, take care of the children, take care of the sheep. They do not understand what good it will do to stay in bed and take certain foods and medicine.

All this must be explained. Such foods as vegetables, fish, chicken, or pork are not part of the regular Navaho diet; so this is something else they must learn. The value of these foods must be explained, as well as the value of the drugs and treatment the doctor recommends.

The Navaho does not understand why the doctor in the sanatorium does not come to see him every day the way he does in a general hospital. The patients like to see their X rays to see if they are "making their way to a cure."

It is the responsibility of the health committee to help the Navaho people understand about diseases, how they are spread, and how they can be prevented. The only way this can be done is through people who are interested and dedicated.

The members of the health committee talk to the doctors in the sanatoriums, so they can explain the progress to the patients. The patient who must stay longer must be encouraged in a way he understands. We explain to him that it will take a lot of effort on his part, as well as on the part of the doctors, to accomplish the cure.

Part of our job is to remind families that patients like to get letters from home, to know about how the children are getting along, and who is looking after the sheep. We tell them that patients like happy letters.

The ones who receive all kinds of complaints from their families want to go home to take care of the problems. When families write such letters, we explain why happy letters are needed.

When patients must be persuaded to return to the sanatorium, we point out what improvement has already been made. The patients admit they feel better in the hospital. They say, too, that they would like to return and will return after the problems at home have been cared for. The health committee emphasizes the danger to the family and how, in the long run, it will be better to be cured of tuberculosis.

It is important to listen to and understand the patient's problems, how he feels about being so far away from home, and just what it means to him to be in the sanatorium.

Another thing that must be clearly explained to the Navaho is that tuberculosis is not a disease peculiar to the Navaho but that it is a world problem, a community disease, and that all health services such as the U.S. Public Health Service are working very hard to stamp out this dreadful disease. We explain that tuberculosis is a disease of long standing and that it is the duty of the Navaho people to help cure themselves.

In the past, the Navaho were not told about tuberculosis in just this way. They were never warned or taught about this disease or that it could be prevented. The only things Navaho patients learned were that, if they were sick, they went to the hospital, got treated, and came home.

I have made films on tuberculosis with the narrative in the Navaho language, which we have shown in many communities. These help to teach the Navaho about tuberculosis, what can be done about this dreadful disease that is killing off our people. The Navaho are interested and active in planned programs throughout the reservation. Through the health committee, they are learning more of what we need to do to raise our children in better health and to safeguard them from disease.

The Blessing Way

When a Navaho patient returns from the sanatorium, a ceremony called "The Blessing Way" is performed. It is a beautiful ceremony performed for those who have been away for months or years, perhaps in the hospital or even in the armed forces. The Blessing Way gives them moral support; it is a happy reunion with a happy spirit. The Navaho knows he is home, that he is welcome, and that he and his family are on a happy journey and wished every prosperity and good health.

I am glad to report that tuberculosis has decreased from first to seventh place as a leading cause of death among the Navaho people. We still have patients who should go to the sanatoriums, who still need to have it explained that tuberculosis is actually caused by a bug discovered by the white man, and that the white man has also discovered the medicine to cure it.

The Navaho patients learn many lessons in the sanatorium and, when they return home, improve their homes because they know that in the hogan with a dirt floor with its uncleanliness, tuberculosis can be developed again. They also bring the message of better health teaching to their families and communities. Now attitudes are changing.

10

Concepts of Disease in Mexican-American Culture[1]

by Arthur J. Rubel

Arthur J. Rubel, Ph.D., is currently serving as Program Advisor for the Ford Foundation. He is Associate Professor in Anthropology at Notre Dame University. Other outstanding contributions have been his service as Consultant, U.S. Public Health Service *(1963–67) and his anthropological research (with emphasis on health behavior and attitudes) among Mexican-American and Indian groups of Mexico. His publications include:* Across the Tracks: Mexican-Americans in a Texas City, University of Texas, *(1966); "Epidemiology of a Folk Illness,"* Ethnology, *(1964); "Role of Social Science Research in Recent Health Programs in Latin America,"* Latin American Research Review, *(1966); and (co-author) "Perspectives on the Atomistic Society: Introduction,"* Human Organization, *(Fall 1968). His article "Concepts of Disease in Mexican-American Culture" is reproduced with permission of the author and of the American Anthropological Association from the* American Anthropologist, *Vol. 62, pp. 795–814 (Oct., 1960).*

Background

This paper discusses some traditional concepts of health and disease found among the Spanish-speaking people of the Texas-Mexican border, and the manner in which these concepts contribute to the maintenance of the social system of that group.

In 1957 a study of the changing concepts of health and disease among the Mexican-Americans of Hidalgo County, Texas, was inaugurated. This is one of a series of publications resulting from that study and describes some aspects of life in Mecca,[2] the largest and most heterogeneous of the three communities studied.

Mecca is a small city of approximately 15,000 inhabitants located on the delta of the Rio Grande. Three-fifths of the total population is made up of persons of Mexican descent, a great number of whom are native-born American citizens.

The overwhelming majority of the Spanish-speaking people of Mecca trace their roots to isolated, rural hamlets which lie on either side of the Rio Grande—south to the Rio Pánuco in Mexico and north to the Nueces River of Texas. The life histories of the present older generation Mexican-Americans portray the lives of their parents as spent from birth to death in isolated, familial hamlets, which were seldom visited by strangers.

In the era which followed the overthrow of Porfirio Diaz in the Republic of Mexico, the usually oppressive living conditions in the arid, northeastern section of the Republic were made worse by the furies of the revolution and counterrevolution, of banditry and punitive government expeditions which swept across the land. This is the area from which the Mexican-American population of Mecca came. The poverty and the general insecurity of the times caused many thousands of emigrants to seek improved conditions on the United States side of the boundary.

At the time of the surging unrest in the Republic to the south, all the previously undeveloped semidesert delta lands, from Brownsville to Mission, Texas, were changing hands from the heirs of Spanish and Mexican recipients of eighteenth-century grants (*porciones*) from the Spanish Crown to Anglo-American speculators. From 1910 until 1930 the speculating land companies gained control of all irrigable land along the lower Rio Grande in Texas. By means of intensive systems of irrigation and emergency floodways the semidesert region was transformed into a vegetable- and citrus-producing region of primary importance. After their development the tracts were resold to English-speaking investors and "home-seekers" brought from small towns and cities in the north central and northeastern sections of the United States and several Canadian provinces.

Each of the land companies then erected a town on its development tract to serve the immigrant population. The land boom and consequent enormous amount of construction activities required the labor of many thousands of unskilled and semiskilled laborers. This was supplied entirely by immigrants from Mexico and by displaced Spanish-speaking American citizens of the ranchos. One of the many towns erected on the delta of the Rio Grande in the early decades of the twentieth century was Mecca.

The differences in custom, language, and standard of living of the two ethnic groups which migrated to the new urban site were perpetuated by a well-recognized policy of separatism. In Mecca, those of Mexican culture were assigned residence, schools, and church on the side of town which lay to the north of the bisecting railway, and the non-Mexican population was assigned residence, schools, and church to the south of the tracks.

Each of the two new communities which comprised the town of Mecca succeeded in transplanting its customary way of life to the new town. Those of Anglo-American small town background quickly formed voluntary associations of a service club and fraternal nature which were designed to unite unrelated individuals with common interests, e.g., by type of vocation, or state of provenance. Today, the 6,000 residents of Anglo-American background are organized into more than seventy social, civic, and fraternal organizations. What remains of their time is further devoted to the social and religious activities of sixteen major churches which include within their framework many study groups, women's circles, and other types of formal organizations. The lives of Anglo-American children are mirror images of their parents', and the youngsters are trained in the group way of life by a succession of organized activities which range from school clubs to associations such as Girl Scouts, Boy Scouts, Sea Scouts, 4-H Clubs, Future Farmers of America, and Little League baseball clubs, to name but a few.

In contrast to the highly organized society on the south side of the tracks, the 9,000 Mexican-Americans have transplanted to the urban environment a customary way of life formed in the familial tradition of isolated ranchos. The religious life of this community is represented by a large Catholic church to which the great majority of people remain faithful. However, some fifteen small missions of different Protestant sects are present, the largest of which ministers to about fifty families who regularly attend services. Efforts by the Protestant churches to organize ongoing incorporated groups such as women's circles, Bible study groups, and discussion groups have been singularly unsuccessful. An active chapter of the Knights of Columbus (which includes both Anglo- and Mexican-Americans) and a small council of the League of United Latin American Citizens represent the only significant current efforts to organize the Mexican-American community into formally constituted associations. Among the children a Boy Scout troop functions as the only voluntary association. The transference of a familial type of life from the hamlet to the city is suggested in the often quoted explanatory axiom: "You can take a ranchero from the rancho, but you cannot take the rancho from the ranchero!"

Given their distinctive sociocultural backgrounds, it is not surprising to find that although both groups share certain illnesses, e.g., measles and pneumonia, other ills are restricted to one or the other of the groups. Five illnesses which are confined to the Mexican-Americans are *caida de la mollera* (fallen fontanel), *empacho, mal ojo* (evil eye), *susto* (shock), and *mal puesto* (sorcery). The first four of the illnesses are categorized as *males naturales*—sickness from natural cause—and thus within the domain of God. *Mal puesto* is considered "one of the others," *mal artificial* or outside the realm of God, the work of the devil. Further, a discussion which concerns any one of the first four illnesses invariably leads to reference to the other three of the *males naturales*. The four illnesses: *caida de la mollera, empacho, mal ojo*, and *susto* are conceptually tied together by the Mexican-Americans of Mecca. Verbalization of this concept takes a highly patterned form: "Doctors do not understand *caida de la mollera, empacho, mal ojo*, or *susto*." It is universally averred by Mexican-Americans that Anglo-Americans are not afflicted by any of these conditions; Anglo-Americans speak of the illnesses as "Mexican superstitions."

Etiology and Healing

A description of the four illnesses which are conceptually bound together by the Mexican-Americans follows, but first a word of caution: we shall follow the practice of Mexican-American culture bearers and not dichotomize psychic or emotional ills and somatic diseases. To do otherwise would be to do violence to the logic of the system.

Caida de la mollera is the only one of the four illnesses which is restricted to the very young. Infants are conceived of by the Spanish-speaking population as possessed of a fragile skull formation. The skull includes a section which in this immature stage easily slips or is dislodged from its normal position. The *mollera* (fontanel) is that part of the skull pictured as sitting at the very top of the head. It is normally sustained in proper position by the counterpoised pressure of the upper palate. A blow upon the youngster's head usually caused by a fall from a height, is believed to dislodge the fontanel, causing it to sink. The sinking of the dislodged fontanel forces the upper palate to depress, in turn blocking the oral passage. A mother or other adult witnessing the fall of an infant from a high place, e.g., a bed or chair, runs an examining finger over the skull in search of an unusual declivity. If such a depression is encountered, a treatment is commenced to correct the relationship of the parts to the whole.

It is more often true that the mother of a child does not witness the fall. Her first indication of trouble is the appearance of the universally recognized syndrome of *caída de la mollera*. Symptomatic of a fallen fontanel and palate are the inability of the youngster to grasp firmly with its mouth the nipple of a bottle or of the breast, loose bowels (*correncia*), and unusual amounts of crying and restlessness. Usually the case is accompanied by high temperature.

Although most women understand the causes and control the curing techniques for fallen fontanel, the delicacy of the corrective operation is such that many young women seek the aid of more experienced older women. Usually one of the child's grandmothers is requested to aid the younger woman to cure the child.

The infant is held in the arms of the curer, face up. The healing is commenced by the recitation of prayers in sets of three. The requisite prayers in this operation are the well-known Catholic Credo, Ave Maria, and Padre Nuestro, respectively. During prayers the healer places a thumb inside the mouth of the little patient, pushing upward three times against the upper palate. An external pull of some sort is applied at the same time, against the depression left by the fallen *mollera*. Whereas there is a universal method of applying internal pressure upward against the palate there are several alternative fashions utilized to apply an external pulling power. The most common of the alternatives is for the curer to fill her mouth with water and to suck (*chupar*) at the depression. Another of the alternative methods is also based upon the principle that the blocking of the digestive processes has caused imbalance in the wet-dry ratio of the organism. A pan of water may be put upon the floor and the child lowered, head first, in such a manner that the tips of its hair lightly brush the surface of the liquid three times. Some women prefer taking an unused bar of soap which they wet. The tips of the child's hair are then gently sudsed and the soapy hair lightly pulled three times by the curer. In cases which are considered more grave the contents of an egg are rubbed into the hair of the patient above the depression to form a "patch" there. The egg is permitted to remain for several moments so that it may draw upward the fallen fontanel and palate. In such instances where the egg is utilized there is no necessity to apply pulls by other means.

Following the procedures designed to push and pull the fallen parts back to position, the treatment is terminated by shaking these parts securely into their normal position. The child may be held upside-down by the ankles and shaken three times in a brusque manner, or else he may be turned in the arms of the curer to rest on one side. The body is then brusquely shaken toward the head. After the third shaking the balls of the patient's feet are lightly tapped by the hand of the curer, three times.

Caída de la mollera can eventuate in the death of the patient if it is not promptly and correctly treated. The blocking of the oral passageway prevents the ingestion of food and liquids, causing the gradual desiccation of the organism. A failure of the treatment to effect a positive response usually causes the family to seek the aid of a physician, for it is then recognized that the original diagnosis was faulty.

Empacho is an infirmity affecting child and adult. An *empachado* condition is believed to be caused by the failure of the digestive system to pass a chunk of food to the intestinal tract. There are emotional facets to *empacho*, however. Regardless of the original cause, *empacho* is conceived as a manifestly physiological condition in which a chunk of food clings to the intestinal wall causing sharp pains. Previous to diagnosis, a condition of *empacho* is often confused with other common indispositions, such as "gas on the stomach," or "indigestion." A clear-cut diagnostic procedure factors out *empacho* from other digestive difficulties.

The patient is made to lie on a bed face down, and the back is bared. The woman in attendance lifts a piece of skin in the rear waist region of the patient between two of her fingers. This skin particle is pinched between two fingers of the diagnostician, who listens attentively for a telltale snap or crack emanating from the abdominal region; such a noise clearly diagnoses the condition as *empacho*. The nature of the illness once established, the curing procedure commences to break up and disengage the offending piece of food from its clinging position. In the course of the treatment the body is used as if it were a beaker as the curer attempts to redress the imbalance between opposing qualities of "hot" and "cold" within the sick organism. The back of the patient is carefully pinched, stroked, and kneaded along the spinal column, as well as around the waist. The massage is interrupted only enough to permit the healer to administer an oral dosage of lead protoxite sold in the pharmacy as *la greta*. *La greta* is useful to penetrate the chunk of food, softening and crumbling it. Although valued for its penetrant abilities, *la greta* is disvalued for its recognized toxicity; furthermore, the "cold" quality assigned this medicinal in the local pharmacology disturbs the "hot-cold" balance of the organism. The toxicity of *la greta* causes some, more timid, women to prefer another penetrant, equally cold, but less dangerous—*asogue* (quicksilver). In order to regain the lost "hot-cold" balance which had been disturbed by the administration of "cold" *la greta* or *asogue*, "hot" epsom salts are administered. In many cases an additional purge in the form of castor oil, also attributed a "hot" quality, is taken by the patient. In such instances "cool" fruit juices (citric) provide a counterbalancing effect to the "hotness" of the castor oil. Throughout these dosages the patient is kneaded, pinched, and rubbed along the spinal column and waist. *Empacho*, though potentially fatal by desiccation of the organism, is clearly enough understood and easily enough treated so that prayer is not mandatory.

When a Mexican-American suffers from an *empachado* condition, it is often suspected that the illness has been caused by the individual having been required to eat against his will. Informants mention hypothetical instances such as a parent calling a son away from play in order to partake of a meal. The unwillingness of the child to desist from his play in order to eat is expected to cause the youngster to have *empacho*. Another typical instance in which one might predict the occurrence of *empacho* is that in which guests at someone's home are invited to eat. Although the guest is not hungry, to refuse such an invitation would be considered insulting to the host. Eating in such a case would likely result in *empacho* for the guest. In each of these hypothetical instances proffered by informants, the afflicted individual had been placed in a situation of conflict and stress. The youngster could not refuse the demand of the parent without showing disrespect; on the other hand obedience conflicted with the ideal behavior of the independent male. The guest is likewise placed under some constraint to accept the bidding of his host, particularly in the latter's home; contrariwise, if one has recently eaten, he may well wish to refuse such an invitation. The context of the situation in which the individual must choose between alternative behaviors, none of which will adequately resolve the immediate problems, are indeed stressful.

Among the Mexican-Americans, social relationships are conceptualized as bearing inherent dangers to the equilibrium of the individual. All individuals are regarded as susceptible to the virulence of *mal ojo,* but the weaker nature of women and children makes them more receptive than mature males. Certain persons in the community are considered to possess particularly "strong power" over "weaker" individuals. The seat of the power is located in the visual apparatus. Strong glances, covetous expression, or excessive attention paid one person by another exposes the actors to the dangers of an unnatural bond portrayed as the afflicted being drained of the will to act, and the entrance into his body of the "stronger power" of the other. As we sat discussing *mal ojo,* old José explained:

Once I went hunting for rabbits with my compadre. It was he that wanted to hunt, although the area was swarming with rattlers. Anyway, we arrived at the grounds where we had planned to shoot and soon saw a rabbit running across our path, first in one direction, and then in another. I pointed out the running animal to my compadre and told him to shoot it. He fired once and then a second time, but each time the bullets skittered harmlessly by. I told my compadre: "Don't shoot again! There must be a snake nearby that has the rabbit in his charm (*liga*)." Sure enough! In a moment we saw a tremendously long rattler coiled by a rock, with its jaws wide open. That snake had the rabbit in his charm and was bringing it closer and closer until finally it could devour the creature. That's what mal ojo is like!

A relationship containing elements of covetousness is the classic cause of *mal ojo* in Mecca, but this is generalized to include any kind of special attention—*El ojo es de bello y de feo* (evil eye affects the beautiful and the ugly in equal measure) —paid an individual. It is manifested by sudden severe headaches, inconsolable weeping (in the case of children only) , unusual fretfulness, and high temperature. The careful person in *el pueblo mexicano* recognizes a situation in which he or she has coveted someone, usually a child, by the appearance of a pain on one of the agent's temples, and will attempt to prevent the occurrence of serious disability by symbolically rupturing the bond between himself and the other. As this stage of the infirmity the linkage may be ruptured by simply passing a hand over the forehead of the child, or by patting it about the temples.

The syndrome of *mal ojo* appears abruptly. At its first signs the family of the patient attempts, in anxious fashion, to retrace the child's social activities of the previous few hours in the search for a significantly affective relationship. If the family is fortunate enough to recall such a relationship, the suspected agent is hurriedly recalled to the patient's side to attempt a rupture of the charm by which one of the actors is held to the other. Ideally, no stigma attaches to an agent of *mal ojo* unless he refuses the family's request to break the charm; in fact, we found no such instance of a refusal.

In those many instances in which the actual agent cannot be recalled to the patient's side, for example when the child has associated or been seen with a great number of strangers during the course of the day ("Every time my wife goes downtown to shop with the children, the littlest child suffers from *mal ojo* when they get home") the bond is broken and the intrusive power of the other is drained from the subject by means of sympathetic magic and religious prayers. Most of Mecca's women of Mexican descent understand the premises, diagnosis, and treatment of *mal ojo;* those who do not control such knowledge easily learn from others.

A hen's egg is taken and rubbed whole over the patient's body to absorb some of the heat and power which has disturbed the balance of the youngster. A water glass half-full of liquid is brought close to the sufferer and the egg tapped three times on the edge of the glass. On the third blow the shell is broken open, symbolizing the rupture of the bond between the patient and the stronger individual. The egg is emptied into the water glass where it is permitted to settle and assume a diagnostic form. If the form assumed by the egg in the glass suggests a "cooked" shape, i.e., sunny side up, the condition is diagnosed as one of *mal ojo.* An elongated shape bespeaks a male cause, a round shape a woman agent. Whatever the result of the diagnosis, all patients who have had the preliminary stages of the treatment, the combined forces of the calm rubbing of the whole egg on and about the body and the quietness of prayer and conversation in a therapeutic atmosphere of tenderness and concern, usually with one's most warm relative (the mother or grandmother) report a suffusing relaxation of body and mind. Many report they ". . . are asleep by the time the first curative stage is completed."

If the egg presents a diagnosis of *mal ojo* as cause of the condition, a treatment follows which is designed to drain the intrusive power of the stronger individual from the patient. The egg-water mixture is placed under the head of the bed, remaining there throughout the night. By morning the mysterious draining powers of the egg are presumed to have drawn the alien power from the subject's organism. In the early morning hours the mixture is supposed to be removed from its position beneath the head of the bed and carefully disposed of by burying in the yard, or flushing in a commode. This potent mixture now contains some essential properties of the self of each of the actors; consequently, "One must not throw the mixture on the usual garbage pile subject to the rays of the sun or the scavenging of the insects or animals, for to do so would be to dry up the eyesight of each of the persons as surely as the mixture is desiccated by the sun or devoured by the scavenger!" Thus we are warned by a knowledgeable older woman.

Mal ojo, unless it is improperly diagnosed or treated, is not considered of fatal nature. However, a faulty treatment—such as a physician is unwittingly likely to attempt—postpones proper treatment and allows the infirmity to advance to grave stages—*ojo pasado. Ojo pasado* is often fatal, due to the severity of coughing and vomiting that are symptomatic of that critical period. The violence of the seizures cause the bile sac (*hiel*) to break, voiding the green bile. Rupture of the *hiel* is mortal and there is no known cure effective at this stage of *ojo pasado.*

A mother permitted one of her young children to accompany a male friend of the family on a trip to a town in northern Mexico. Shortly after their return from Mexico the friend brought the child to its home. In several hours the youngster developed a high fever and became most restive. This initial condition was followed by a severe cough and vomiting. Before the family could organize itself to meet the crisis the child had died. The mother of the child diagnosed the cause of death as *mal ojo,* the coughing and vomiting having ruptured the *hiel.* It is her belief that on the trip to Mexico the family friend had played and romped with the child, but had failed to touch it upon the forehead when taking his leave.

Rafael, who has begun to doubt the realities of such things as *ojo* in the past few years, related an incident which would convince anyone:

> You know, the other day before I came to work I shaved, took my whiskers and all off. When I was outside I met a woman who looked at me and said, "You just shaved, didn't you? Took your whiskers off?" Well, I went on to work, and pretty soon I was feeling sick, and then I felt real hot. Well, I went up to Mrs. Brown, my boss, and said, "You know, I don't think I'm going to make it today!" So she put her hand up to my head and said, "Wow!" Boy, my head was really burning! I went on home and got into bed and around nine my brother came home and said, "Come on, let's go see the doc." So I went to see the doc and he gave me a shot, and gave me some pills, and I went on back to bed. I wasn't feeling any better, so I told my wife to go on over to that woman's house and bring her over here. She came over with my wife, and she ran her hands over my face and said, "Well, you looked so young and so cute that I guess that's why I noticed you." Well, she went away then, and pretty soon I began to feel better. I went back to work the next day and Mrs. Brown said, "Well, you sure were sick yesterday!"

A young woman described how she suddenly became sick after her husband arrived home from his army service: "I was working around the house, and then I turned my head and saw my husband staring at my back from the doorway."

Gilberto described the latest instance of *mal ojo* in his family:

> Last week my cousin's cute little baby had *ojo*. In the hours of the late afternoon my cousin was holding her child out in their front yard. One of the neighborhood men returning from work stopped to talk with the couple, remarking on the child's cuteness. Then he went on his way. That night when they put the child to bed, it began to cry and remained

inconsolable through most of the night. Even though I slept in the other part of the house I could hear them moving about with the child. Very early the next morning I could hear my cousin leave the house as she went next door to speak to our neighbor who is a relative of the man with whom they had chatted the evening before. She asked the neighbor to do her the favor of requesting the man to stop at our house on his way to work. The neighbor went and roused the man with strong eyes. On his way to work that man stopped at our place and went into the other room where he ran a hand over the child's face and forehead, cooing to her and talking to her. He didn't remain any longer than about five minutes. When he left the baby had stopped crying.

A young mother recounted the following in one of the interviews held at the Well-Baby Clinic:

One morning my son—the middle one—awoke with a cold and fever. I had to go downtown to run an errand and left the child with his father. My husband took some cardboard from the house and spread it out on the ground for the child. The child was cutely dressed in checked shirt and shorts, I remember, and looked very handsome. My husband went across the street to chat with one of our neighbors and the little boy followed his father. When the boy and his father returned to our house the child began to tremble and had convulsions. My husband recalled that during his conversation with the neighbor, the latter had commented favorably on my boy's appearance. With this in mind, my husband returned to the other house and asked our neighbor to accompany him to the child. Our neighbor agreed to come, saying, "I guess I can *really* cause *ojo!*" My neighbor then took the boy in his arms and fondled him, touching him upon the forehead.

Mal ojo "is like electricity," said old Marcos. He went on to explain that if someone was walking down a street in town with his child and a passer-by came up to request permission to touch the child about the head and permission was not granted that *mal ojo* would result.

You never see *mal ojo* work on an adult, but then . . . one time I was working on the loading platform of the Green Garden shed. I was sitting there with Mr. Ronald and another, equally bald. The other workers were laughing at the picture presented by the three *pelóns* (bald ones) sitting together. One of the onlookers approached me and suggested that I have the others touch me about the head to protect me from *mal ojo;* but I told him that something like that wouldn't affect me, for I was an adult and too strong for *ojo.* But when I got home that night and started to go to sleep I had a terrible ache in the head. Someone from the house went right out and called one of those fellows who had been staring and laughing at me over at the shed and brought him over to the house. He rubbed his hands all over my forehead, and above the eyes, and within five minutes I was no longer bothered by the pain.

In Mecca an incident having an unstabilizing effect on an individual often causes a part of the self, the *espiritú,* to leave the body. A person who suffers long continuous periods of langour, listlessness, and lack of appetite is presumed *asustado.* The causal experience may be that of a frigtthening nature, or it may be the patterned reaction of the afflicted to the vexations of everyday social life. The various forms of the verb *mortificar* are often heard used by Mexican-Americans to describe a traumatic personal reaction to upsetting situations.

A shock sufficient to disengage one's *espiritú* may be caused by the yap of a dog at close hand when least expected, a fall from a horse, or a fall occasioned by tripping over an unnoticed object in the path. A particularly unpleasant sight, such as a highway accident or the knowledge that one has shared a hospital ward with a patient who had died during the night, is unbalancing and makes the person liable to the loss of his *espiritú.* Equally jarring is a nighttime encounter with an apparition. The most common cause of the loss of one's *espiritú* and consequent physical disability is the impingement of society upon the individual. Social situations which engender a disquieting condition of anger or fear in the individual are avoided for they, too, cause one's *espiritú* to wander. (The volatile anger of the child is contrasted with the proneness of adults to bear malice over longer periods; correlatively, only the adult type of malevolence is perceived as unstabilizing and causally interrelated with *susto*.)

Simple *susto* is easily treated and most older women of Mecca's north side understand the curing procedures. The patient is made to lie down with arms outstretched so as to resemble a cross. Nowadays the healing of *susto* takes place on the wooden floor of the house or on a bed, but informants recall the older custom of the patient being made to lie on a mat on the packed-dirt floor of the home. The patient's body is swept with a branch of the herb *pirul*. The sweeping commences from the chest and stomach proceeding in lateral directions, and also upwards and downwards toward the extremities. Before sweeping, however, the curer and patient talk over matters of a personal nature such as might throw some light on the reason for the condition. As the cure progresses with the sweeping motions, the curer prays in calm quiet tones, and the patient hopefully calls out to his wandering *espíritu* to return. Sometime during the calm-enveloped treatment a sudden sputter of liquid, either water or liquor, is emitted from the mouth of the healer, shocking the patient and bathing him about the face. Both patient and curer recognize when the treatment has succeeded in reuniting the wandering *espíritu* with the body. The patient for his part "feels" that his *espíritu* has rejoined the body; he begins to feel whole once again, as his voice changes from the plaintive insistence of *"¿Donde andas, donde andas?"*—where are you, where are you?—to the electrifying *"Hay voy, hay voy"*—I'm coming, I'm coming! The curer realizes the passing of the critical period when a drop in body temperature and a lessening of fitfulness is ascertained. A treatment may last for three days in more serious cases of *susto pasado*. At the conclusion of the treatment, the patient is instructed to drink the water from a special receptacle in which are floating herbs and palm leaves blessed during Easter services.

An alternate procedure, portraying the same general principles as the preceding treatment, was expounded by middle-aged Mrs. García.

> Until I was fourteen I lived with my family on a rancho just outside the northern town of Cadereyta Jimenez in Mexico. In those days either the family cared for its sick or else they died. There were no doctors for *us* to run to whenever we felt sick! Every house was furnished with a copper pot in those days, and when *susto* occurred to a member of the family that pot would be put on the kitchen fire to heat until its surface became red hot. The patient would lie on the dirt floor of the house and his mother would dig holes under his head, his feet, and each of the outstretched hands. Some water would be poured into the holes, and then the muddied water would be scraped up and put into a vase. Mother would then place a bit of red ribbon, some *alvaca* [an herb], and a gold ring into the vase, as well as four crosses of palm leaf. After the patient had been swept with the pirul branch he was led to the fire where he began pouring the cold liquid from the vase into the red-hot copper pot. The terrible hiss given off by the copper as it received the cold mixture frightened the patient terribly. He leaped back away from the fire and shrieked, and a tremor ran through his body (*se chilló*). At that moment the *susto* he had suffered ran from his body into the copper pot. Then for two nights following, the patient was swept and prayed over, sweated at night, and had to drink from the copper receptacle before eating in the morning (*en ayunas*), and before retiring for the night.

There is a great number of instances in which neither the patient nor his family recognizes soon enough the nature of the affliction. In those instances in which *susto* is not recognized quickly enough, its debilitating advance reaches alarming proportions and requires more potent treatment. Advanced cases—*susto pasado*—are generally brought to the attention of the Catholic clergy with the urgent request for an *ensalme*. The *ensalme* is the regular blessing of the sick person performed by the priest as described in Father Simon's compilation of the ritual used in this region (1948). Father Simon recognized the singular extension of the use of the blessing by the Mexican-American laity to include conditions caused by other than physical disturbance. He said:

> . . . people come quite often to the priest and ask him to pray over them. They say, "Padre, *quiero que ud. [usted] me ensalme.*" ["Father, I want you to bless me."] It is always good to find out when they have been to confession the last time. If they have been away from the sacrament for quite a while, it will offer us a golden opportunity to induce them to go to confession and to receive Holy Communion in order to be better disposed to obtain from God the grace they are asking for. In many cases they will come and then the blessing can be given after Mass.

The use of the blessing for the sick to include cases of *susto* is attested to by local priests who report that "many people come who are not *really* ill" (italics ours). Attempts by the clergy to dissuade the petitioners have proved to be of little avail. We submit that the difference between the calm chatting behavior followed by prayer in the home of the patient with the attendant mother, or the *curandero,* and that of the relationship between patient and father-confessor in more serious cases is, therapeutically speaking, one of degree rather than of kind.

Cases of *susto* which are permitted, either through undue postponement of proper treatment or making use of a practitioner not equipped to handle such conditions, e.g., a physician, eventually prove to be fatal. Death is caused by the slow wasting of the organism due to desiccation. The wasting effects of *susto pasado* lend the condition its other names, *mal de delgadito, tis,* or tuberculosis. The practical considerations that the confusion of *susto* with tuberculosis present to professional health personnel and public health administrators treating the Mexican-Americans of the border region will be dealt with in forthcoming papers of the Hidalgo County Project.

The Montalvo family went to a nearby lake for a picnic

one Sunday in April. It was young Ricardo's first experience in a body of water and though coaxed and entreated by his family to venture into the water, he refused and remained an anxious onlooker. As the family continued to frolic in the lake, five-year-old Ricardo went to the car and fell asleep in the heat of the sun. He slept long and heavily throughout the afternoon and was carried, still slumbering, to his bed when the family arrived at home after dark. Several times during the night Ricardo was fitful and talked aloud in his sleep. The next morning the family assumed that he had been *asustado* the previous day, though not out of fear of the water. Rather, it was the family's insistence that he enter the water, demands to which he could not accede, as the father explained, which was causing the syndrome of *susto*. The day following the outing saw Ricardo brought to a neighboring woman to be cured.

Mrs. Benítez is a thin, distraught woman of about forty-five years of age. For the past six years she has been suffering from attacks brought on by an *asustada* condition. Mrs. Benítez's aura consists of severe, painful headaches, and a strange tingling sensation as if she were being pierced by numerous pins and needles. Following the aura she "goes out of her senses" and although able to hear those attending her, is unable to respond. Her limbs become taut and convulsive in movement, the jaw clamps shut, and the teeth clench in ironbound fashion. Upon regaining her senses she has no recollection of the seizure but is exhausted and has an overpowering urge to be completely free from the social world about her. Although Mrs. Benítez has several times been advised by physicians that she is an epileptic, her own diagnosis and that of her friends run counter to medical opinion.

Mrs. Benítez traces her condition from the vexatious (*mortificada*) period during which she lived with her husband, a man who has since deserted her and the children. "When I lived with my husband he used to beat me at regular intervals. On some mornings following a beating I could not lift my arms to eat with or in order to do the housework. I lived in an upset state all of the time (*vivia asustada*)." The first seizure she recalls caused her to go to an old man then living in Mecca with a local reputation for his effectiveness in the cure of *susto*. (This *curandero* is an unusual example as his cure for *susto* depended solely upon prayer, whereas all others contacted relied upon several therapeutic techniques to combat *susto*. Parenthetically, Mrs. Benítez relied to such a great extent upon the Mecca *curandero because* of his stressing the role of prayer.) At the time of the first seizure she was living with her husband and she visited the old man several more times following seizures caused by her *asustada* condition.

In December of 1958, Mrs. Benítez suffered a particularly severe seizure occasioned in general by the presence in her one-room apartment of the troubled relationship between her daughter and the daughter's husband, and in particular by an altercation between herself and the son-in-law. One night in an angry mood the young man came home in search of a revolver which he had left in the care of his mother-in-law. The young man was quite intent on murdering a drinking companion with whom he had had words at a local bar. Mrs. Benítez refused to relinquish the weapon, which further incensed the youth. The son-in-law then proceeded to assault the informant verbally, at the same time knocking his wife about the house. On the following morning, in the early pre-dawn hours, Mrs. Benítez suffered a severe headache which awakened her, presaging the terrible seizure which followed. The violence of the scene during the night had caused her a *susto nuevo* which, combined with her older *susto,* created the very dangerous *susto complicado* or *susto pasado*.

An older woman of the town recalled how, many years ago, when her family had just arrived in the region, her brother was practicing the art of baking. Every day he used to go to the loading platforms of the warehouses to sell his newly baked breads and cakes. One day as he walked across the platform he failed to notice an open hole through which ice was poured to cool the stored crates of vegetables. The brother's foot caught on the edge of the open passage and he fell forward, doubling his leg underneath him, and then fell backward hitting his shoulder. The men who were engaged in the crating operation saw him fall and began to laugh as his breads and cakes scattered in all directions. The brother, unable to extricate himself from the ludicrous position into which he had fallen, and suffering great pain from his injured leg, was incensed at the laughter of the onlookers. (The informant thought the laughter of the workers and the consequent anger and mortification of the victim important enough to repeat three times during the course of the narration.) However, when the men noted that her brother had been injured by his fall they rushed over to help. The victim was carried home by two of the men and others collected his goods for him and brought these to his home.

The first thing that the mother of the injured brother did when he was brought into the house was to ask him if he could straighten his leg, which he was able to do though only with great difficulty. His mother then called a neighbor, a close friend of the injured, and requested him to go out of town to gather the "flesh" of the *huisatche chino* tree just under the bark. When this was brought it was boiled and fed to the victim for eight days, a period during which the leg was rubbed down.

As soon as possible the brother was laid on the dirt floor of the home and curing for *susto* was begun.

In Mecca the treatment of the ill is logically consistent with the premises upon which a diagnosis is made. A fallen fontanel is assumed to carry with it the upper palate which blocks the oral passage. A diagnosis is based upon symptoms suggesting that the child is unable properly to ingest food, particularly liquids. The cure attempts to elevate the palate to which is attached the fontanel, thus clearing a passage for food to pass to the stomach. *Empacho* is perceived as an indisposition caused by the clinging of a hard "ball" of food to the wall of the intestine. Certain penetrants are administered orally to attack the offensive chunk of food, breaking it into smaller pieces. The penetrants possess qualities of toxicity and "coldness." Consequently, treatment is continued in order to purge the toxic substance from the body, and then to balance the "cold" quality with a "hot" quality. Each time that an imbalance of "hot" and "cold" is created, an adjustment is made to redress the essential balance. Throughout the cure the area of the waist is massaged to help crumble the offensive "ball" of food.

In the case of the other two high-incidence illnesses, *mal ojo* and *susto,* an essential part of the self of an individual is believed to be overcome or lost due to the power of a stronger alien force, eventuating in the loss of the individual's equilibrium. The loss of balance is manifested by somatic illness. In each of these illnesses the treatment procedure attempts first to quiet the patient and to envelop him in a therapeutic atmosphere containing highly concerned people, generally the closely related female members of the family. The low-pitched monotone of prayer, and the relaxed ministrations of the healer, are accompanied by an attempt to recapture the occasion on which the traumatic loss was sustained. In the treatment for *mal ojo,* the agent and subject are brought together, if possible, and the agent symbolically ruptures the bond between the two by caressing the patient, demonstrating thereby that the condition was unwittingly caused and without malice aforethought. The ideally poised state of an individual, that is, before having been *asustado,* is re-created by the slow, languorous sweeping of the patient with a medicinal herb, the low pitch of the healer's prayers, and relaxed conversation between healer and patient. This ideal harmony of a person and the world about him is rudely shattered by the sudden, frightening spurt of alcohol or water about the face, or else the shrill hiss of steam which rises from the red-hot copper pot. The original shock which caused the *susto* is recalled in conversation and recaptured in its intensity by either of the two shock treatments described. The treatments for *mal ojo* and *susto* then proceed to make the individual whole once again. In the case of the former ailment, an intrusive foreign force is drained from the patient, enabling him or her to act in an ideally independent manner. In the treatment for *susto*, an essential part of the self—the *espiritú*—must be returned to the host organism before the illness, product of such a loss, can be cured.

The traditional framework of knowledge about health and disease of the Mexican-Americans of Mecca is integrated by a conceptualization of the individual as a sum of balanced parts and qualities. A healthy individual is one whose entire being is in balance. The concept is, in some measure, couched in a framework provided by the so-called Hippocratic system in which the body is visualized as healthy when sets of contrasting qualities, hot and cold, wet and dry, are balanced (Madsen 1955). Structurally, the members and parts of the body are conceived as having specific place and functionally change in the manner in which any of these parts relate to the whole is presumed to cause illness.

We have seen that in two of the conditions, *mal ojo* and *susto*, illness is caused by stressful interpersonal relations; and, also, that in some instances *empacho* may be due to the nature of a role relationship in which the prescribed behavior of one player is that of unresisting compliance to the will of another, e.g., child-parent, guest-host. In each case of which we have record in the field materials, the person suffering *ojo* or *susto* has been caused to lose an essential part of the self. In the case of *mal ojo* a "weaker" person is overcome by the strength of a "stronger" individual. All persons in Mecca are susceptible to *mal ojo*, but women and children, inherently weaker in the nature of the case, are more receptive than adult males. Anyone may cause another to have *mal ojo* irrespective of the nature of the relationship, although strangers are far more dangerous than relatives, due to the ease with which the latter may be recalled to the side of the patient to rupture the unnatural bond between them.

The Mexican-Americans of Mecca perceive the individual as a sum of complementary parts and qualities. The arrival of a large number of doctors and medical facilities in the delta region since 1916 has removed much of the healing from the household and has seriously eroded a number of traditional concepts. The four illnesses discussed in this paper present a hard core of resistance to modern medical practice, none of them being amenable to the care of a physician. We hypothesize that the persistence of the beliefs in the illnesses *caida de la mollera, empacho, mal ojo,* and *susto* is due to the fact that they support certain core values and ways of behavior in the Mexican-American community.

Cultural Values

Certain aspects of Mexican-American culture are of far greater importance than others to its perpetuation as a unique entity. These aspects may be said to provide a core for the way of life of the people; if the core is affected by change the traditional way of life is vitally affected. The three generation family of socialization among the Mexican-Americans is a focal point of dominant or prescribed values, the ramifications of which deeply influence other areas of the social life (Kluckhohn 1951:415).

Any study of the social system of the Mexican-Americans leads to the family of socialization within the bilaterally organized kinship group. That shallow and narrow unit stands out in sharp relief from the rest of kin and is characterized by denotative kinship terminology in contrast with the general, classificatory usage of the system. Ego's essential social unit is comprised of his parents and his parents' siblings, in particular his mother's sisters. In the second ascending generation both sets of grandparents are respected members of ego's extended household, but not the siblings of the grandparents. In ego's own generation his siblings (*hermano, hermana*) are conceptually separated from others, as are also his first cousins (*primos hermanos*) separated from cousins (*primos*) further removed; in all contexts, references to first cousins on both sides pointedly distinguish them from other classes of relatives. *Primos hermanos* are said to be somewhat like one's sisters or brothers and one is expected to have especially affective relations with them; particularly is this true between female first cousins. The unity of the female sibling group is of great importance to women of all ages and perdures throughout a woman's married life. The strength of the relationship between sisters is such that sisters' husbands are conceptually brought together in a special bond and known by the self-reciprocal term *concuño;* thus the sisters' husbands are separated from all other relatives-in-law in one's own generation. There is no similar usage for the feminine equivalent, *concuña,* and the term itself is flaggy and almost unknown in Mecca. In the first descending generation one's own children (*hijo* [m], *hija* [f]) are separated from others of their own generation who are known as *sobrinos* (m) or *sobrinas* (f). Thus the distinction observed between first cousins and all other degrees of cousins in one's own generation is lost in their children's generation. In Mecca the importance of the relationships found to obtain in the three generation family is equalled only by the bonds between an individual and his baptismal sponsors—*padrinos de pila*—or by the relationship between one's self and the sponsors of one's children's baptisms—*compadres de pila*. Persons who fill statuses within the close family described above are enmeshed in a network of behavior and attitudes which are sharply defined by cultural values which prescribe sentiments of restraint and respect between the individuals concerned.

With few exceptions those who regularly visit one's home are persons whose prescribed behavior toward members of the household is of a respectful nature. A man's home is his castle, but the home is also a sanctified place in which one's womenfolk are safe. At the head of the household is the father or, in the event of his death or absence, the oldest son. "In my home," says one of Mecca's patriarchs, "I am judge, jury, and policeman." Although the mother asserts a good deal of authority with the younger children and with the older daughters, she is expected to be naive about worldly matters and to occupy herself fully with the wants of her children and her husband. Both the father and the mother are figures toward whom conduct is enveloped in terms of extraordinary respect, but the restraint shown in relation to each is derived from different sources. The father must be respected because of his authoritative position at the head of the household, the mother due to her saintly qualities. The organization of the Mexican-American household has been most succinctly described by a young married woman of the community: "In *la raza* the older order the younger, and the men the women."

In a number of households the nuclear family is expanded by the presence of the mother of either of the parents. In such instances a great deal of friction exists, particularly if the older women is the husband's mother. All of those with whom the question of residence was discussed stressed the desirability of the young married couple establishing their residence apart from that of either of the parental sets. Indeed, friction is considered inherent in a permanent arrangement in which the parent of one of the spouses resides in their home. *El cuerpo y el arrimado en tres días se pesten* (after three days a corpse and a guest begin to smell), it is maintained. The values which order behavior within the household unit proscribe levity or frivolous behavior such as jocularity, dancing, smoking, drinking, or discussions of sexual relations, especially in the presence of one's parents or elder brother.

The condemnation of random visiting between the members of unrelated households precludes the formation of friendship relations between unrelated women of the community. "*We are your best friends,*" the daughter is likely to hear her parents advise. Many times the observer hears women express the value-laden statement: "I don't like to visit with my neighbors. If we have something to discuss it is better done out in the yard." In fact, during the two years in which the author was in Mecca only two cases were discovered in which a woman regularly visited the home of another to whom she was not related. In both instances the visiting was nonreciprocal, i.e., only one of the pair was the visitor, the other was always the visited. Neither of the visitors had any kin in town other than affinals; one of the visitors had been deserted by her husband many years ago. Each of the visitors conceived of herself as a social isolate for whom life was meaningless, hopeless, and without order; one of these anomic women was contemplating suicide at the time of our acquaintanceship. Both of the visitors regularly suffered from seizures diagnosed as epileptic by local physicians. In each of the instances of irregular visiting the husband of the visited woman peremptorily forbade his wife to admit the visitor any more, an action which resulted from the gossip which surrounded the unusual pattern. In one case the visiting continued and the husband's sister carried the case to Commissioner's Court, the charge: trespass. The cultural values of Mexican-American society prescribe the place of the woman as within the protection of the home provided by her parents or her husband; her proper companions are restricted to her husband and children, as well as her mother, sisters, female first cousins, and ritual kin.

Highly congruous with those values which provide the home a sanctified air are others which direct that the men pursue their social activities away from the household. In Mexican-American society a man is expected to pursue the pleasures of the flesh for as long as he is able; it is considered most desirable that a male function in as untrammeled a fashion as possible—*a cada cabeza un mundo* (each head is a world unto itself) says the *chicanos*.[3] An individual whose attachment to his home is such as to interfere with more manly activities engaged in which his age-set—*palomilla*—causes serious concern to his family and the others of the *palomilla*. Too close an attachment to one's wife detracts from the regard in which one is held by the community and causes negative sanctions to come into play. In one instance a mother expressed her concern over the fact that her married son tended to remain at home at night with his wife and children. The older woman accused the wife of refusing him permission to leave the house during the night hours. Said the son querulously, "I *like* to stay at home nights."

Young men in Mecca's Mexican-American society move about in informally organized age-sets, or *palomillas*. A *palomilla* may contain men who are married, unmarried men, or a mixture of both. With the exception of the very close, confidant-type relationship—*amigos de confianza*—found in the *palomilla* between two men no other structured form of relationship exists; members of a *palomilla* are brought together by mutual interests and the need for companionship. The last factor is extremely important in a society in which the core of the social system is the close family, the values of which proscribe conversation about the very type of behavior which other values demand of younger men. The *palomilla* spends the hours in which the members are not at work telling stories, drinking, discussing one another's amorous adventures, arranging barbecues, and discussing problems of common interest. Often one member of the *palomilla* will recommend a discarded girl friend to another, particularly if they are *amigos de confianza*. It is only with his *palomilla* that the young Mexican-American man may "display the full social personality of an adult male" (Pitt-Rivers 1954:90) ; consequently, two brothers are never found habitually associating in the same *palomilla* no matter how close their ages.

A number of core values of Mexican-American culture have been described. These highly regarded norms select a narrowly defined group of kinsmen of three generations as persons whose relationship to ego is of the greatest importance. Supplemented by one's baptismal sponsors and the sponsors of one's children's baptisms, this group is considered the only social unity upon which an individual may rely. Relationships within this group are sharply defined and expressed in behavior characterized by respect and restraint. Within the culture the greatest emphasis is placed upon the differentiation between the expected role behavior of male and female.

The cases of *mal ojo* which have been included in this article describe a number of situations in which behavior considered highly irregular, as measured by the cultural values, took place. All the cases were believed caused by an unusual amount of attention having been paid an individual by a person whose relationship to the subject was not one permitting such familiarity. (The exception is the young wife whose husband had recently returned from military service. Not enough is known about the context in which the incident occurred to venture a reason for its nonconformity to the general pattern.) In each case in which a child was involved as subject of *mal ojo,* the accused agent was from outside the close family group. In Rafael's case the passing woman accused of causing him *mal ojo* had reversed the expected sex roles, making him the passive partner. Old Marcos' illness was caused not so much by the attention that he had received while on the loading platform but the humiliating nature of that attention.

Although *empacho* is always believed caused by the failure of the organism to digest a piece of food properly, often the failure is attributed to tension caused by contradictory role demands made by the society upon the individual. The value which stresses the independence of the boy is in conflict with that one which prescribes filial obedience; the independence of the individual is also in conflict with the respect behavior enjoined upon a visitor in the home of another.

The five-year-old Montalvo boy found himself unable to enter the water as a little man should in spite of the coaxings and jeers of his sister and parents. The vexations suffered by the distraught Mrs. Benítez were due not to her earlier fear of the husband, nor a present fear of her son-in-law, but rather, as she put it, to her inability to defend herself and her daughter ". . . even in my own home." Mrs. Benítez lays the general blame for her illness upon the vexations (*morti-*

ficaciones) of everyday life; a life which, at best, is unhappy. The man who had fallen in the open hole had his leg cured by potions of boiled huisatche chino bark, but his equilibrium was restored by treatment for a lost *espíritu*.

Other students of cultures in Latin America (Gillin 1948; Adams 1956, for examples) have suggested that fright is a common denominator in cases of soul-loss, and that generally the soul has been captured by magico-spiritual forces which must be placated by the victim and the curer. The material from Mecca indicates that fright is not a necessary condition of soul-loss. On the other hand, the material in this paper is supported by all other reports on the incidence of soul-loss in the claim that personal or social stress *is* a necessary, but not a sufficient, condition of loss of soul (see Gillin, 1948).

The case histories of those who have been reported as suffering from *susto* or soul-loss in Mecca are devoid of the belief, found elsewhere, that loss of the soul is associated with its capture by magico-spiritual forces. The absence of the theme of magical capture among this non-Indian group of south Texas lends support to Adams' impression (1956:197) that the capture of the soul is a peculiarly Indian variation on a general theme of soul-loss.

Conclusions

It has been shown that the four illnesses herein described have remained firmly embedded in the socio-cultural framework, despite the introduction of an alternate system of belief and competing healing ways. It has been argued that three of these four illnesses function to sustain some of the dominant values of the Mexican-American culture, those which prescribe the maintenance of the solidarity of a small, bilateral family unit; and others which prescribe the appropriate role behavior of males and females, of older and younger individuals. We are unable to demonstrate such an association between one of the four conditions—*caida de la mollera*—with the configuration of values. We submit that probably this lack of association is related to the fact that *caída de la mollera* occurs only in children under three years of age, and generally in those younger than six months. It is here contended that children of such a young age are not yet socialized to appropriate role expectations, a contention which seems plausible from other observations of behavior and expectations in the group.

We are still confronted with the question: What are the implications of the empirically observed aggregation of the four illnesses in the conception of the Mexican-Americans? One of the threads which runs through all four illnesses is that they are not amenable to the understanding or treatment of the technically trained physician, be he Anglo-American, Mexican-American, or Mexican. They, furthermore, share the characteristic that only people of Mexican background are afflicted.

The pathologies described above are an area of high anxiety for all sectors of the Mexican-American population. Those whose orientation is toward adoption of Anglo-American socio-cultural behavior—particularly those persons who are now attending, or have once attended, high schools together with Anglo-Americans—tend to disparage these concepts of illness as ingenuous beliefs, survivals of an unsophisticated past. The more credulous, on the other hand, seize upon every available opportunity to vouch for the authenticity of the illnesses. Invariably, informants in the latter category will volunteer information about an incident in which a patient was brought to a physician only to be told that there was nothing wrong with him. The patient was subsequently brought to a lay curer who not only diagnosed the illness but successfully healed the condition. The successful effort of the lay curer is always related triumphantly in a manner to suggest that much more has been at stake than a simple matter of the curing of an individual patient. It is submitted that each success of a traditional healing procedure is a vindication of traditional modes which are beset by pressures to change. The four illnesses described in this article have attained a significance which goes far beyond their importance as pathological conditions. They have become highly symbolic of a traditional way of life. It is predictable that the greater the number of Mexican-Americans who adopt new behavior and values, the more value will the traditionally oriented invest in the aggregate of *caída de la mollera, empacho, mal ojo*, and *susto*.

Notes

1. The author conducted the research upon which this paper is based from September 1957 to September 1959. His indebtedness is acknowledged to the Hogg Foundation for Mental Health University of Texas, for its financial support during the field work; and to William Madsen, Assistant Professor of Anthropology, University of Texas, the director of the Hidalgo County Project. The Institute for Research in Social Science, University of North Carolina, kindly assisted in the preparation of the final manuscript. Jerrold Levy, William Madsen, Duane Metzger, and Ralph C. Patrick all contributed to the improvement of earlier drafts of this paper.

2. The names of all places and persons in this paper are pseudonyms in order to permit maximum privacy to those who aided so much by their cooperation in the study of Mecca.

3. *Chicano* is from the Spanish *Mexicano*. It distinguishes Mexican-Americans and Mexican nationals from all other groups.

References

Adams, Richard N., Encuesta sobre la cultura de los Ladinos en Guatemala. Seminario de Integración Social Guatemalteca 2. Guatemala City, Editorial del Ministerio de Educación Pública, 1956.

Foster, George M., Relationships between Spanish and Spanish-American folk medicine. Journal of American Folklore 66:201–218, 1953.

Gillin, John, Magical fright. Psychiatry 11:387–400, 1948.

Kluckhohn, Clyde, Values and value orientations in the theory of action. *In* Toward a general theory of action, Talcott Parsons and E. A. Shils, eds. Cambridge, Harvard University Press, 1951.

Madsen, William, Hot and cold in the universe of San Francisco Tecospa, Valley of Mexico. Journal of American Folklore 68:123–129, 1955.

Pitt-Rivers, J. A., The people of the sierra, Weidenfeld and Nicolson, 1954.

Simon, Alphonse, A Spanish-Latin ritual, with directions in English. Paterson, N. J., St. Anthony Guild Press, 1948.

Part III

LATIN AMERICANS—MEXICANS, CENTRAL
AND SOUTH AMERICANS

Introduction

Scientists contend that folk medical beliefs and practices play crucial roles in human life and, to some extent, exist in all cultures. However, they contend that these beliefs and practices seem to be more widespread in cultures of low technology and among individuals of the lower status groups.

The information included in Part III of this volume relates to individuals of Spanish heritage whose beliefs and practices (as recorded by Kenny and Foster) reflect socio-cultural values of today's rural Spaniard.[1,2] These researchers suggest that Spanish socio-cultural values, prototypes of many Latin socio-cultural values, inculcate various religious dogma and conceive the "individual as an integral being—body and soul" with specific social roles, *honorable manhood* for the male and *immaculate motherhood* for the female. Conversely, health (or the lack of health) is based on the extent to which the individual fulfills his ideal social role. So, illness represents a moral crisis invoked by the supernatural and cure is thought to be affected directly or indirectly by supernatural forces. Likewise, agents of cure, folk or scientific, are generally conceived of as agents of God or the supernatural.

The selections which follow describe beliefs and practices

1. *Michael Kenny, "Social Values and Health in Spain,"* Human Organization *21, no. 4 (Winter 1963), pp. 280–89.*
2. *George Foster, "Relationships between Spanish and Spanish-American Folk Medicine,"* Journal of American Folklore *64 (1953), pp. 201–17.*

of folk medicine in certain lower status groups in areas of Latin America. In general, the findings show the germ theory of disease holds little significance. And, indigenous systems of folk medicine in these areas represent not a rejection of scientific medicine but an effort to seek the therapy conceived to be best suited to the particular malady. Hence, maladies thought to be caused by supernatural forces are taken to folk curers, since scientific medicine (Western) often is believed to have little or no effect on such maladies. Scientific medicine is sought for maladies against which folk medicines have proven ineffective and for which scientific ("doctor") medicine has been shown to provide immediate and/or dramatic cure.

In an article "Health Behavior in Cross-Cultural Perspective: A Guatemalan Example," appearing in *Human Organization*, Volume 25, Summer 1966, Gonzales asserts that the nonindustrial Guatemalan culture has a tri-ethnic composition of Mayan Indian, Ladino (Colonial Spanish), and the Black Carib. Each of these subcultures was found to embrace its own native symptom of medicine which reflected certain characteristic disease concepts. However, certain parallels were seen to traverse all three systems as follows: (1) The Indian concept attributed disease to some "outer" condition, possibly involving natural causes and/or supernatural powers (natural elements, witchcraft, evil spirits) acting in conjunction with an inner weakness of a physiological or psychological nature. The various curers—midwives, herbalists, diviners or shamen—use such remedies as herbs, magical devices and rites to eliminate the fundamental cause of illness. (2) The Ladino concept includes the hot-cold dichotomy and/or inner weakness which predisposes individuals to disease. Also, such factors as fear, anger, envy and fright are believed to have the potential for causing disease independently of an external stimulus. Other disease influences were such natural causes as filth, air, germs and bad food. Native curers use both scientific and folk medicines. The assistance of spiritualists is sometimes used to determine causes and suggest cures for illnesses. The Catholic priest and various saints are often implored in a search for relief from disease. (3) The Black Caribs consider illness a misfortune caused by such factors as malevolent spirits, living enemies, or jealous dead ancestors. These factors are thought to use such agents as bad air or germs to invoke illness. Charm wearing, social good behavior, and making offerings to ancestors are preventive measures used. Curative measures involve the use of medicines and magical practices. The shaman, priest, and the Western doctor are employed, depending upon the observed symptoms.

In the research which follows, Gonzales contends that folk medicine among the Guatemalans provided (a) some means of explanation when cure is impossible and (b) psychological effect which is realized immediately. Also, according to Gonzales, some Guatemalans often exposed the same maladies to both "folk" cures and "doctor" medicine. Among the disease concepts found to exist were (1) hot-cold dichotomy, (2) contact contagions, (3) susceptibility—understood to be "strong" in adults as against "weak" in children, (4) *ojo* (evil eye), and (5) *aire*.

In the Mestizo communities of coastal Peru and Chile, Simmons found popular medicine centered around the concept of disease causation, categorized as: (1) severe emotional upset, (2) contamination by ritual uncleanliness (3) gastrointestinal obstructions, (4) *mal aire*, and (5) hot-cold dichotomy. The curing techniques employed were either magical or empirical.

Open practice of popular medicine is outlawed in Peru and Chile, though Simmons found it very much in evidence. He feels that the partial acceptance of scientific medicine by the recipients is based less on recipient understanding and more on pragmatics.

Folk medical practices are thought to be designs which assist man in biological and social adjustment to his environment and it is mentally stimulating to project on the origin of the practices. Currier uses psychological theory in his attempt to explain the origin of folk medicine. He offers the hot-cold principle as the theoretical basis of folk medicine and explains that it originates in child-rearing practices and social relationships of individuals.

11

Beliefs and Practices Concerning Medicine and Nutrition Among Lower-Class Urban Guatemalans

by Nancie L. Solien de González

Nancie L. Solien Gonzalez, Ph.D., is Associate Professor of Anthropology at the University of New Mexico. She is currently engaged in research in the Dominican Republic, as a result of a National Science Foundation Grant for 1967–69. She was Professor at the University of San Carlos, Guatemala, summers of 1957 and 1961. Her published works include: The Spanish Americans of New Mexico: A Distinctive Heritage, *University of California, (1967);* "Family Organization in Five Types of Migratory Wage Labor," *American* Anthropologist, *(1963); and* "Health Behavior in Cross-Cultural Perspective," *Human* Organization, *(1966).* "Beliefs and Practices Concerning Medicine and Nutrition Among Lower-Class Urban Guatemalans" *is reprinted with the permission of the author and of the American Public Health Association, Inc. from the* American Journal of Public Health, *Vol. 54, No. 10 (Oct. 1964), pp. 1726–1734.*

This paper attempts to describe current medical and nutritional beliefs and practices among lower-class urban Guatemalans. A study based upon questionnaires and intensive interviews was conducted in fifty-seven lower-class Ladino[1] families living in Guatemala City and its immediate environs. The majority of the samples studied were born in rural areas and had moved to the city in early youth. The sophistication of urban life has impinged upon this group in many ways, but most of their basic values remain similar to those of the folk societies from which they have sprung.

Characteristics of the Group

The person observed are completely dependent upon wage labor for a living. None own land upon which they might plant crops, and although most have a small space near the house in which a garden might be planted, none do so for various reasons, the most important being lack of water. In addition, vegetables, the only items for which the available space might be adequate, form a small part of the total diet and are relatively cheap. Therefore, it is not worth their time and effort to plant such gardens. Although some of the families keep a few chickens, ducks, and pigs, these are relatively rare and serve as a kind of insurance against emergencies when cash is desperately needed.

Many of the women make and sell tortillas or candies to supplement their husbands' incomes, and a few work by the day as domestics or take in laundry. One woman makes cigars and another wraps firecrackers on consignment for local factories. But for the most part, these families are dependent upon the money brought in by the men, who have a variety of occupations. The highest in the wage scale are chauffeurs, weavers, and tailors. The majority work as day laborers at anything they can find, and many reported they worked only irregularly. No family reported an income of more than $80 per month, and this figure was quoted by the wife of a policeman, whose house and obvious standard of living were somewhat better than that of any other family encountered. Incomes of some families are also supplemented by charitable donations of food and/or medicines from churches and public health services.

Literally all the necessities of life, as well as the luxuries, must be purchased. Most of the families are heavily in debt to a small local store, from which they buy all foods (except meat and milk), as well as soap, candles, some medicines, and various household items such as brooms, needles, thread, and the like. Clothing is usually purchased in the center of town, either at one of the large markets, or at cheap general stores. Some articles are ordered from local tailors and dressmakers. Nearly all families must buy water daily from the few persons in the community who have wells. I encountered only one family which had its own well. Only one house visited had electricity; the others depended upon candles or kerosene lamps for illumination. Cooking is done over an open wood fire built on top of an adobe platform—a typical Ladino cooking arrangement.

Meat markets are plentiful, and meat is available daily to those who can afford it. There are several dairies which make door-to-door deliveries in the area. The people supply their own bottles or containers, and the milk is ladled out to them from large cans. A few families reported using powdered milk, which is bought in one pound cans from the small stores. Occasionally a woman reported doing the bulk of her shopping at one of the large city markets once a week, but the majority are unable to buy in this more economical way because they never have enough cash on hand. They are therefore dependent upon the credit offered by the small "corner stores." Most shop throughout the day, running out several times to obtain what they need. Convenience and saving the 10 cents round-trip bus fare to the larger markets are also factors which determine where these women buy. Because incomes vary tremendously from week to week, and even from day to day in most cases, expenditures also vary. It was always extremely difficult, therefore, to make an estimate of the household's financial status.

People in this social class are rarely able to eat as they would really like. They are aware of and place great value on those items eaten by upper classes in Guatemala, but their actual consumption seems to vary little from that of the poor rural Ladinos. The basis of the diet is tortillas, most often made by the housewife, but occasionally purchased. Bread is also consumed by most families at least once a day. Aside from tortillas, black beans and rice are the standard fare; noodles or macaroni are occasionally used, more as an accompaniment rather than a substitute for the rice. Beets, cabbage, güisquil (*Sechum edule*), güicoy (*Cucurbita pepo*), and green beans are liked and eaten in small amounts two to three times per week. Tomatoes and onions are used more frequently, primarily as flavorings for rice and meat—often in the form of a sauce called "chirmol." On the average, meat is consumed about once a week, each family member receiving from two to three ounces of edible meat. Most families with children want to include milk in their diet, and in some cases they will sacrifice to buy it for the children, but rarely does a child receive more than one glass per day either as a supplement to the breast or as the only source of milk. A few families reported that they used Incaparina[2] as a gruel for young children. In all cases they had heard of this vegetable protein mixture through the health center in their area. Pregnant and nursing women often described milk as a food they should have, but which most often they were unable to afford. These people like eggs very much, and those who have chickens usually consume their hen's produce, rarely more than one or two eggs per hen per week. Many times, on the other hand, the 5–6 cents for which an egg may be sold makes it desirable to trade the eggs at their small local store for other items more desperately needed.

A large amount of money is expended by these families for doctor's services and for "medicines" of various types. Most of these are patented syrups and pills, but they also purchase antibiotics and steroids, as well as dried herbs, roots, and seeds, for making "teas" and compresses. Many seek the services of private physicians and others buy medicines on the advice of friends, relatives, and neighbors. There are untrained persons within a few blocks of all houses who give injections for a small fee. All of the women interviewed had heard of vitamins, and although they did not have a clear idea of what vitamins are, they were convinced of their health-giving value. In all cases, however, vitamins were considered as medicines and were administered only to the sick.

There is a wide range in the use of the free health facilities offered in the nearby health center and the local hospitals. At one extreme are the mothers who take their children regularly to the well-baby clinic at the health center. Many others have never visited any of these institutions, and the majority go only after a prolonged illness has failed to respond to home treatments. Among the latter group, a great deal of dissatisfaction with the treatment received was expressed to me. For example, one woman said, "When my husband was stricken with 'attacks' I took him there for treatment, but they said he wasn't really sick." She consequently "cured" her husband by taking him to a spiritualist. Except in the cases of women who had gone to the hospitals for childbirth, similar comments were made in regard to hospital services. The women were extremely pleased and satisfied with their experiences in the maternity wards and most indicated a desire to return there for their next child. However, it is interesting to note that even these women generally do not go to the hospital for pre-natal examinations until the final month of pregnancy, and some even arrive for their first examinations after labor has begun. Most of the women in the area still prefer a midwife for assistance in delivery, even though the expense is greater[3] and the physical comfort less. The only reason given for this is embarrassment at being examined by a male doctor.

The study of this urban group has suggested several points which seem to me to be worthy of further emphasis and discussion. First, there is tremendous variation in verbal expression of certain beliefs and practices, due, in part, to the diverse origin of the people. In addition, some people are simply more interested in accumulating knowledge concerning health and nutrition, and as such serve as advisers to their neighbors and friends. In spite of this apparent variation, I believe it is possible to generalize concerning the entire body of lore available to this segment of the population, and also concerning the attitudes of these people toward nutrition and medicine. The following classification is offered as an attempt to describe and reduce these concepts to some order.

Concepts Relating to Nutrition

Negative Value Emphasis

Hot-Cold Dichotomy: Anyone familiar with Latin-American culture will immediately recognize the widespread belief in hot and cold foods.[4-7] Both extremes are felt to be dangerous under certain circumstances. All persons in a "delicate state," including small children and infants, sick persons, and pregnant and lactating women, should be careful to balance their diets in accordance with their own needs and sensitivities. Cold foods are generally considered to be more dangerous than hot, but it is interesting to note that most cold foods may be altered in some way so that they are safe to eat. Thus, milk boiled with cinnamon is no longer "cold," and pork cooked for a long period of time with cloves and black pepper becomes "regular," in fact, much of the art of cookery concerns not only the flavor given foods by additions of herbs, spices, and condiments, but also the manipulation of the hot or cold qualities of the foods. Contrary to what has often been reported, it appears that among this population the process of cooking, which of course involves changes of temperature, is important in determining the ultimate classification of the food. For example, "thrice-cooked gruel" is, by virtue of its number of cookings, very "hot." Leftover foods which have once been cooked are "cold," but heating them on the fire renders them safe to eat. Boiled water is "hot," but if it is left standing overnight it becomes cold and must be boiled again before one can drink it with impunity (for parallel case see Wellin[8]). I am not suggesting that there is no difference between the concepts of heat as defined by temperature and "hotness" as a natural quality of food. I am suggesting, however, that there is some relationship between the two concepts—at least among the Ladinos studied in the poor urban sections of Guatemala City. It is possible that the observed ideas and practices concerning "hot" and "cold" foods are results of ongoing acculturation which has led to a reinterpretation of former beliefs.

Further investigation on this point in nonurban, relatively unacculturated centers of population should help clarify the matter.

Strong Food: Far more important than "hot" and "cold" foods to the average woman interviewed, are those which she classifies as "strong." As in other cases, the particular foods which a given person will include in this category vary according to his or her own physical and mental constitution. The following foods, among others, however, are considered to be "strong" by many persons: meat, lard, chili. "Too much" of any of these foods is bad for anybody, but some persons can take more than others. In other words, a person with a "strong" constitution (which usually includes personality traits) can safely eat larger quantities of such foods. Children, especially younger than two years, cannot handle strong foods well and most often do not receive them; but when they do, as in the case of meat, they are given very small amounts just to chew and spit out. Occasionally, a child below this age is allowed to eat meat, and the mother's explanation is that that particular child is stronger than most. Sometimes mothers also express the child's unusual ability to tolerate strong foods in terms of the number of teeth he has or the precocious development of his stomach and internal organs. Strong foods differ from cold or hot foods in that their qualities are inalterable—one must simply eat less of them or avoid them altogether. It is of interest to note here that milk is sometimes placed in this category—especially goat's and donkey's milk. On the whole, however, the people in this study group place a high positive value on cow's milk (see below) and are not overly worried about its possible harmful effects.

Indigestible Foods: This should more properly be termed "foods which are more difficult to digest than others." There is some overlapping here with the two classes discussed above, for "cold" foods and "strong" foods may also produce indigestion. However, apart from the former qualities, some foods are thought to be "heavy" or simply indigestible for some persons. For this reason, potatoes and rice are commonly excluded from the diet of very young children. Whole black beans and corn on the cob are also considered to be indigestible for the obvious reason that they sometimes appear in the feces. Powdered milk is sometimes claimed to be indigestible because it does not readily dissolve in water and sometimes lumps remain after mixing. As with the strong foods, there is nothing to be done about these foods except to avoid them in infancy, early childhood, or sickness.

Positive Value Emphasis

Growth-Promoting Foods: The concept of growth as an index of health is not only very prevalent, but seems to be the only area in which food is directly and positively related to good health. The people constantly refer to the healthy child as being big and fat. Thin children, although otherwise healthy, active and alert, are worried over, and the mother will claim that such a child "doesn't eat a thing." Diarrhea is considered dangerous for children because "it keeps them from growing," and "it keeps them from getting fat." Conditions of the skin, eyes, mucous membranes, and hair are *not* related to either qualitative or quantitative food deficiencies. In fact, changes in the condition of the body which may actually be evidence of dietary deficiencies *may* be attributed to the eating of a particular food or class of food.

Everyone has his or her own ideas as to what constitute nourishing foods, but in general the following list is agreed upon: milk, bread, tortillas—especially if made with yellow corn—noodles, oatmeal and other starchy gruels, vegetables, black beans, eggs, and sometimes beef.

Some people equated "hot" foods with "nourishing" foods, but in such cases they also expressed the belief that since these foods were so potent and so nourishing, one needed to eat them only in small quantities.

The Diet of Infants and Sick Persons: In addition to those foods which are generally nourishing, there are some that are thought to be particularly efficacious in treating sick persons and in rearing infants. Gruels of cornstarch, rice, and yuca are most important here. In addition, soft-boiled eggs and meat broths are frequently mentioned as being good for this class of persons.

The Diet of Pregnant Women: In order to ensure the health of the mother, proper growth of the fetus, and an easy delivery, the pregnant woman should also be careful of her diet. Milk, especially when fresh from the cow, and raw eggs, often mixed with sweet wine or beer, are recommended. Needless to say, most women in the group are unable to buy milk and eggs in sufficient quantities to feed both themselves and their children. That which money can buy almost always goes to the children first. It might be interesting in this regard to check possible differences in the prenatal health of primiparas and multiparas. "Hot" foods have a positive value emphasis in helping to avoid being "chilled," one of the dangers to be encountered during pregnancy, when the body is abnormally "hot."

Lactating Women: It is thought that for successful lactation a woman must eat well, and that she must consume larger quantities than usual of certain foods to ensure a good milk supply. Chocolate is the most frequently mentioned lactagogue, and ideally it should be drunk three times a day for forty days after birth. In addition, gruels of oatmeal and of *masa* (ground lime-treated corn), boiled milk, and beer are often recommended. Also included are special herbal teas which may be drunk to increase the flow of milk.

Neutral Foods

Snack Foods: A large number of foods, not eaten regularly, but enjoyed occasionally or even frequently, by most persons, even by quite poor families, include candy, soft drinks, potato chips, and fruits, either fresh or in syrup. Interestingly enough, the people seem to consume fruit as a snack more often than any other item. Fruits are proscribed, however, for lactating women, because of the fear that the mother's milk will become sour, rotten, acid, or will decrease in quantity. Sometimes fruits are thought to be "cold," and under certain conditions they may not be consumed because of this quality. In general, however, fruits are thought to be neither especially nourishing nor especially harmful.

These snack foods are seldom, if ever, consumed at mealtimes, and if the family income drops to the survival level, they disappear entirely from the diet.

Classification of Diseases and Causative Agents

Physical Causes of Disease

Contagion: It is commonly understood that a sick person may pass on his disease to others through bodily contact or through a secondary agent such as bedclothes or eating utensils. The concept of contagion seems to apply especially to those diseases involving eruptions of the skin, such as measles, chicken pox, boils, dermatitis, and so on. There is also a corresponding concept of immunity which holds that some persons are not susceptible to diseases because they are particularly "strong." Children, who are in general "weak," are more susceptible than adults.

People have great faith in the power of vaccines as a preventive measure, but they think that vaccines are equally effective before and after exposure. Furthermore, many people believe that modern medicine has vaccines against all diseases. This misunderstanding often leads to great dissatisfaction with the services of local health facilities. For example, a woman whose child has been exposed to chicken pox may go to the clinic demanding vaccine as a preventive. If she does not obtain a shot of some sort, and especially if her child later develops the disease, she blames the clinic and feels the personnel are withholding medicine from her for personal reasons.

The concept of contagion described above, although colored by ideas garnered from modern medicine, has its roots in older folk beliefs regarding "contagious magic." Another commonly held notion, and one widely distributed in European and American cultures, is that congenital deformities are caused by the pregnant woman's having come into contact with similarly deformed persons. In a very real sense, this type of contagion is not different from that described above, at least to the people involved. The only difference is that a vaccine is not considered helpful in this case.

The idea of contagion seems also to apply to conception. That is, a woman "catches" a baby by having intercourse with a man. Several women told me that they have heard that there were injections as well as pills which one could take to prevent conception. Even the terms used in discussing this matter indicate its relationship to disease; for when a woman becomes pregnant, she gets "sick," and the injections mentioned above are said to "cure" her. It is clear, however, that these injections are sought as a preventive measure, and not as an abortifacient, although it is also assumed that modern medicine has ways of "curing" pregnancy in the latter sense as well. It is commonly believed, though the exact mechanism remains vague, that there are ways of "curing" a man so that his wife will not become pregnant.

Filth: Although many people have heard of "microbes," there is no real understanding of what they are. They are invariably associated with visible dirt, dust, droppings of animals, and spoiled food (garbage). If one is present, so is the other. On the other hand, if things look clean, they are clean. A soiled dish may be washed in dirty water, wiped with a dirty cloth, and considered clean if it appears to be clean (for a parallel example from Peru, see Wellin[8]). Similarly, a glass used by several people in turn may be wiped clean after each user with any handy rag.

Flies are considered to be disease bearers because they leave visible specks of dirt, especially on foods such as sugar. Also, dust in the air, as occurs often in the dry season in areas with unpaved streets, is considered to be unhealthy as well as unpleasant. The mouth and nose are frequently protected by handkerchiefs to avoid inhaling the dust when people venture out in the dry season. It is also thought that dust may cause eye irritations, especially conjunctivitis.

The occasional child who eats dirt is worried over, punished, and frequently purged for fear of sickness. A crawling baby may be restricted in his movements by placing him inside a box. He is seldom allowed to crawl about on the floor or in the yard without constant attention. Mothers frequently attribute diarrhea in young infants to their having eaten dirt or having sucked dirty objects.

"Spoiled" food is that which smells bad or which has become moldy, and it is considered unfit for human consumption (although it may be thrown to the dogs or pigs). Actually, in these poor households where food is most often purchased and prepared each day, there are few leftovers to become spoiled.

In only two instances did I encounter beliefs concerning cleanliness in which visible dirt did not play a part. The first of these involved the scissors used by midwives to cut the umbilical cord of the newborn baby. One woman told me that her midwife was not careful to boil the scissors before using them and that this could cause infection of the umbilicus. Other women also stated that "dirty" scissors might be responsible for such infections, but they did not mention boiling as a preventive measure. They merely thought that the midwife should have a special pair of scissors used only for this purpose, and that they should be washed each time.

In general the idea of sterilization is linked only with hypodermic needles. Most persons interviewed knew that doctors and pharmacists boil the needles each time after use, and occasionally a disease was attributed to the "doctor's" not having boiled the needle before an injection, but this concept does not transfer to other items, such as baby bottles, for example. I found no women who boiled their bottles, although some said they rinsed them with boiled water. I highly suspected, although I have not enough data to confirm it, that the idea of boiling is more related to the hot-cold dichotomy discussed above, than to killing bacteria. Boiling may remove dangerous coldness not only in foods, but also in other objects. Other anthropological reports from Meso-America[9] indicate that metal objects (such as knives and scissors) are often considered to be "cold" and therefore unfit for cutting a baby's umbilical cord.

Psychological Causes of Disease

These have been well outlined by other authors[4, 7, 10] and the present field work has provided only confirming data. The most important and frequently mentioned psychological cause for disease is fright. An individual may be frightened by either natural or supernatural events which cause a variety of symptoms. Actually, any disease may be attributed to fright if the family is able to remember that the sick person had a bad experience shortly before the onset of symptoms. Fright is commonly given as a cause for the lactating mother's milk diminishing or disappearing. Anger may also be the causative factor here.

Embarrassment (*vergüenza*) is another possible cause for disease. This does not seem to be so important a factor as fright, and in this field study it was mentioned only in regard to children who were having difficulty learning bladder control. It was said that accidents in public led to apathy, sadness, and other symptoms of disease. On the other hand, shaming is a technic often used to "cure" such children—especially in the case of nocturesis. In such cases the embarrassment is not thought to produce other sicknesses.

The only other physiological disturbance related to psychological factors found in this study was spontaneous abortion. This is said to be brought about by a woman's not satisfying her food cravings. It is thought that the unborn child demands these substances and becomes angry if the mother does not provide them.[11] The cravings can be successfully stifled in most cases by taking a pinch of salt with a glass of water.

Magical Causes of Disease

Ojo (evil eye): This concept does not require extensive treatment here since it has been well described by many others. The complex as encountered among the urban lower class is virtually the same as that in other Latin-American groups, but it does seem to be diminishing in importance. Babies and small children frequently wear amulets of one kind or another to prevent the possible ill effects of *ojo* but ascription of a disease or symptom to this cause is often only a last resort. The symptoms most commonly attributed to *ojo* are vague and generalized aches and pains, apathy, madness, and so forth. *Ojo* is a serious thing, since it may cause death, but actually there are many other things more to be feared than *ojo*.

Aire: This concept, also fairly well described in the literature, is still highly important to the urban folk. There are various kinds of *aire* which may bring about disease symptoms. The most usual type is "cold" air, which may or may not be literally cold. Night air always has a magical cold quality, as does strong wind. These kinds of air are thought to cause colds, inflammation, whooping cough, edema, and occasionally diarrhea. In addition, there are the "bad airs," which usually have a bad odor and may be derived from decaying organic matter. The nose and mouth may be protected with a handkerchief when bad or cold airs are likely to be encountered. Small babies are also especially susceptible to air, and they are usually well wrapped in blankets and their heads are protected with hats or bonnets even in fairly warm weather. The air is not considered dangerous because it carries illnesses, but because in and of itself it is harmful to the body.

Summary

This paper has reported the results of a field survey of the medical and nutritional beliefs among the lower-class urban population of Guatemala City. Although this presentation is not exhaustive, some of the more general characteristics of practice and belief have been outlined. That the majority of the older rural folk beliefs still survive in the city is evident, even though many new ideas have been adopted from the more sophisticated middle and upper classes. In some cases, the newer practices and modern terminology have simply been applied to or incorporated into the older patterns of folk medicine and nutrition.

References

1. Persons of Latin, as opposed to Indian culture. See reference 1. below for definitions and discussions.

2. A low-cost vegetable protein mixture developed by INCAP.

3. Empirical midwives, as well as a few trained by the Public Health Department, deliver babies for fees ranging from $1.50–$15, depending upon the family income and the experience and reputation of the midwife.

4. Adams, R. Cultural Surveys of Guatemala, El Salvador, Honduras, Nicaragua, and Panama, Washington, D.C.: Pan American Sanitary Bureau, 1957. Scientific Publ. no. 33.

5. Gillin, J. Moche, a Peruvian Coastal Community. Washington, D.C.: Smithsonian Institution, 1947. Institute of Social Anthropology. Publ no. 3.

6. Foster, G. "Relationships Between Spanish and Spanish-American Folk Medicine." J. of American Folklore LXVI:201–217, 1953.

7. Adams, R. N. Un análisis de las creencias y prácticas médicas en un pueblo indígena de Guatemala. Guatemala, C. A.: Editorial del Ministerio de Educación Pública, 1952. Publicaciones especiales del Instituto Indigenista Nacional no. 17.

8. Wellin, E. "Water Boiling in a Peruvian Town." In Health, Culture and Community. Edited by Benjamin Paul. New York, N. Y.: Russell Sage, 1955, pp. 71–103.

9. Tax, S. Heritage of Conquest. Glencoe, Ill.: Free Press, 1952.

10. Foster, G. "Relationships Between Theoretical and Applied Anthropology." Human Organization XI:5–16, 1952.

11. ———. Culture and Conquest. New York: Wenner-Gren, 1960. Viking Fund Publications in Anthropology no. 27.

12

Popular and Modern Medicine in Mestizo Communities of Coastal Peru and Chile[1]

by Ozzie G. Simmons

Ozzie G. Simmons, Ph.D., is Program Adviser for the Ford Foundation. He has served previously as Field Director, Institute of Social Anthropology, Smithsonian Institute; Staff Anthropologist, Institute of Inter-American Affairs, Chile; Associate Professor of Anthropology at Harvard; and, most recently, Professor of Sociology and Director, Institute of Behavioral Science, University of Colorado, Boulder. His research and writings indicate a profound interest in health, culture, and the social structure. His most recent publications include: (co-author), The Mental Patient Comes Home, Wiley (1963); (author) Work and Mental Illness, Wiley (1965); and (co-author) "The Role Path: A Concept and Procedure for Studying Migration to Urban Communities," Human Organization, (Summer 1968). "Popular and Modern Medicine in Mestizo Communities of Coastal Peru and Chile" is reprinted with the permission of the author and of The American Folklore Society, Inc. from Journal of American Folklore, Vol. 68 (1955), pp. 57–71.

The present paper represents an attempt to delineate the key patterns of Mestizo popular medicine and to analyze their implications for the reception accorded modern medicine by examining the nature and degree of acculturation to the latter that has already occurred. In working with professional personnel—doctors, nurses, and health educators—engaged in action programs of public health in Peru and Chile, the writer encountered a pervasive preconception that the task of educating local populations in the concepts and practices of modern medicine is largely a matter of filling a mental vacuum, of providing information for the "uninformed." There seems to be little awareness on their part that the need for emotional adjustment and cognitive orientation to the anxiety-arousing situations produced by such frustrating experiences as disease and death has characteristically led to the development and elaboration in all known societies of beliefs and practices for coping with these uncertainties. Popular medical beliefs and practices are ordinarily deeply rooted in the basic assumptions of a culture and provide more or less complete explanations of illness and of the appropriate means for dealing with it. Consequently, any serious attempt at converting so-called "underdeveloped" peoples to modern health practices will require not only some knowledge of their popular medicine but an assessment of its most receptive and resistant points with regard to modern medicine.

Magic and the Supernatural in Popular Medicine. For present purposes, the distinction between magical and empirical idea and action patterns will be drawn on the basis of orientations to the supernatural and natural "worlds."[2] The magical patterns of popular medicine are those which manipulate intangible entities, symbolically represented aspects of nonempirical reality, while empirical patterns are those which deal with tangible entities. Both are utilized for the achievement of empirical ends, but magical patterns are neither verifiable nor understandable in terms of the criteria established for defining empirical knowledge in Mestizo culture, while empirical patterns are subject to these standards. An empirical idea or action pattern of popular medicine may be inadequate and erroneous if tested by the standards of modern science, but it is nevertheless empirical if the criteria of empirical knowledge in Mestizo culture can be applied to it. The empirical lore utilized by popular medicine is largely of folk origin, was developed in response to immediate needs stemming from the problems posed by illness, and, despite the fact that it is empirically grounded, has been severely limited in its development by a tradition that also sanctions recourse to magic and the supernatural for solution of the same problems. The empirical knowledge utilized by modern medicine, on the other hand, represents an application of results obtained by scientific investigation dedicated to the abstraction and generalization of knowledge rather than to the solution of immediate problems, investigation carried on under conditions that do not involve competition with nonempirical cognitive orientations.[3]

A convenient departure point for a discussion of Mestizo popular medicine is Malinowski's theory of the function of magic, which has been further elaborated by Parsons, Homans, and most recently Vogt.[4] In brief, Malinowski stated that the use of magic is prominent in enterprises whose success is emotionally important to the group and where there is great uncertainty as to the outcome, and is resorted to as a means of control over the incalculable and dangerous that cannot be eliminated solely by use of the empirical techniques available to the group. The magical techniques take over, as it were, where the empirical techniques leave off in order to insure the success of the enterprise, and the employment of magic provides the necessary optimism and confidence in a successful outcome that would otherwise be lacking. In his studies among the Trobrianders, Malinowski found that, where it was employed, magic was considered as indispensable to the success of the enterprise as was empirical activity. The magical and empirical were dedicated to the realization of a common empirical end, and performed complementary functions.[5]

In general, the relationship between anxiety and ritual that Malinowski has demonstrated for Trobriand culture, holds, for the most part, for Mestizo culture in Peru as well. The greatest elaboration of magical beliefs and practices seems to be associated with those aspects of culture that involve the greatest uncertainty. The highest concentration is apparently to be found in connection with illness and its treatment, but ritual is commonly employed during crop planting to insure a successful harvest, at various stages in the technology of elaboration of alcoholic beverages, in practices connected with birth, toilet training, and weaning of children, in the inauguration of any new commercial enterprise, and for warding off landslides, earthquakes, and other calamities of nature.[6] However, detailed consideration of the distribution and employment of magical elements in the popular treatment of illness reveals the existence of patterns not always consistent with Malinowski's views. The treatment of many important illnesses makes no use of magic at all, magic is not always considered indispensable where it is employed along with empirical curing techniques, and, more often than not, although utilized for the achievement of a common empirical end, magical and empirical techniques perform equivalent rather than complementary functions. As will be seen, all these considerations have important implications for the problems involved in inducing acceptance of modern medicine.

The peculiar way in which magic is used in Mestizo popular medicine is in part due to the fact that the fundamental assumptions on which the latter is based are couched more in natural than in supernatural terms. The attribution of most or all illness to action by supernatural forces, either benign or malign, is characteristic of a wide variety of nonliterate cultures.[7] Such different groups as the Berens River Salteaux of Canada, the Azande of Central Africa, the Maya Indians of Quintana Roo and Chan Kom in Yucatan and of Santiago Chimaltenango in Guatemala, and the Quechua and Aymara Indians of Highland Peru,[8] adhere to a theory of disease that makes the maintenance of health contingent on the observance of the moral and religious imperatives of the society, and illness a retribution by supernatural forces for lapses in such observance.[9] In all these societies, no matter how supernatural-ridden they may be, there is some recognition of empirical or natural causation of disease and a more or less elaborate repertory of empirical curing techniques and pharmacopoeia, but either the empirical cause is always derived from an ultimate supernatural cause and the empirical cures are secondary or supplementary to the utilization of magical and supplicatory techniques, or empirical causation and cure are reserved for minor illnesses while supernatural considerations predominate in explaining and coping with serious illness. Most of these societies recognize a wide variety of illnesses and utilize an impressive number of curing techniques for coping with them, but the fact that there is only one possible ultimate cause for illness decisively determines the nature of therapeutic principles and severely limits the variation in ends sought by therapeutic techniques. In those societies where illness is principally the result of supernatural visitation for violation of religious or moral rules, medical beliefs and practices seem to be well integrated with the religion and morality of the group and play a prominent role among the mechanisms of social control.

Patterns of Etiology in Popular Medicine. The patterns of popular medicine adhered to by Mestizo groups in coastal Peru and Chile differ considerably from those dominated by a belief in supernatural causation, just as they do from those of modern scientific medicine.[10] Mestizo etiological conceptions seek no support or sanction from religious or moral considerations, although a few are defined nonetheless in supernatural terms. Consequently, there is no single all-embracing causative factor, such as incurring the displeasure of the benign or malevolent gods, that can provide a central integrated theory of disease. Instead, there are five major etiological categories that embrace all of the serious illnesses and the vast majority of the minor ones. Illness is caused by severe emotional upset, contamination by ritually unclean persons, obstruction of the gastrointestinal tract, undue exposure to heat or cold, or exposure to *mal aire*, bed air.[11] Exposure to heat and gastrointestinal obstruction are sometimes cited as the causes of the same illnesses, but with this exception there are no significant interrelations between the several etiological categories. The single common thread that runs through all popular medicine is the distinction between "hot" and "cold." There is a pervasive tendency to classify illnesses, as well as foods and remedies, as hot or cold, a classification that sometimes refers to actual temperatures but more often to innate qualities that have no necessary relation to warmth or coldness. The hot and cold distinctions are empirical and provide a set of general rules, not always observed and often inconsistent, that prescribe a proper balance between hot and cold in consumption of food, hot remedies for cold illnesses, and vice versa. This distinction has an etiological aspect in that violation of the dietary rules can be a direct cause of illness, while failure to observe the rule of opposites in curing will certainly aggravate the illness and may be fatal.[12]

Only the briefest description of the etiological and curing patterns of popular medicine will be attempted here, sufficient to illustrate their considerable divergence from those of modern medicine and their utilization of magical and empirical elements. Peruvian patterns will be described first and then compared with those encountered in Chile.

It is generally believed that severe emotional upset may directly cause organic disorders most of which are potentially fatal. *Susto*, fright, results from encountering an apparition, which always involves soul-loss, or from a sudden and unexpected experience such as being startled or attacked by an animal, falling, particularly falling into water, a loud noise or clap on the back perpetrated by a person whose presence was hitherto unsuspected, and so on, which may or may not involve soul-loss. Symptoms of fright include wasting away, fever, diarrhea, sleeplessness, loss of will, malaise, and general "nervousness." There are no important differences in the syndromes identified with those cases where soul-loss does or does not occur. Embarrassment can result in *chucaque*,[13] whose symptoms are severe aches in the head, stomach, and abdomen, vomiting, diarrhea, fever, and chills. A fit of anger can lead to *colerina,* characterized by severe stomach ache, diarrhea, vomiting, and fever. *Celos,* jealousy, is an illness contracted by the youngest child when its mother becomes pregnant and the child is jealous of the sibling to come. In one version, the jealousy occurs only if the nursing child and the fetus are of opposite sex, but in another, just as common, this is not a requisite. A nursing child learns of the expected infant through the taste of his mother's milk, while one already weaned can "sense" it through contact with the mother. *Celos* can also be postnatal, when a child feels jealous of the new-born sibling who has supplanted him as the youngest. Children suffering from *celos* exhibit regressive and aggressive behavior by wishing to be fed or refusing to eat, annoying the mother constantly, having temper tantrums, and so on. The pre- and postnatal syndromes differ only in that in the latter the newborn child is added to the objects of aggression. Anger or grief experienced by a woman during the postpartum period of forty days will result in *sobreparto,* an illness characterized by severe colic, fever, and general debilitation. None of these syndromes have exact equivalents among those recognized by modern medicine; however, jaundice is included in this category as caused by severe disillusionment or grief, and "heart trouble" is attributed to the same cause or to fits of anger. With the exception of the supernatural apparition that may cause fright, there are no nonempirical elements in the etiologies that fall into the category of severe emotional upset.

Contamination by "ritually unclean"[14] persons is an etiological category of an entirely magical nature. The most important and pervasive cause in this category is *el ojo,* evil eye. A person who possesses a "strong glance" will contaminate a child when he demonstrates affection for it since the force of this glance passes into the child. Contamination by evil eye is usually unwitting on the part of the person who is the causal agent, and is most apt to occur when the latter is agitated for some reason or has "hot blood" due to recent exertion. The most common symptoms of evil eye, to which only children are vulnerable, are constant crying, irritability, vomiting, diarrhea, fever, loss of appetite, and nightmares. Pregnant or menstruating women who look at or pick up an infant when they are thus "ritually unclean" may cause an illness variously called *pujo* or *quiebra del niño*. The infant thus contaminated cries and screams hysterically and is subject to severe heaving from the abdomen that results in a protruding navel. The evil-eye syndrome has no parallel in modern medicine, but part of the *pujo* syndrome corresponds to that found in umbilical hernia.

Obstruction of the gastrointestinal tract, described as a "loaded" or "dirty" stomach from which food will not pass into the intestine, provides the etiology for all gastrointestinal illnesses, chicken pox, measles, and smallpox. The popular syndromes for these illnesses do not vary significantly from those of modern medicine. This etiological category is wholly empirical.

Undue exposure to excessive cold or heat, with reference to environmental temperatures, is the cause ascribed for a variety of important illnesses, including the common cold, cough, whooping cough, bronchitis, influenza, pneumonia, and tuberculosis. All muscular and neuralgic ailments, including rheumatism, sciatica, and arthritis, are ascribed to cold, as are malaria and conjunctivitis. Heat causes sunstroke, and was cited by a few informants as the cause of all the illnesses indicated above as due to gastrointestinal obstruction. Like the latter category, that of heat and cold is wholly empirical. Popular syndromes said to be caused by heat or cold conform, on the whole, to those recognized by modern medicine for these illnesses.

"Bad air" is usually described as a current of air that enters any part of the body, especially through the openings, lodges there, and results in aches, pains, and malfunctioning in the area affected. Any sudden change in environmental temperature, as when one emerges from a house with a "heated" body, will make one vulnerable to *aire*, as the illness is called. Contact with something hot immediately after handling something cold, or vice versa, such as taking hold of a hot iron right after washing clothes, will bring on an *aire* called *pasmo*, characterized by swellings and eruptions. The source of bad air may be the atmosphere itself, or it may emanate from the graves and ruins of the pre-Columbian peoples when one tampers with them or is near them. This latter source may involve a nonempirical element, but bad air is otherwise an empirical etiological category. The syndromes said to be caused by bad air, when these involve more than mere aches or pains, are usually rather vague, and are peculiar to popular medicine for the most part.

These five etiological categories embrace practically all illnesses in Chile as well as coastal Peru, but there are a number of important differences in popular syndromes and in the attribution of illnesses to causes between the patterns of popular medicine in the Chilean communities and those in the Peruvian. As in Peru, the hot and cold classification of foods, remedies, and illnesses is pervasive and constitutes a major characteristic of Chilean popular belief. The most prominent illness caused by severe emotional upset is *pension*, brought on by grief due to separation from or loss of a loved one, as parents from children and lovers from each other. The victim is usually a child, but may be an adult. In the former case, *pension* may also be incurred because of the advent of a new sibling. Symptoms, for both children and adults, are sadness or profound depression, loss of appetite, irritability, insomnia, crying, and brain "upsets." Children also manifest regressions in toilet training and eating. Grief may also cause anemia and jaundice. Fright or a fit of anger during the forty-day postpartum period causes *sobreparto*, whose syndrome is similar to that described for Peru. If the fit of anger is strong enough, the woman may die instantly. The concept of fright as a cause of illness is, however, little developed in Chile. Experiencing fright may cause a temporary indisposition, and a severe fright may affect the heart, but there is no idea of soul-loss as a consequence of fright nor any elaboration of syndromes and curing techniques such as exists in Peru.

In the category of ritual uncleanness, only evil eye is recognized, a concept as well developed and pervasive as in Peru. Chileans attribute large, bulging eyes and "heavy," "thick," or "fat" blood, as well as the "strong glance," to the person who possesses the evil eye. The act, always unintentional, of casting the evil eye relieves the person of the pressure of his "heavy" blood. Chilean and Peruvian syndromes are, with slight variations, very similar.

Gastrointestinal obstruction is the cause of only one illness, *empacho,* mainly a children's disease although adults are also vulnerable. *Empacho* is as pervasive and considered as dangerous as evil eye, and is caused by an object such as green fruit, soft bread, or half-cooked food becoming stuck in the stomach or intestine. Its symptoms are depression, paleness, loss of appetite, diarrhea, fever, vomiting, and stomach or abdominal pains.

Excessive cold or heat are believed to be the causes of the vast majority of major and minor illnesses in Chile. Cold causes asthma, the common cold, cough, whooping cough, influenza, bronchitis, pneumonia, tuberculosis, liver ailments, diarrhea, dysentery, chicken pox, measles, mumps, smallpox, and meningitis. Heat is the cause of cataracts, sunstroke, and heart trouble, while kidney ailments, conjunctivitis, and rheumatism may come from either heat or cold. Popular syndromes of all these illnesses do not differ essentially from those recognized by modern medicine.

The concept of bad air is the same as in Peru except that the only source of bad air is the atmosphere. In Chile, it is believed that a current of bad air may also be the cause of pneumonia, tuberculosis, and infantile paralysis.

Of the principal etiological categories defined by Peruvian and Chilean popular belief, only that of ritual uncleanness is wholly magical. All other etiological categories, in both Peru and Chile are essentially empirical. The only important exception is that of fright in Peru as caused by encounter with an apparition or spirit, but fright by living beings and material objects seems to be at least as common, and may result in soul-loss with similar symptomatic manifestations to those resulting from encounter with an apparition. Thus the nonempirical and encounter with an apparition. Thus the nonempirical and empirical versions of the cause of fright may be considered functional equivalents.

Patterns of Curing in Popular Medicine. Although popular concepts of illness are framed largely in empirical rather than supernatural terms, the only consistency to be found between etiology and cure is that an illness attributed to supernatural causes will always have at least one magical cure. Magical ritual and supplication are often considered appropriate methods for curing illnesses that fall within an empirical etiological category, an empirical curing technique may be believed effective for an illness thought to be of supernatural origin, and ritual, supplication, and empiricism may all be employed in curing an illness regardless of the nature of its cause. Empirical curing techniques include infusions taken orally, massages, poultices, inhalations, syrups, laxatives, enemas, pomades and ointments, baths and cupping. The most common ingredients used in all but the last of these are herbs and other plant varieties but alcohol, fats and inner organs of animals, cooking oil, and various other items are also utilized. Magical techniques are extraction of the illness by passing a live guinea pig, egg, or other object over the patient's body; exhortation and calling of the patient's spirit to return to the body; utilization of formulae and objects with ritual potency, such as the form of the cross, numbers, and charms; and "holy remedies," also called "secrets of nature," which are ritual acts for curing specific illnesses. Prayers to the saints sometimes accompany empirical or magical cures and may be complete cures in themselves, as in curing evil eye and fright by blessing (*santiguar*). For the most part, these empirical and magical curing techniques are available to all laymen and may be performed by anyone. Knowledge of them is general, and only rarely is a magical cure so esoteric that it requires performance by a folk specialist (*curandero*). The latter is most often resorted to for curing fright and evil eye, but these are also treated at home. In general, folk specialists are employed when "lay" curing fails or the knowledge of the layman is not adequate for the case.

Consideration of the curing techniques deemed applicable for specific illnesses in Peru and Chile reveals that practically all magic and supplication are employed in treating the illnesses that fall into the etiological categories of severe emotional upset, ritual uncleanness, and bad air. Except in the case of fright and evil eye, popular medicine offers magical and empirical cures, each complete in itself, as alternative means of coping with each of these illnesses. Cures for fright involving soul-loss, always magical, are variations of the basic pattern of calling to the spirit of the patient to return to the body. The exhortations, performed at a certain hour (usually midnight), and a certain place (where the fright occurred), follow a standard formula addressed to the errant spirit, and are accompanied by invocations to the saints and ritual acts with the patient's clothes, all of which are repeated three times. Three cures, on successive days or Tuesdays and Fridays, are considered necessary. Other cures consist of passing a guinea pig or a piece of alum over the patient's body or of suspending a rooster's crest or a piece of beef from the neck of the patient, whereby the illness passes into the animal or object employed. These techniques are also performed three times, on specified days, and accompanied by exhortations and prayers. The administering of infusions and massages form part of all three cures, and if the fright does not involve soul-loss, ritual and prayer may be omitted, thus making the cure entirely empirical. To cure *chucaque,* the patient's palms are placed flat against his face and he is lifted by the elbows until his bones make a cracking noise; the operation is repeated holding the patient around the waist; and finally hairs are pulled out of the patient's head until one makes a cracking noise, which "breaks" the *chucaque*.[15] This is followed by drinking an herbal infusion. *Chucaque* may also be cured empirically by massages and infusions. *Colerina* is cured magically by heating the canvas potholder used in the kitchen and placing it on the patient's stomach, empirically by herbal infusions. *Celos* has a magical cure that consists of dressing the jealous child in red clothes turned inside out, while empirical cures are baths prepared with herbal infusions or attempts to distract the child from his jealousy, such as separating him from his mother by sending him to live with a relative, or serving him his food at the grinding stone rather than at the table.

Cures for evil eye are mainly magical, since they have as their end the elimination of the ritual contamination that is the basis of the illness. The classic cure for evil eye is to pass a freshly laid egg over the patient's body in the form of a cross, break it into a dish of water, and beat the mixture in the form of a cross with the hands and feet of the patient following a prescribed order. If the egg curdles, the illness is believed to have passed into it. The ritual is accompanied by special prayers recited three times, the egg mixture is disposed of in the form of a cross at a street corner (which has the form of a cross), and the cure must be performed three times on specified days. An alternative cure consists of massages with rue soaked in brandy and then with *ají,* hot peppers soaked in rose oil. The principle is the same as in the egg cure, and is ritually performed. *Pujo* or *quiebra del niño* is cured magically by placing the afflicted infant on the floor and having a female virgin walk over it lengthwise and then sidewise in straddling fashion, thus forming a cross, reciting a prayer at the same time; or by placing the navel binder always worn by infants around the waist of the pregnant or menstruating woman who has caused the illness, then replacing it on the infant while still warm from the woman's body. Empirical cures include applications to the navel of the milky sap of the fig tree or of a species of the comfrey plant.

The aches and pains that result from bad air are most often cured empirically, with massages, infusions, and inhalations. There is a magical cure that consists of passing a hot coal wrapped in cotton over the affected part. The coal is then thrown to the ground, and if it makes a loud sound, as though it were heavy, the bad air has passed into the coal.

Popular medicine provides a cure for every one of the illnesses listed above believed to be due to gastrointestinal obstruction or heat or cold. All of these cures are empirical, utilizing one or more of the empirical techniques already indicated, although they may sometimes be accompanied by a ritual element. It should be emphasized that in these cases the accompanying ritual is not considered indispensable to the effectiveness of the cure. Added insurance may be provided by giving three drops of a liquid medicine as a dose rather than any other number, by cutting a lemon, onion, or other item in the form of a cross when preparing it for use in a home remedy, or by reciting a prayer when administering an empirical cure, but omission of these procedures is not considered decisive in rendering the empirical remedy ineffective.

Empirical curing techniques utilized by Chilean popular medicine are the same as those in Peru, but magical techniques differ somewhat. The extraction of illness by passing a guinea pig, egg, or other object over the patient's body is not known in Chile, and since fright does not result in soul-loss, there are no techniques for exhortation or calling of the spirit. Of the illnesses said to be due to emotional upset, *pension* is cured magically by having the patient throw flower petals into a river and as the current carries away the petals, the grief goes with them. Empirically, *pension* is cured by infusions and distracting the patient from his grief. A magical cure for jaundice is to moisten a piece of sugar with one's saliva and throw it with pretended anger into running water. Jaundice is also cured with infusions.

The classic cure for evil eye in Chile is praying over the patient and blessing him with the sign of the cross (*santiguar*) .

Special prayers are recited and at the same time three branches of *palqui* (a tree of the solanaceous family) or three hot peppers are waved in front and then in back of the patient in the form of a cross. This is followed by fumigation with incense (*sahumerio*) of the patient to ensure the elimination of contamination. If the *palqui* branches or hot peppers remain fresh until the next day, it means the cure has been effective. Infusions administered orally may accompany this cure.

The remedy for *empacho* usually comprises three operations: a laxative is administered of grated potato, salt, lemon, and cooking oil to "loosen" the object causing the *empacho*. The *empacho* is "broken" by massaging the small of the back with ashes and then lifting the skin until a cracking noise is heard. Finally, herb infusions are given. This cure is magical-empirical, but the "breaking" of the *empacho* is not always believed to be necessary, in which case only the empirical parts of the cure are performed.

The pains and malfunctionings brought on by bad air are cured empirically by inhalations, massages, cupping, or poultices, and magically by placing a piece of crystallized sulphur on the afflicted part so that the bad air will pass into it. If the sulphur falls apart, the cure has been effective.

As in Peru, there are popular cures for all the illnesses believed to be due to heat or cold. All of these draw only upon the empirical curing techniques, although they are occasionally accompanied by one or another ritual element.

In both Peru and Chile, there are "secrets of nature," ritual acts, for curing hernia, warts, sties, and ringworm, as well as empirical cures. None of these ailments are ever included within the principal etiological categories of popular medicine.

Acculturation to Modern Medicine. In assessing the influence that modern medicine has exerted on popular medicine, it is evident that the latter has borrowed nothing from the former in the way of etiologies. Everyone has heard of *microbios*, germs, but no one explains illness in terms of the germ theory of disease. On the other hand, the adherents of popular medicine have accepted a great deal from modern curing practices. Popular medicine provides no techniques for major surgery, so doctors are resorted to for all cases of major surgical intervention. The use of injections has become common and widely diffused among the people of Peru and Chile. Anyone with a little experience in administering injections is thought to be qualified. Drugstore preparations and patent medicines are also very popular with the people, while sulfa and penicillin are enthusiastically accepted as wonder-working drugs. However, it is important to note that these modern remedies are utilized mostly for the illnesses whose etiologies fall within the categories of gastrointestinal obstruction and heat or cold. Moreover, the modern cures have not replaced popular remedies but have simply been added to the popular repertory. They are regarded as alternative cures, not necessarily as better ones, and are used along with household remedies.

In all the communities studied, the people maintain an evident dichotomy between popular and modern medicine. The dichotomy is made most explicitly between those illnesses that must be treated by *remedios caseros,* household remedies, and those that may also be treated by *remedios del medico,* the doctor's remedies. It is believed that the doctor's remedies are ineffectual for certain illnesses or may actually aggravate them because the doctor does not "know" these illnesses or does not "believe" in them. The illnesses said to be amenable only to popular curing techniques are those which fall within the etiological categories of severe emotional upset, ritual uncleanness, and bad air, the illnesses with syndromes peculiar to popular medicine. In Peru, e.g., fright, *chucaque, colerina, celos,* evil eye, *pujo,* and bad air are always cited as illnesses the doctors cannot cure. It is interesting to note that the only two illnesses within these etiological categories whose syndromes do not vary significantly from those of modern medicine, namely jaundice and "heart trouble," are said to be curable by either household or doctor's remedies. Illnesses due to gastrointestinal obstruction or heat or cold are usually cited as curable by household or doctor's remedies, or both, but one or another of these is occasionally classified as an illness the doctor does not "know."

The explicit delimitation of the domain of popular medicine by the people is in part a defensive reaction to their acculturation experience. The illnesses placed in this domain and defined as inaccessible to the ministrations of modern medicine represent precisely those popular medical beliefs that have been ignored or attacked most consistently by the representatives of modern medicine with whom the people have come in contact, beliefs which the former in no case have taken seriously. The etiological patterns of emotional stress, ritual uncleanness, and bad air, and the syndromes they are believed to produce comprise the core of the fundamental assumptions on which popular medicine is based. They are definitions of a cultural and psychological reality, peculiar to Mestizo thinking, in which the proponents of modern medicine do not share. So long as modern medicine denies this reality the Mestizo has no choice but to reaffirm his own beliefs by denying the doctor's competence to pass judgment on them. Given the Mestizo's fundamental assumptions, these core patterns have a functional value for which modern medicine can provide no equivalent even if the Mestizo were to relinquish them. They may be symbolic expressions of tensions and conflicts to which the Mestizo is subjected in the various roles he enacts in his society, or culturally patterned mechanisms for escape from such tensions.[16] Consequently, they cannot be eliminated or even modified simply by ignoring their existence, or by labeling them erroneous.

There is an evident functional division between these core patterns and those patterns related to the etiological categories of gastrointestinal obstruction and heat and cold. The latter, like the former, provide explanations of disease which have no parallel among those of modern medicine, but the syndromes of the illnesses they are said to cause are for the most part in accord with those that prevail in modern medicine. Moreover, the popular curing techniques considered appropriate for these illnesses includes no wholly magical cures and utilize very little magic at all. The etiological categories of gastrointestinal obstruction and heat and cold may be regarded as performing a residual role. The categories of emotional stress, ritual uncleanness, and bad air provide specific causes for specific illnesses, while the other two major categories provide generalized causes to account for all the other illnesses the people recognize but cannot explain in terms of the core concepts. From the point of view of modern medicine, gastrointestinal obstruction and heat and cold are no more acceptable as explanations for disease than are the core categories, but their generalized nature, as well as the fact that they are employed for syndromes recognized by modern medicine, syndromes that define illnesses for which the latter also offers cures, makes it possible for the people to find equivalents in modern medicine for this residual area that are not available for the core area. Thus, although popular medicine offers etiologies and cures for most of the illnesses recognized by modern medicine, these are defined as also within the competence of modern medicine, while the illnesses explained by the core categories are only within the competence of popular medicine. The functional division described here has been the basis for the people's dichotomy between popular and modern medicine, and their experience in acculturating to modern medicine has provided the occasion for making the dichotomy explicit and for sharpening it.

This dichotomy should not be taken at its face value, however, as determining the circumstances under which the people will seek the services of the doctor and modern medicine. Popular medicine offers cures for all the illnesses believed to be amenable to the doctor's treatment as well, and in many cases priority is given to home therapy and the folk specialist, while the doctor is consulted only as a last resort. More important, however, is the fact that the illnesses classified in the popular domain as outside the competence of the doctor have syndromes broad and diffuse enough to conceal and assimilate a wide variety of "modern" illnesses that have high incidences in Peru and Chile. Public health nurses cited a number of cases encountered in home visiting where people suffering from severe respiratory and gastrointestinal ailments had diagnosed their illness as fright or bad air. To take one example, emaciation, weakness, anemia, fever, and sweats are common to nearly all forms of tuberculosis, and this is a syndrome that bears marked resemblance to that of fright. Since the doctor does not "know" fright, his remedies are considered ineffectual and even dangerous, and where tuberculosis masquerades as fright he has no access to the case.

In general, the core illnesses are still thoroughly believed in even by those who have become skeptical of, or have given up, other aspects of popular beliefs and practices as "superstition." However, although no complete modern cures have been accepted for these illnesses, popular curing techniques have not been entirely immune to modern influence in that drugstore preparations have penetrated, in the form of "waters" and "spirits," as elements of even the most esoteric cures practiced in popular medicine.[17] Beyond the core patterns, the people manifest a dominant tendency to utilize modern therapeutic techniques as readily as popular ones once they have demonstrated their pragmatic value. The usual pattern is to take the modern cure along with its popular counterpart, regarding it as an additional measure for insuring a successful outcome to the treatment. In both Peru and Chile, interviewing revealed dependence on popular remedies in many families who also had splendid records of attendance at the local health center. The writer encountered a number of cases of mothers simultaneously administering home remedies and those prescribed by a health-center doctor for children ill with diarrhea. In one case in Chile, a woman who had enthusiastically supported the local health center since its inception and had volunteered her services for many center projects turned out to be a specialist in curing core illnesses and one of the best informants on popular curing techniques in general.

For reasons that should by now be evident, the doctor is not the most effective innovator in promoting the acceptance of modern medical practices by the people. However, attitudes toward doctors are commonly ambivalent, characterized on the one hand by skepticism, suspicion, and even hostility, and on the other by the grudging admission that doctors may be competent in curing a variety of illnesses. The increasing prestige accorded doctors is manifested in a tendency to buttress popular beliefs and practices by giving them the doctor's sanction. For example, it is said that doctors have taken to prescribing home remedies because they are so effective, and that various popular remedies are effctive because the "doctor says so." Apparently more effective as an innovator of modern medicine is the druggist, whose role as a practitioner of medicine epitomizes whatever rapproachement has occurred between popular and modern medicine. In both Peru and Chile, many druggists have built up substantial practices as curers of a wide variety of illnesses, including a few considered within the special domain of popular medicine such as *empacho, pujo,* and bad air. The druggists are usually thoroughly familiar with popular beliefs, and instead of attacking them, accord them the supposed sanction of modern medicine. The druggists utilize both popular and modern remedies in curing, and their prestige is enhanced by their professional status as representatives of modern medicine. The most popular druggist in Valparaiso manufactures patent medicines and herb teas for every conceivable kind of illness which are sold not only to the local population but to the country at large on a mail-order basis.

Summary and Conclusion. This analysis of the patterns developed by Mestizos to cope with the problems posed by health and illness has revealed a vigorously functioning set of popular beliefs and practices for explaining and treating illness rather than the mental vacuum commonly assumed to exist by those dedicated to dissemination of modern medical practices among the people of Peru and Chile. Where the innovators have encountered medical beliefs and practices among the people, they have retreated from the vacuum assumption to another which labels these beliefs and practices as "magical superstition," and have conceived their task to be one of eradicating the superstition by "rational" education. Magic far from dominates popular medicine, however, and such a point of view reduces the issue to one of "magic versus science." The fundamental assumptions upon which popular medicine is based, as expressed in its etiological conceptions, are mainly naturalistic rather than supernaturalistic, while therapy may be either magical or empirical in nature. For those illnesses where magic is utilized at all, the dominant pattern is one of regarding magical and empirical techniques as alternative ways of curing an illness. Either magical or empirical knowledge may be resorted to with equal facility, or if one is unsuccessful the other may be employed, but they represent separate cures, not complements of the same cure. Mestizos can of course distinguish between magical and empirical knowledge, and know when they are applying one or the other, but many magical cures stand alone, as functional equivalents of empirical cures, and include no empirical elements.[18] Since magic is rarely indispensable for curing illness, it can hardly be said that the conflict between popular and modern medicine is one of a supernatural versus a natural world view, or of magic versus science. Whatever resistance to modern medicine has occurred has been due not so much to any incompatibility, from the Mestizo's point of view, between magical and empirical knowledge as to incompatibility between the differing empirical beliefs regarding the causation of disease characteristic of popular medicine on the one hand and modern medicine on the other.[19] In this connection, it may be pointed out that modern medicine has exerted least influence on popular etiological conceptions, which are mainly empirical, and most influence on therapeutic techniques, where magic is most prominent. The core etiological conceptions of popular medicine, and the illnesses attributed to them, present the greatest differences from modern medicine, and these differences have been enhanced by the negative or disparaging attitudes displayed by representatives of modern medicine. Other etiological conceptions are residual, and explain illnesses whose syndromes do not vary significantly from those of modern medicine, so that acceptance has not been nearly so limited in this area. Borrowing from modern medicine has been consistent with the old pattern of juxtaposition and interchangeability of magical and empirical cures in that modern cures have simply been added to the popular repertory as another means of coping with illness and have not supplanted it. That modern cures have supplemented rather than replaced their popular counterparts is in large part due to the persistence of the old etiological concepts. If illnesses are "really" caused by gastrointestinal obstruction and heat or cold rather than germs, the old remedies lose none of their value despite the acceptance of the new ones.

Since the adherents of modern medicine do not admit the reality of the core illnesses of popular medicine, it might be argued that no serious limitations are imposed by popular medicine on the acceptance of modern medicine. According to their point of view, all the "real" illnesses would fall into the residual categories, where acceptance has been greatest. However, the people are far from according priority to modern over popular cures for these illnesses, and the tendency to diagnose many of the "real" illnesses as core illnesses presents another serious limitation. Moreover, the acceptance of modern therapy must of necessity be piecemeal rather than integral due to orientation to popular etiological concepts rather than the germ theory of disease.

The present analysis points to the conclusion that attempts to introduce modern curing practices will have a higher probability of success than attempts to modify basic causal concepts, at least in those cultures which have patterned the theory and practice of medicine in ways similar to those described here.[20] It is apparent that the people have considered their own theories of disease more useful and adequate than the one advanced by modern medicine, but at the same time they have been willing to accept modern remedies as still another means of curing illness, once they have demonstrated their pragmatic value. The conclusion advanced here may seem discouraging to public health people, who are formally dedicated to preventive rather than curative medicine, but it is certainly a consideration that must be taken into account in the planning of action programs for "underdeveloped" countries. On the encouraging side, it has been shown that popular orientations are mainly empirical, and therefore do not necessarily channel selection of means into the magical sphere. The fact that acceptance of modern medicine is largely governed by pragmatic considerations certainly provides a more substantial wedge for the introduction of change than would be the case if magical orientations were dominant. Moreover, the present fundamental assumptions of popular medicine are themselves not immutable. If medical personnel were to concede the possibility of the reality defined by popular core beliefs, and went ahead to treat for the actual malady involved, substantial strides might be made in gaining the confidence of the people with regard to the core illnesses. This would eventually lead to the breakdown of the popular-modern dichotomy and subsequent modification of the basic etiological conceptions.

References

1. The author is indebted to William Caudill, Charles Erasmus, and Lyle Saunders for reading the original manuscript, and to Grete Mostny for assistance in collecting the Chilean field data. The data on which this paper is based were obtained in the course of field surveys made by the writer in 1951 and 1952 of public health programs for the Institute of Inter-American Affairs in selected communities of Peru and Chile where the Institute operates health centers. In Peru, the communities surveyed were the Rimac district

of Lima and the seaport town of Chimbote, population about 15,000, on the north coast. In Chile, Valparaiso, the principal seaport, and Temuco, a southern city of about 50,000, were the survey sites. The material was obtained mainly through interviews with people in the low and middle income brackets, representative of population groups served by the health centers. The writer has also drawn upon the data collected in an extended field study of Lunahuaná, a community of about 10,000 on the south coast of Peru. The groups studied are all of Mestizo culture. All field work was done as field representative, from 1950 to 1952, of the Smithsonian Institution's Institute of Social Anthropology. More complete treatment of the material dealt with here may be found in the writer's two unpublished manuscripts, "A Survey of Aspects of Health Center Activities in Lima and Chimbote in Relation to Local Populations" and "A Survey of Aspects of Health Center Activities in Valparaiso and Temuco, Chile," on file with the Institute of Social Anthropology, Smithsonian Institution, Washington, D.C.

2. On the distinctions made in this paragraph, see Talcott Parsons, *The Social System* (Glencoe, Ill., 1951), pp. 326 ff.

3. Applied science, however, is not always free of such competition. Modern medical practice contains a number of pseudo-scientific elements. See Parsons, *The Social System,* pp. 466 ff.

4. Talcott Parsons, *The Structure of Social Action* (Glencoe, Ill., 1949), esp. pp. 432–433; Parsons, *The Social System,* pp. 468–469; George C. Homans, *The Human Group* (London, 1951), pp. 321 ff.; Evon Z. Vogt, "Water Witching: An Interpretation of a Ritual Pattern in a Rural American Community," *The Scientific Monthly,* LXXV (1952), 175–186.

5. Bronislaw Malinowski, *Coral Gardens and Their Magic* (New York, 1935), I, 435–451; *The Dynamics of Culture Change* (New Haven, 1945), pp. 48–49.

6. This statement is meant to apply only to Peru, since the writer's research in Chile was limited to the study of medical beliefs and practices. Investigation of other aspects of Chilean Mestizo culture may reveal a similar pattern.

7. This theory of disease has not been confined to nonliterate cultures, however. In *Human Society* (New York, 1949), pp. 572–573, Kingsley Davis states that it is also characteristic of ancient Egyptian, Babylonian, Jewish, and Greek cultures, in which modern medicine had its beginnings. Parsons, *The Social System,* p. 432, cites the examples of traditional China and our own Middle Ages.

8. A. I. Hallowell, "Some Psychological Characteristics of the Northeastern Indians," *Man in Northeastern America,* ed. Frederick Johnson, Papers of the Peabody Fdn. for Archeology (Andover,

Mass., 1946), pp. 195–225; E. E. Evans-Pritchard, *Witchcraft, Oracles and Magic Among the Azande* (London, 1937), p. 479; Robert Redfield, *The Folk Culture of Yucatan* (Chicago, 1941), pp. 308–309; Charles Wagley, *The Social and Religious Life of a Guatemalan Village*, Memoris of the American Anthropological Assn., LXXI (1949), p. 76; Bernard Mishkin, "The Contemporary Quechua," *Handbook of South American Indians*, ed. J. H. Steward, Bureau of American Ethnology, Bull. 143 (Washington, 1946), II, 469; Harry Tschopik, Jr., "The Aymara," *Handbook of South American Indians*, ed. J. H. Steward, Bureau of American Ethnology, Bull. 143 (Washington, 1946) II, 568; Tschopik, *The Aymara of Chucuito, Peru*, Anthropological Papers of the American Museum of Natural History (New York, 1951), XLIV, 301.

9. Illness is not always a direct retribution by the benign spirits. In some cases failure to keep on good terms with benign spirits is punished by withdrawal of their protection, thus permitting the malevolent spirits to send illness, and the latter may sometimes cause illness regardless of the state of grace of the individual either through being called upon by a sorcerer or through sheer caprice. See Mishkin, "The Contemporary Quechua," p. 465.

10. It should perhaps be noted that modern medical practice is a good concern in Peru and Chile, comparable to that in our own culture, and that this represents the "official" definition of medicine in both these countries. The popular medicine of folk origin that is the subject of this paper is descredited by "official" sources, and its practice by folk curers, the *curanderos*, is outlawed. Nevertheless, as will be seen, popular medicine has a vigorous and more or less self-sufficient life of its own.

11. In his discussion of popular medicine in the Peruvian community of Moche, Gillin attaches a great deal of importance to the role of witchcraft in explaining and curing illness (John Gillin, *Moche: A Peruvian Coastal Community*, Publications of the Institute of Social Anthropology, Smithsonian Institution, III [Washington, 1947]). Although varying degrees of preoccupation with witchcraft were manifested by informants in both the Peruvian and Chilean communities, it was never advanced as an etiology for the illnesses discussed here, or as a curing technique. Data collected on witchcraft indicate that it performs a residual role in that it is considered as a possible explanation for mental and physical disorders whose syndromes do not square with those known to the people. No one offered witchcraft as an etiology for any specific illness either peculiar to popular medicine or shared by the latter with modern medicine. There is evidence to show that the role attributed to witchcraft has

considerable regional and local variations in Peru. In Lunahuaná, e.g., witchcraft plays no significant role in connection with any aspect of the culture. In any event, if further investigation in the other communities were to disclose that witchcraft is deserving of greater consideration in connection with illness than is granted it here, this would not necessarily require modification of the writer's interpretation of popular medicine. Since popular etiological conceptions account for all illness without resorting to witchcraft as a necessary source, the latter could at best serve only as an alternative explanation, functionally equivalent to the patterns of etiology described here.

12. For parallels in Mexico and Guatemala for this and other beliefs described here, see Redfield, *The Folk Culture of Yucatan;* Ralph L. Beals, *Cheran: A Sierra Tarascan Village,* Publications of the Institute of Social Anthropology, Smithsonian Institution, II (Washington, 1946); Charles Wisdom, *The Chorti Indians of Guatemala* (Chicago, 1940); Wisdom, "The Supernatural World and Curing," *Heritage of Conquest,* ed. Sol Tax (Glencoe, Ill., 1952), pp. 119–141; and Richard N. Adams, "Un analisis de las enfermedades y sus curaciones en una poblacion indigena de Guatemala," Instituto de Nutricion de Centro America and Panama (Guatemala, 1951, dittoed). For Peru, see Gillin, *Moche;* Tschopik, "The Aymara;" and Hermilio Valdizan and Angel Maldonado, *La medicina popular peruana,* 3 Vols. (Lima, 1922).

13. This term and others that are not translated have no English equivalents.

14. This phrase is borrowed from Wisdom, "The Supernatural World and Curing," p. 131, who uses it to refer to an etiological concept in Middle America similar to the one described here.

15. Cf. Gillin, *Moche,* reference footnote 63, p. 138.

16. In a subsequent paper, the writer plans to analyze the functional interrelations between the childhood illnesses of fright, evil eye, and especially *celos,* child training patterns, and sibling rivalry in the Mestizo community of Lunahuaná.

17. See the description of fright in Gillin, *Moche,* p. 132.

18. As noted above, the magical cures for some illnesses, e.g., fright and *chucaque,* are always accompanied by infusions or massages, but these are regarded as minor elements in the cure.

19. It should perhaps be made clear that there are factors other than those given prominence in this paper that may have importance in determining the reception accorded modern medicine. The writer has focused on the limitations imposed by the cultural orientations of the recipient group, but equally important as limiting factors.

where action programs are attempting to introduce change in medical beliefs and practices, are the orientations and objectives of the acculturating agents, and the nature and degree of interaction between members of the recipient culture and acculturating agents. These aspects have hardly been touched upon here, but research by the writer, as yet unpublished, indicates that they may have strategic bearing on the reception accorded modern medicine.

20. William Caudill arrives at a similar conclusion on the basis of findings contained in forthcoming studies by John Whiting and Irvin Child, and by Francis L. K. Hsu (William Caudill, "Applied Anthropology in Medicine," *Anthropology Today*, ed. A. L. Kroeber [Chicago, 1953], pp. 771–806).

13

The Hot-Cold Syndrome and Symbolic Balance in Mexican and Spanish-American Folk Medicine

Richard L. Currier

Richard L. Currier, Ph.D., is Professor of Anthropology, University of California, Berkeley. His article "The Hot-Cold Syndrome and Symbolic Balance in Mexican and Spanish-American Folk Medicine" is reprinted with the permission of the author and of the Department of Anthropology, University of Pittsburgh from Ethnology, an International Journal of Cultural and Social Anthropology, *Vol. 5, No. 3 (July, 1966), pp. 251–263.*

In contemporary Mexico (and Spanish America as well), one important aspect of folk medical belief and practice is a simplified form of Greek humoral pathology, which was elaborated in the Arab world, brought to Spain as scientific medicine during the period of Moslem domination, and transmitted to America at the time of the Conquest (Foster 1953: 202–204). According to this classical pathology, the basic functions of the body were regulated by four bodily fluids or "humors," each of which was characterized by a combination of heat or cold with wetness or dryness (blood—hot and wet; yellow bile—hot and dry; phlegm—cold and wet; black bile—cold and dry). Proper balance of these humors was considered necessary for good health, and any imbalance resulted in illness. Curing of disease consisted of correcting such imbalances by the addition or subtraction of heat, cold, dryness, or wetness (Taylor 1963: 15).

In Latin America today, most foods, beverages, herbs, and medicines (and some other substances as well) are classified as "hot" (*caliente*) or "cold" (*fresco* or *frío*). This classification is usually independent of such observable characteristics as form, color, texture, and physical temperature, and it is descriptive only of the effects which a substance is thought to have upon the human body. As in classical humoral pathology, illness is often attributed to imbalance between heat and cold in the body, and curing is likewise accomplished by the restoration of proper balance. On the other hand, there is no corresponding classification of substances as "wet" or "dry," nor do the concepts of wetness and dryness appear in folk medicial belief and practice. Why has the hot-cold syndrome persisted for centuries as the basis of folk medical beliefs, while the wet-dry syndrome, equally important in classical theory, has long since been lost? The following functional hypothesis is offered as an explanation of this phenomenon.

In the process of weaning, the Mexican child is subjected to a prolonged period of acute rejection. As a result of this experience he forms strong subconscious associations between warmth and acceptance or intimacy on the one hand and between cold and rejection or withdrawal, on the other. In adult life these associations appear in those beliefs intimately concerned with the problem of personal security: theories about nourishment and about the prevention and cure of disease and injury. On a conscious level, then, the hot-cold syndrome is a basic principle of human physiology, and it functions as a logical system for dealing with the problems of disorder and disease. On a subconscious level, however, the hot-cold syndrome is a model of social relations. In this case, disease theory constitutes a symbolic system upon which social anxieties are projected, and it functions as a means of symbolically manipulating social relationships which are too difficult and too dangerous to manipulate on a conscious level in the real social universe. In this latter sense the hot-cold syndrome is the kind of secondary institution which Kardiner (1945: 39) called a projective system. Finally, the nature of Mexican peasant society is such that each individual must continuously attempt to achieve a balance between two opposing social forces: the tendency toward intimacy and that toward withdrawal. I propose, therefore, that the individual's continuous preoccupation with achieving a balance between "heat" and "cold" is a way of reenacting, in symbolic terms, a fundamental activity in social relations.

Unless otherwise indicated, the data on Mexican folk medicine presented in this paper was gathered in Erongarícuaro, Michoacán, during the summers of 1963 and 1964.[1]. Erongarícuaro is a peasant village on the southwestern shores of Lake Pátzcuaro in the Central Mexican Highlands; it has a population of about 3,000. Although it is surrounded by several smaller villages in which Tarascan is still the principal language spoken, Erongarícuaro is a mestizo village. All my informants were Spanish-speaking Mexican peasants.

The Hot-Cold Syndrome as Medical Belief

The hot-cold syndrome in Latin America has been reported for Mexico (Beals 1946; Foster 1948; Lewis 1960; Redfield 1934), for Mexican-American communities (Saunders 1954; Clark 1959; McFeeley 1949; Rubel 1960), for the Guatemalan Highlands (Gillin 1951; Adams 1952), for coastal Colombia (Reichel-Dolmatoff 1958; Velasquez 1957), for the Colombian Highlands (Reichel-Dolmatoff 1961), and for coastal Peru and coastal Chile (Simmons 1955). It appears in a discussion of Inca medical practices at the time of the Spanish Conquest (D'Harcourt 1939). A more thorough investigation would doubtless reveal its presence elsewhere, but for the purposes of this paper the above references suffice to establish that the syndrome is widespread among the Latin-American peasantry. That, in addition, it often forms the basic theoretical foundation of indigenous folk medicine is illustrated by the following sample quotations:

> [T]here is one important concept which enters into the ideas
> of disease and its treatment . . . [and] constitutes a sort of
> physiological principle of the folk. This concept is the dis-
> tinction between things "cold" and things "hot" (Redfield
> 1934: 161).

> A strict observation of the rules imposed by these categories
> of "cold" and "hot" is imperative in the treatment of all
> illnesses (Reichel-Dolmatoff 1958: 236; my translation) .

> The single common thread that runs through all popular
> medicine is the distinction between "hot" and "cold" (Sim-
> mons 1955; 61) .

Any cultural institution which survives with such vitality for
so many centuries can hardly be a relic, stubbornly but use-
lessly buried in the matrix of a traditional culture. The concept of hot and cold qualities in Latin-American folk medicine
must have functional significance in peasant culture, or it
would have suffered the same fate as its counterpart, the
concept of wet and dry qualities.

Although to the casual observer the hot-cold syndrome is
most conspicuous in the classification of foodstuffs, several
facts point to the conclusion that it derives its ultimate importance from the problem of disease and injury. First, its
historical roots are in medicine, not in the culinary or agricultural arts. Second, the "temperature" (henceforth I will use
the Mexican term *calidad,* literally "quality") of a foodstuff
is relevant only to its effect on the human body, and then only
because it might have an adverse effect on health. Third, the
qualities of heat and cold play an important role in numerous
situations that have nothing whatever to do with food (for
example, it is considered dangerous to expose oneself to the
night air when one's body is warm) . Fourth, the only way of
determining the *calidad* of a food or other substance is by
observing the effect it has on an illness known to be hot or
cold. Finally, there is relatively little agreement as to which
foods are hot and which are cold, not only between one
geographical area and another but even among the members

of a single community. In a study of Mexicans living in the
United States, McFeeley (1949: 41–53) prepared a list of
plants and foodstuffs and asked several informants to identify
the *calidad* of each. Of the first 52 items which more than one
informant identified, the informants agreed on the *calidad* of
25 and disagreed on 27. Foster (1948: 51), Saunders (1954:
147), and Lewis (1960: 12), each reporting from a different
Mexican community, found substantial disagreement among
the members of each community as to the *calidad* of various
items. This evidence suggests that what is important is only
that foodstuffs be assigned a *calidad,* and that, ultimately, it
makes little difference which particular substances are classified
as hot and which as cold.

Although these qualities affect the body only through the
agency of the substances in which they reside, the people blame
the damage on the qualities themselves and not on the substances involved. If, for instance, a person eats green peaches
and develops stomach cramps, he does not complain that
"those green peaches made me sick" but that "the cold of the
peaches has gotten me in the stomach."

Some of the illnesses believed in Erongarícuaro to be caused
by cold entering the body are listed below:

Chest cramp. Cold air enters the chest when a person is overheated.
Earache. A cold draft of air enters the ear canal.
Headache. The coolness of mist or of the night air, called
aigre (a localism corrupted from Spanish *aire,* "air"),
penetrates the head.
Paralysis. A part of the body is "struck" by *aigre.* Stiffness,
considered a partial, temporary paralysis, is ascribed to
the same cause.
Pain due to sprains. Such "cold pains" are the result of cold
entering the damaged part.
Stomach cramp. When the body is warm, and not adequately
covered, cold can enter from the air or from a body of
water.
Rheumatism. Cold from some outside source lodges in the
afflicted bones.

Teething. The pain of teething is a "cold pain," originating in the coldness of the white new teeth that are growing in.

Tuberculosis. Cold enters the body from water or carbonated beverages, especially when the body is overheated from work or travel.

The following are some of the illnesses believed to be caused by an over-abundance of heat in the body:

Algodoncillo. Heat rises from the center of the body to the mouth, causing the gums, tongue, and lips to turn white.

Disipela. Overexposure to the sun can cause the sun's heat to collect in the skin, resulting in an outbreak of red spots on the hands, arms, or less commonly the feet.

Dysentery. Since it is accompanied by bloody stool, and since blood is intensely hot, dysentery is classed as a hot disease, and may be caused by consuming too much hot food.

Sore eyes. A person may overstrain his eyes, causing them to "work hard" and thus to heat up, or, alternatively, cold wet feet can cause the body heat to rise to the head, overheating the eyes.

Fogazo. Heat rising from the center of the body causes the mouth and tongue to break out in tiny red spots. In contrast to *algodoncillo,* this is not a serious disease.

Kidney ailments. Any pain in the kidneys is a hot pain; most kidney ailments are accompanied by itching feet or ankles, a reddening of the palms of the hands, and fever.

Postemilla. An abscessed tooth results from heat concentrating in the root of the tooth, evidenced by the fact that when the abscess bursts it releases blood.

Sore throat. Wet feet cause sore throat by driving the body heat up into the throat.

Warts and rashes. Whatever their cause (a subject upon whilch my informants refused to speculate) , these ailments are the result of heat. This is a conclusion from the fact that warts and rashes are irritating, and irritation is always ascribed to heat and never to cold.

Another group of illnesses may be caused by either heat or cold. In other words, each has a hot and a cold form, to which, of course, different remedies must be applied. The following are examples:

Diarrhea. Diarrhea is usually cold—caused by "cold in the stomach"—but it may also be hot. In the former case the feces are merely loose; in the latter they are green, and steam when fresh.

Enteritis. A case of diarrhea, if not checked, may develop into a case of *torzón* or enteritis, a more serious ailment. *Torzón* may be of either the hot or the cold variety, and these types are again distinguished by the appearance of the feces—hot if these are streaked with blood, cold if they are white and covered with mucous (the cold-wet humor of classical theory).

Toothache. Pain in the molar teeth are hot, caused by improper diet. Those in other teeth are usually cold, in which case they are allegedly caused by a draft of air.

Cold maladies are principally phenomena of disablement, in which sensory and motor functions of the body are disrupted or entirely stopped. In almost every case the illness is caused by the intrusion of a quantity of coldness into a part of the body; in many cases this intrusion is made possible by the fact that the body, or a particular part of it, is more than usually warm. To be warm in any excess at all is to be vulnerable to attacks of cold which may come suddenly and unexpectedly, leaving the individual in crippling pain. For this reason, the people of Erongarícuaro are constantly on guard against the threat of cold and are unusually sensitive to the possibility that a given activity will produce warmth and, with it, vulnerability.

Maladies which are the direct result of excessive heat are, in contrast to cold maladies, often generated from within the body itself. Heat which resides in the outside world is never unpredictably threatening; illness caused by overexposure to the sun or overconsumption of hot foods is, in some ways, perfectly predictable and easily avoidable. The most dangerous aspect of the quality of heat is its ability to be displaced upward in the body. Normally, the stomach is the focus of warmth in the body, the head and extremities being relatively cool. When, however, the feet and legs come into excessive contact with coldness, either by being wet or by being too long in contact with the cold ground, body heat withdraws from them and begins to extend upward into the throat and head, destroying the balance of various temperatures within the body and prejudicing the eyes and mouth.

While sensations of pain are usually cold, sensations of irritation are hot. All skin ailments I know of are caused by excess heat on the surfaces of the body. It is thus a general principle of this system of pathology that cold harms the individual by invading his body from without, while heat harms the individual by expanding (or being displaced) from the center of the body outward to its surfaces. Finally, hot illnesses are not only visible but conspicuous to the outside world, taking the form of skin eruptions, fever, coatings, and hoarseness. Cold illnesses, on the other hand, are often not at all visible to the outside world; their principal symptoms are pain and immobility.

Digestive disorders account for virtually all of those illnesses which may be due either to hot or to cold.[2] This makes perfect sense, since inherent in the notion of achieving a balance between hot and cold foods is the premise that an excess of either quality will be damaging. The words for diarrhea, enteritis, and dysentery seem to connote the intensity of an intestinal disorder rather than its specific variety. The fact that these illnesses are defined broadly enough to include hot and cold varieties makes it possible to express the degree of imbalance without having to specify its nature. This implies that both heat and cold must be taken into the body to insure good health.

I will not burden the reader with long lists of foodstuffs and their corresponding *calidades,* at least partly because such information adds little to an understanding of the problem to which this paper is addressed. There are, however, some generalizations which it is possible to make about classification of foodstuffs in Erongarícuaro. Bearing in mind that there is substantial disagreement among villagers as to the exact classification of the available foodstuffs, the following characteristics are generally true.

Cold foods include most fresh vegetables, the ancient Indian staples (maize, beans, and squash), most tropical fruits (including citrus fruits), dairy products, and low-prestige meats such as goat, fish, and chicken. Hot foods include most (but not all) chili peppers, most temperate-zone fruits, goat's milk, cereal grains, high-prestige meats such as beef, water fowl, and mutton, most oils, hard liquor, and aromatic beverages. A given foodstuff is often both hot and cold, depending upon whether and how it is cooked. Examples of foods that can be either hot or cold are beans, rice, wheat, pork, and peaches.

Warm foods are believed to be more easily digested than cold foods. Other things being equal, a person will often identify a food as warm simply because it is easily digested, and vice versa. Villagers explain this fact by pointing out that, since the stomach is warm, all foods must become warm in the body before they can be digested. Warm foods are, therefore, ready to be digested as soon as they reach the stomach. Cold foods, on the other hand, must first be warmed in the stomach, a process requiring more effort on the part of tthat organ. It would seem logical to conclude that if a person ate nothing but warm foods he would have no digestive problems, but, in fact, this is not the case. A partial answer to this paradox is that a diet consisting largely of warm foods will not necessarily make a healthy person sick, whereas a diet consisting largely of cold foods would sicken even the most healthy individual in a few days. Tepoztecans also believe that cold foods are less easily digested than warm foods (Lewis 1960: 12).

The qualities of hot and cold are related to aspects of life other than those of nutrition and disease. It is in these other contexts that the symbolic meanings of warmth and cold are most clearly revealed: cold is associated with threatening aspects of existence, while warmth is associated with reassurance.

The two main sources of cold in Erongarícuaro are air and water, and both are threatening elements. Air can physically enter the human body, causing the same kind of damage as the attacks of cold described above.[3] Night air is especially threatening, and almost every man who ventures outside the house after dark keeps a corner of his blanket or serape pulled up over his nose and mouth, to prevent the night air from entering his body. A virtually identical belief and preoccupation has been described by Simmons (1956: 62) for Peru and Chile. Water is approached with great circumspection, for it is the most intensely cold substance in the natural world. No one will approach the shore of Lake Pátzcuaro, venture out in the rain, or take a bath when his body is warm from working, traveling, eating, or sleeping. Most people will not wash their hands immediately after they have handled physically or qualitatively hot substances. One villager, after having gotten oil of eucalyptus (a "hot" substance) on his hand, lost an entire night's fishing, being convinced that his hand would be paralyzed if he went out on the lake before an entire day had passed. Finally, villagers associate water with death, believing that when a person dies his blood turns to water. Adams (1952: 49) reports that in Guatemala coldness is a more threatening quality than warmth. Rubel (1960: 799, 807) describes the use of a remedy among Mexican-Americans, the toxicity of which is associated with its coldness.

Warmth, on the other hand, is closely associated with some of life's most reassuring activities; the human body is believed to grow warmer during work, digestion, sleep, and travel. Blood is both the primary source of life in the body and the primary agency of warmth. The presence of blood in any of the symptoms of an illness is usually sufficient to identify it as a hot illness. Blood can become weak by becoming watery, but strengthening foods and fresh blood itself (drunk at the slaughtering yard) can usually remedy this condition.[4]

The symbolic significance of heat and cold is most obvious in their effects upon the processes of reproduction and in the role they play in folk theories about the nature of these processes. In this realm, warmth most clearly assumes the symbolic significance of support and affection, while coldness most clearly symbolizes rejection and withdrawal.

In Erongarícuaro, a woman believes herself to be unusually warm during menstruation. For this reason, most women avoid cold foods until menstruation has ceased. Many women will not bathe during menstruation, for fear that they will be harmed by the coldness of the water. In Colombia, Velasquez (1957: 227) reports that menstruating women should eat hot foods in preference to cold ones, and in Yucatán a cold wind is believed to halt menstruation (Redfield 1934: 162).

Notions about fertility are equally bound up with the hot-cold syndrome. Redfield (1934: 161) reports that cold foods are said to cause sterility in Yucatán. In the Valley of Mexico sterile women are thought to have cold bodies, and "bad airs" can sterilize a woman (Madsen 1962: 117). Clark (1959: 170) discovered that Mexican-American women in California attribute barrenness to a "cold womb." In this connection, there is almost complete correspondence between fertility and warmth on the one hand and barrenness and coldness on the other.

A pregnant woman has an unusually warm body during the entire course of her pregnancy. This makes it necessary for her to avoid cold foods, a fact noted also by Velasquez (1957: 228), Gillin (1951: 32), and Madsen (1962: 120–121). People in Erongarícuaro believe that pregnant women should take slow walks and bathe often, in order to dissipate the large amounts of heat which they accumulate in their bodies. If a mother fails to do this, a fatty membrane will form on the baby's back, cementing him to the inside of the womb, with the result that the mother will experience a long and difficult delivery. In a curious way this belief is a small drama, for it symbolizes the mother's experence of relinquishing her child to the world later in life.

Let me now suggest that the intimate association of warmth with the reproductive cycle, fertility, and pregnancy is due to unconscious associations between the idea of warmth on the one hand and the notion of intimacy, epitomized in the relationship between mother and fetus, on the other. The drama can then be interpreted as follows. A mother must periodically slough off the natural feelings of protective intimacy generated by her relationship to her child, because there will come a time when she must give up the child to the world. If she fails to take such precautions, she will be virtually incapable of breaking the strong attachment she has allowed to form, and relinquishing her child will be a far more difficult, dangerous, and traumatic experience.

On the other hand, it is always possible that a pregnant woman will so strongly resent the dangers and difficulties involved in the birth of a child that she will want to reject this new burden on her life. In fact, there are indications (such as the reluctance of many women to nurse their children adequately) that women in Erongarícuaro have strongly ambivalent feelings about their children; they are often both overly possessive of their children and, at the same time, resentful of the burdens which their children impose. For this reason, a pregnant woman is unusually susceptible to the emotionally based illness called *bilis*, a cold disease (normally a person afflicted with *bilis* is immediately wrapped in several layers of blankets) characterized by symptoms of physical and psychological withdrawal. Although in all other cases *bilis* is a dangerous and harmful disease, it is harmless to a pregnant woman herself; instead, the child will be permanently injured and will suffer from chronic headaches throughout his life. Headaches are cold maladies, and they are often attributed to insufficient sleep and, especially, to insufficient nourishment. If we consider cold to be symbolic of withdrawal and rejection, we can easily interpret this kind of *bilis* as the expression of the rejection of the fetus by its mother. Hence there is nothing strange about the fact that an attack of *bilis* harms, not the woman afflicted with it, but rather the child whom she rejected. It is reasonable that such a child should grow up to display symptoms of chronic malnourishment, since the nourishment of a child by its mother is one of the primary human acts of affection and support.

Nursing, one of the most expressive symbols of intimacy and support in human life, is also closely bound up with the qualities of heat and cold. Exposure to cold diminishes the flow of milk, while warmth increases it. On the other hand, too much warmth within the mother may cause the child to become *enlechado*, a condition in which milk curdles inside the child and cannot be digested. Normally a baby will drink no more milk than it can assimilate, but if the mother is especially warm, e.g., from sitting near the fire, the baby will accept all the milk that she can give it and not reject any excess by vomiting. The remedy for this affliction involves treating the baby with cold substances, the purpose of which is to induce it to reject the excess milk.

Women in Erongarícuaro believe that it is dangerous and harmful to continue nursing a child after the onset of the next pregnancy. They say that the mother's milk becomes "weak" and "watery" and will sicken the nursing child. This implies that a woman should nourish only one child at a time, and that when it comes to a choice between a nursing child and a developing infant the former must be rejected in favor of the latter. Hence, as soon as a woman knows herself to be pregnant, she weans her nursing child abruptly and completely. At this point a child is expected to develop a children's disease called *chipil*. Villagers explain that the child is jealous of the unborn sibling and needs a great deal of affection from the other members of the family, who should hug him and sleep with him. *Chipil* is a hot disease, and, since a woman's body is believed to be especially warm during pregnancy, the pregnant mother must not hug him, pick him up, or sleep in the same bed with him. This is, of course, the moment when the child experiences the most traumatic rejection of his life. In the space of a few days he is deprived of a constant source of nourishment, security, and affection. The intimate ties that bound him to his mother have been shattered, and he is forced to turn to a host of poor substitutes in his search for the security he has lost. Mexicans interpret this increased need for affection as a disease of heat excess, and treat it with heat-diminishing remedies.

The Hot-Cold Syndrome as a Projective System

From birth until weaning Mexican babies are in continuous contact with another human body, usually that of the mother. In Erongarícuaro, a baby is usually wrapped up in his mother's *rebozo* (a long, wide shawl worn over the upper body) during most of the day. At night he sleeps in bed next to his mother. Consequently, every Mexican peasant spends the first year or two of his life in close contact with a warm human body, during which time he never experiences physical abandonment, isolation, or lack of warmth. Lewis (1960: 73), Clark (1959: 134), and Redfield (1943: 188–189) have all commented on this fact. Nevertheless, at about the age when he begins to walk the child is both weaned and deprived of all but the most perfunctory physical contact with his mother. He is rarely carried or held, and he no longer sleeps with his mother. Instead, he is left to crawl or walk on the earth floor of the house and yard and must usually sleep on the cold (and often damp) floor of the house, protected only by a layer of reed mats. Undoubtedly one of the most novel experiences of his life is the discovery, after weaning, of the strong sensation of physical cold. To make matters worse, he has had little previous experience in coping with this situation.

The period immediately after weaning is usually characterized by rage, acute depression, and psychological withdrawal on the child's part, and he usually displays severe symptoms of protein malnutrition (no doubt owing to the almost complete absence of milk in his diet). Villagers identify this behavioral syndrome as *chipil*, a disease from which all children are expected to suffer immediately after weaning. Some children display the symptoms of *chipil* for as long as a year before recovering; many never recover, but sicken and die. This is evidence enough that weaning is a traumatic experience of some duration in the lives of the villagers. It is therefore difficult to see how most children could fail to make an intense and indelible association between the unanticipated and concurrent experiences of rejection and deprivation of physical warmth. It is to be expected that such an association be carried into adult life by almost every member of Mexican peasant society; it is further to be expected that this association become institutionalized in cultural mechanisms for the protection and support of the individual in daily life.

Recent work in Latin-American ethnography indicates that peasant life is characterized by lack of social cohesion, by distrust of social bonds, by instability in social relationships, by anxiety over intimacy, and by fear of abandonment (Guiteras-Holmes 1961; Lewis 1960; Paz 1961; Reichel-Dolmatoff 1961). In a series of articles, Foster (1961, 1963, 1964) has emphasized the importance of informal contractual relations between individuals in Mexican peasant society. Since these contracts are easily terminated, and are maintained only with deliberate effort, a number of social forms have arisen which stress social engagement and protect the individual against rejection (Foster 1961: 1186–1187; 1964: 110). Yet at the same time there exists a fear of intimacy, lest it render the individual socially and psychologically vulnerable to those who might use him (Foster 1964: 115). Foster (1963: 1280) notes that individuals hope to avoid social entanglements but that such entanglements are essential to both social and economic security. In such a world the individual survives by virtue of his ability to manipulate his social relationships so that he is rendered neither vulnerable because of over-involvement with others nor insecure because of lack of involvement with others. This encourages the attitude that social relations are means to an end and must be capable of rapid adjustments in strength or, if necessary, of abrupt termination. When all the members of a society are trying to manipulate their social ties in this manner, some people end up as losers while most others live in fear of losing. The two principal ways of losing are (1) being rejected and left without the security of friends and (2) being taken advantage of through too great a commitment to another.

We recall that cold in the outside world poses a threat to individual well-being as a result of its ability to pass through the skin into the body. I submit that in this case cold symbolizes rejection from without. Like rejection, it is an ever-present danger, and, since peasants are especially sensitive to rejection, it may cause great psychological pain to the individual by penetrating his psychological defenses. Cold is harmless to the individual when directed outward, for rejection directed outward merely reflects the necessary capacity to reject others for one's own benefit.

We may further recall that heat in the outside world poses no such threat, but that heat moving outward from the center of the body to its extremities is harmful. I further submit that this internal heat is a symbol of the need for intimacy, affection, and support, but that when this need becomes so imperative as to show itself in a conspicuous way the individual jeopardizes his position in society. Advances made by others, represented by heat directed toward an individual from outside, do not normally constitute a threat since they can usually be parried or turned to personal advantage. Finally, the increased vulnerability of the body, when warm, to attacks of cold seems symbolic of the increased vulnerability of the individual, when unusually intimate with another, to the misfortune of rejection.

Conclusion

The biological relationship between man and his environment, and the threat of disease (which is a part of that environment), are reflected in a set of beliefs which also functions as a model of the individual's relationship to his social environment. This model serves as a symbolic system onto which social anxieties can be projected and within which social desires can be fulfilled. In other words, while it may be difficult or impossible, for example, to protect oneself against social rejection, it is usually easy and possible to protect onself against the "cold" forces in one's diet or environment. In Erongarícuaro, as in most of peasant Mexico, one of the primary needs which society generates in the individual is the need for balance in his social relations. Lacking the luck, initiative, intelligence, or wealth to achieve this, an individual is still free to seek a balance in the world of nature, where it is always easier to find. Burgess and Dean (1962: 68), speaking of food habits in general, make the following observation:

> Other ways of attempting to deal with the internal stress of threats to life or to emotional security are to overestimate external dangers, or to attribute internal threats almost entirely to external influences of various kinds; and, with this, to attempt magically to evade or appease an apparently external threat, or to balance one type of threat against another. *The practice of giving "heating" or "cooling" foods in particular kinds of clinical conditions may be a form of this kind of balancing technique for evading what are regarded as threatening influences—not of a nutritional kind* (emphasis mine).

We make a similar association in English when we identify a "warm" person as affectionate and intimate and a "cold" person as distant and withdrawn. Is it possible that this association is similarly a manifestation in adult life of associations we made as children, though in a manner less traumatic and less emotionally intense? The researches of clinical psychologists may some day provide an answer.

Finally, I do not wish to imply that the hot-cold syndrome can have no other meanings in Mexican peasant culture than the particular symbolic ones to which I have referred in this paper. Like any symbolic system, its use can easily be extended to other aspects of human existence, in which it may acquire additional symbolic significance. I do feel, however, that its primary importance is along the lines I have indicated, and

272 THE CROSS-CULTURAL APPROACH TO HEALTH BEHAVIOR

that its ultimate origin is to be found in the unique combination of the historical background, the child-rearing practices, and the social relationships characteristic of Latin American culture in general and of Mexican peasant culture in particular.

Notes

1. I undertook field work during the summer of 1963 as research assistant to Professor George M. Foster, who supported the work from the Research Committee of the University of California at Berkeley and by the National Science Foundation (Grant No. G7064). Field work during the summer of 1964 was supported by the National Institutes of Health (Training Grant GM-1229). I would like gratefully to acknowledge my debt to Susan K. Currier, who assisted me in both the original field research and the preparation of this paper, and to Professor Foster, without whose advice, encouragement, and support this paper would never have been written. I wish also to thank the Instituto National de Anthropología e Historia of Mexico, and its Director, Dr. Eusebio Dávalos Hurtado, for permission to do ethnological field work in Mexico.

2. Dysentery, which I have listed as a hot illness, may more properly belong to the hot-or-cold category. A "cold dysentery" is recognized in Mexico (Madsen 1962: 106), but I did not encounter it in Erongarícuaro.

3. In fact, there is good reason to believe that villagers do not clearly distinguish between air and coldness. The word for the kind of cold which enters one's body is *aigre,* and some substances are *aigrios,* rather than *fríos* or *frescos.* This word is sometimes used interchangeably with the word *frío,* and it is also used interchangeably with standard Spanish *aire,* "air". Reichel-Dolmatoff (1961: 283) reports that in Colombia " 'winds' are always associated with 'cold,' and often the two terms are interchangeable." Foster (personal communication) points out that *aigre* is, in fact, a corruption of the word *aire.*

4. Also associated with the notion that blood and heat are sources of life is the concept of bodily strength, which is thought to depend primarily on the quantity of blood in a person's body. Foremost among strengthening foods is beef, which is hotter than almost any other food. Adams (1955: 446) found that the Guatemalan Indians conceive of blood as a non-renewable source of strength and life,

and look upon the loss of blood as a permanently debilitating experience. My own experience in Erongarícuaro confirms the widespread existence of this belief in Michoacán.

Bibliography

Adams, R. N. 1952. Un análisis de las creencias y prácticas médicas en un pueblo indígena de Guatemala. Publicaciones Especiales del Instituto Indigenista Nacional 17: 1–105. Guatemala.
———. 1955. A Nutritional Research Program in Guatemala. Health, Culture, and Community, ed. B. D. Paul, pp. 435–458. New York.
Beals, R. L. 1946. Cherán: A Sierra Tarascan Village. Publications of the Institute of Social Anthropology, Smithsonian Institution 2: 1–225.
Burgess A., and R. F. A. Dean. 1962. Malnutrition and Food Habits. London.
Clark, M. 1959. Health in the Mexican-American Culture. Berkeley and Los Angeles.
D'Harcourt, R. 1939. La médecine dans l'ancien Pérou. Paris.
Foster, G. M. 1948. Empire's Children: The People of Tzintzuntzan. Publications of the Institute of Social Anthropology, Smithsonian Institution 6: 1–297.
———. 1953. Relationships Between Spanish and Spanish-American Folk Medicine. Journal of American Folklore 66: 201–217.
———. 1961. The Dyadic Contract: A Model for the Social Structure of a Mexican Peasant Village. American Anthropologist 63: 1172–1192.
———. 1963. The Dyadic Contract in Tzintzuntzan, II: Patron-Client Relationship. American Anthropologist 65: 1280–1294.
———. 1964. Speech Forms and Perception of Social Distance in a Spanish-speaking Mexican Village. Southwestern Journal of Anthropology 20: 107–122.
Guiteras-Holmes, C. 1961. Perils of the Soul: The World View of a Tzotzil Indian. Glencoe.
Kardiner, A. 1945. The Psychological Frontiers of Society. New York.
Lewis, O. 1960. Tepoztlan: Village in Mexico. New York.
Madsen, C. 1962. A Study of Change in Mexican Folk Medicine. M. A. thesis, University of California at Berkeley.
McFreeley, F. 1949. Some Aspects of Folk Curing in the American Southwest. M. A. thesis, University of California at Berkeley.
Paz, O. 1961. The Labyrinth of Solitude: Life and Thought in Mexico. Transl. L. Kemp. New York.

Redfield, R. 1934. Chan Kom: A Maya Village. Washington.

Reichel-Dolmatoff, G., and A. Reichel-Dolmatoff. 1958. Nivel de salud y medicina popular en una aldea mestiza colombiana. Revista Colombiana de Antropología 7: 199–249.

———. 1961. The People of Aritama: The Cultural Personality of a Colombian Mestizo Village. Chicago.

Rubel, A. J. 1960. Concepts of Disease in Mexican-American Culture. American Anthropologist 62: 795–814.

Simmons, O. 1956. Popular and Modern Medicine in Mestizo Communities of Coastal Peru and Chile. Journal of American Folklore 68: 57–71.

Taylor, H. O. 1963. Greek Biology and Medicine. New York.

Saunders, L. 1954. Cultural Difference and Medical Care. New York.

Velasquez, R. 1957. La medicina popular en la costa colombiana del Pacífico. Revista Colombiana de Antropología 6: 193–241.

Part IV

PACIFIC ISLANDS

Introduction

Anthropology asserts that certain factors—natural selection, isolation, social selection, etc.—influence human differentiation and, inevitably, the culture of various populations. The ethnological evidence revealed by the following research indicates that the religious factor, though thoroughly integrated with other aspects of culture, is a definite deterrent to the evolution of culture in these Pacific island territories; yet, the islanders' cultural belief in the inherent capacity of supernatural beings has certain positive and vital effect on the islanders' total well-being.

Spiro's findings reveal that belief in *alus* has certain "vital and crucial consequences for optimal psychological and social function of the Ifaluk population." In these restricted island territories the malevolent beings (*alus*) were reported to be the harbingers of most unexplained phenomena, including all types of illness and disease. Belief in and constant pursuit of these beings provide an outlet (means of expression) for aggressive drives.

Similarly, Lieban found the dangerous *ingkantos* concept to be an important agent of social equilibrium and control in the community of Sibulan, a municipality on the island of Negros in the Philippine Bisayan islands.

Lieban states in

The individual who sees and interacts with an ingkanto can, through fantasy, bring temptation within reach, or succumb to it. However, such experiences are considered haz-

277

ardous and often are thought to lead to illness or death. This pattern of thought and behavior associated with beliefs about inkantos and their influence appears to support social equilibrium in the community by dramatizing and reinforcing the idea that it is dangerous to covet alluring, but basically unattainable, wealth and power outside the barrios. In this way, the value of accepting the limitations of barrio life and one's part in it is emphasized. Furthermore, if someone has a relationship with a dazzling ingkanto and becomes ill, it is the mananambal, a symbol of barrio service and self-sufficiency, who restores the victim to health and reality.[1]

1. Richard W. Lieban, "The Dangerous Ingkantos: Illness and Social Control in a Philippine Community," American Anthropologist, 64, No. 2 (1962), 306.

14

Ghosts, Ifaluk, and Teleological Functionalism

by Melford E. Spiro

Melford E. Spiro, Ph.D., is Professor of Anthropology, Chicago University. Previously, he was Professor of Washington University, (Seattle). He has been recipient of a National Science Foundation Resident Grant, (1961–62); Resident Fellow in Anthropology, Social Science Research Institute, University of Hawaii, (1967–68); and National Institute of Health Resident Grant, (1968–71). *His publications include* Kibbutz: Venture in Utopia, *Harvard, 1955;* Children of Kibbutz: A Study in Child Training and Personality, *Harvard, 1956; and* Burmese Supernaturalism *Prentice Hall, 1967.* (Editor) Context and Meaning in Cultural Anthropology, *New York Free Press, 1965.* "Ghosts, Ifaluk, and Teleological Funtionalism" *is reproduced by permission of the author and of the American Anthropological Association from* American Anthropologist, Vol. 54, (Oct.–Dec., 1952), pp. 497–503.

Ifaluk,[1] a small atoll in the Central Carolines (Micronesia), is inhabited by about 250 people, whose culture, with minor exceptions, reveals very few indications of acculturation.[2] The subsistence economy consists of fishing and horticulture, the former being men's work and the latter, women's. Politically, the society is governed by five hereditary chiefs, who are far from "chiefly," however, in their external characteristics. Descent is matrilineal and residence is matrilocal. Though clans and lineages are important social groups, the extended family is the basic unit for both economic and socialization functions. This culture is particularly notable for its ethic of nonaggres-

sion, and its emphasis on helpfulness, sharing, and cooperation.[3]

Ifaluk religion asserts the existence of two kinds of supernatural beings, or *alus:* high gods and ghosts. The former,
though important, do not play as significant a role in the
daily lives of the people as the latter. Ghosts are of two varieties—benevolent and malevolent. Benevolent ghosts (*alu-
sisalup*) are the immortal souls of the benevolent dead, while
malevolent ghosts (*alusengau*) are the souls of the malevolent
dead. One's character in the next world is thus not a reward
or punishment for activity in this one, but rather a persistence
in time and space of one's mortal character.

Malevolent ghosts delight in causing evil. They are not only
ultimately responsible for all immoral behavior, but, more
importantly, for illness which they cause by indiscriminately
possessing any member of their lineage. Benevolent ghosts attempt to help the people, and with their assistance the shaman
may exorcise the malevolent spirits. These malevolent ghosts
are the most feared and hated objects in Ifaluk by persons of
all ages and both sexes. This fear and hatred, found on both
a conscious and unconscious level, is attested to by abundant
evidence, derived from linguistics, overt behavior, conscious
verbal attitudes, projective tests, and dreams.[4] As a consequence, most Ifaluk ceremonial life is concerned with these
alusengau, and much of their nonceremonial life is preoccupied with them.

We must now ask ourselves, what are the functions of the
belief in the *alus* in Ifaluk?[5] On a manifest level this belief is
both functional and dysfunctional, providing for both individual and group a consistent theory of disease. In the absence
of scientific medicine, this function is not to be lightly dis-
missed. The two areas of life over which the Ifaluk have no
technological control are illness and typhoons, and the belief
in *alus* serves to restrict the area of uncertainty. For it affords
not only an explanation for illness, but also techniques for its
control, minimizing the anxieties arising from intellectual be-

wilderment in the fact of crucial life crises, and the feeling of impotence to deal with them.

Furthermore, the belief serves to explain another problem—the existence of evil and defective people. Native psychological theory has it that man is born "good" and "normal." In the absence of the concept of the *alus*, the people would be hard put to explain such phenomena as aggression and abnormality, for it also serves to explain these inexplicable and potentially dangerous phenomena. All abnormalities—in which the Ifaluk include violations of the ethic of nonaggression, as well as what we would label mental subnormality, neurosis, and psychosis—are termed *malebush*, and are explained by possession by an *alus*.[6] The manifest functions of this belief, however, seem to be outbalanced by its obvious dysfunctions. The *alus* cause worry, fear, and anxiety, as well as sickness and death; and by causing the death of individuals they can, potentially, destroy the entire society. From the point of view of the people, it would be better if there were no *alus*.

We are thus presented with a difficult question: Why does such a manifestly dysfunctional belief continue to survive? To answer this question we must turn to other aspects of Ifaluk culture. This culture, we have observed, is characterized by a strong sanction against aggression. No display of aggression is permitted in interpersonal relationships; and in fact, no aggression is displayed at all. The people could not remember one instance of antisocial behavior, aside from the *malebush*, nor were any examples of it observed in the course of this investigation. To this striking fact another, equally striking, may be added: namely, that the absence of overt aggression in interpersonal relationships is found in persons who may be characterized as having a substantial amount of aggressive drive.[7] But aggressive drives, like other imperious drives, demand expression; if they are not permitted expression they are deflected from their original goal and are either inverted or displaced.[8] Some Ifaluk aggression is inverted; but that all aggression should be turned inward is impossible, assuming even the lowest possible level of psychological functioning. For if this were the case, we would have to predict the probable disintegration of personality, if not the destruction of the organism. This has not happened in Ifaluk, because the Ifaluk have a socially acceptable channel for the expression of aggression—the *alus*.

The *alus*, as already observed, are feared and hated; and this hatred is expressed in conversation, dreams, and fantasies as well as in overt behavior patterns of public exorcism, ritual and ceremony, whose purpose is to drive off the *alus* and to destroy them. Thus, though the intrinsically hated qualities of the *alus* are sufficient to arouse aggressive responses, the belief in their existence allows the individuals to displace his other aggressions onto the *alus*, since all the hatred and hostility which is denied expression in interpersonal relationship can be directed against these evil ghosts. As Dollard, following Lasswell, has put it, in any instance of direct aggression, "there is always some displaced aggression accompanying it, and adding additional forces to the rational attack. Justifiable aggressive responses seem to break the way for irrational and unjustifiable hostilities. . . . The image of the incredibly hostile and amoral out-grouper is built up out of our own real antagonism plus our displaced aggression against him."[9]

Thus, antisocial aggressive drives are channeled into culturally sanctioned, aggressive culture patterns. The possibility for this is important in any society; it is particularly important for the Ifaluk because of their ethic of nonaggression, as well as of the smallness of the land mass which they inhabit. Kluckhohn, for example, points out[10] that belief in witchcraft provides an outlet for Navaho aggression and, as such, serves a crucial function for the Navaho, despite the fact that they have other channels for aggression as well. The Navaho show aggression in interpersonal relationships by quarreling, murder, and violent physical fighting. These avenues are closed to the Ifaluk; indeed, they are inconceivable to them. Furthermore, Kluckhohn points out, the Navaho can "withdraw from unpleasant situations, either physically or emotionally, by drinking. The Ifaluk cannot "withdraw." As Burrows has put it: "The people of Ifaluk are so few (two hundred fifty of them) ; their territory so restricted (about one half square mile of land surrounding a square mile of lagoon); and their lives all forced so much of the time into the same channels by the routine of getting a livelihood, that it would be nearly impossible for any part of them to keep aloof from the rest. So there is next to no segregation. Each individual surely has some face-to-face contact with every other."[11] Nor can they "withdraw" by drinking, since they have no liquor that is genuinely intoxicating.

Given this situation, therefore, as concerns both the physical and cultural reality, there is no way to deal with aggression except to displace it. Hence, a latent psychobiological function of the *alus* is to provide an outlet for Ifaluk aggressions, preventing the turning of all aggression inward, and thus precluding the collapse of Ifaluk personality. That this problem is not unique to Ifaluk, but is found with equal intensity on other tiny atolls, is revealed in Beaglehole's discussion of Puka-Puka. Here, too, we find an ethic of nonaggression in a tiny Pacific atoll, whose culture is similar to that of Ifaluk. And here, too, socially sanctioned channels exist for the expression of aggression, serving the same functions that the *alus* serve in Ifaluk. "Life is such," writes Beaglehole,[12] "that no one may get away from his fellow villagers. Privacy and solitude as we know them are almost nonexistent. Day and night, month in and month out the individual is continuously in contact with others. He cannot get away from them no matter what the provocation. Were it not for certain socially approved ways of expressing otherwise repressed emotions the society would disintegrate under the weight of its own neuroses."

But the Ifaluk must deal with their anxieties, as well as with their aggressions. The Ifaluk experience certain anxieties in childhood which establish a permanent anxiety "set" in the Ifaluk personality.[13] This anxiety is particularly crippling, for it is "free-floating"; that is, its source is unknown or repressed, so that there is no way of coping with it. In this connection, belief in *alus* serves another vital latent function for the individual, since it converts a free-floating anxiety into a culturally sanctioned, real fear. That is, it provides the people with a putative source of their anxiety—the *alus*—at the same time that it provides them with techniques to deal with this fear by the use of time-proven techniques, in the form of ritual, incantations, and herbs, whereby the imputed source of the anxiety may be manipulated and controlled.

Thus we see that the belief in the *alus* has certain consequences for the psychological functioning of the Ifaluk, which though they are unaware of them, are nonetheless vital and crucial for their functioning at an optimum level of psychological adjustment. For the Ifaluk individual, that is, the latent function of the cultural belief in *alus* is to protect him from psychological disorganization. Without this belief—or its *psychological equivalent*[14]—the tensions arising within the individual, as a result of his anxieties and repressed aggressions, could well become unbearable.

But the belief in *alus* has important sociological functions, as well. If there were no *alus* and the people repressed their aggressions, the society, as well as individual personalities, would disintegrate. On this level, then, the consequences for the group follow from the consequences for the individual; if all individuals collapse, it follows that the group collapses. But the probabilities of the repression of all aggression in any society are very small. In all likelihood, the strength of the Ifaluk ethic of nonaggression would be weaker than the strength of the aggressive drives, because of the strength of the tensions created by the latter, so that these drives would seek overt expression.[15] But this is exactly what could not occur in Ifaluk without leading to the disintegration of the entire society. The Ifaluk ethic of nonaggression is a necessary condition for the optimal adaptation of a society inhabiting a minute atoll. The minimal aggression permitted in other societies inhabiting large land masses does not lead to disastrous con-sequences; but here even this minimum cannot be permitted because of the impossibility of isolation. The physical presence of others is a constantly obtruding factor, and the existence of even a modicum of aggression could set up a "chain reaction" which could well get out of control. This fact is recognized by some of the people. Thus, our interpreter told of an in-dividual who had offended others by his unseemly conduct, who had made no attempt to rebuke him. When asked for an explanation of their behavior, it was pointed out that any action on their part would have led to strife, and since "very small this place," other people would become involved, until "by'm-by no more people this place."

Even if the expression of aggression in interpersonal rela-tionships would not lead to the physical destruction of Ifaluk society, it would result in the dissolution of the distinctive aspect of its culture—sharing, cooperation, and kindliness to-ward others. Sharing and cooperation have enabled the Ifaluk to exploit their natural environment to its fullest extent with the technology at their disposal, and to live at peace with one another, in mutual trust and respect. In short, it has given them both physical and psychological security. The breakdown of the Ifaluk ethic of nonaggression, even a minimum of ag-gressive behavior, would destroy this mutual trust. It would create distrust and insecurity and, at the same time, destroy the positive attitudes that make cooperation and sharing pos-sible, which would seriously reduce economic efficiency and psychological security. The disappearance of cooperation, then, would result in a precariously low level of adaptive integration.

With their belief in the *alus,* however, it is possible for the people to turn their aggressions from their fellows and direct them against a common enemy. The common hatred that results not only enables the people to displace most of their aggressions from the in-group to the out-group, but also serves to strengthen the bonds of group solidarity. For all the people may suffer the safe fate—attack by the *alus.* All must defend themselves against this, and all attempt to defend others from it. The resultant solidarity is both expressed and symbolized in the medicine ceremonies, both therapeutic and prophylactic, which are occasions for convening the entire group.

Thus we again see that the belief in *alus* has certain latent consequences of which the people are unaware, but which are vital to the functioning of this society and the preservation of its culture. The absence of this belief, or of some other institution with the same functions, would be disastrous for Ifaluk society, as we know it today.

Having assessed the belief in malevolent ghosts in terms of the total social functioning of one society, it may be instructive to compare this belief with institutions in other societies, which have the same functional importance. Sorcery and witchcraft play the same functional role among the Ojibwa and Navaho, respectively, that ghosts play in Ifaluk. But we can now perceive the superiority of the belief in ghosts over witchcraft and sorcery for the achievement of their common latent end—the release of aggression. For though the latter beliefs serve to deflect some aggressive drives from other members of society onto the sorcerers or witches, they also serve to instigate other aggressive drives. Since witches and sorcerers are members of one's society, and since their identity is usually obscure, one tends to become suspicious, wary in interpersonal relationships, and insecure with one's fellows. Thus, though the belief in witches and sorcerers succeeds in deflecting aggressive drives and contributing to social solidarity, it also increases aggressive drives and decreases social solidarity. Belief in ghosts, however, serves the dual function of both decreasing in-group aggression and increasing group solidarity. It may not be irrelevant to observe in this connection that societies, such as Dobu, Kwoma, Ojibwa, and Navaho, which practice sorcery or witchcraft, are also characterized by individualism and insecurity, whereas Ifaluk is characterized by communalism and mutual trust.[16]

Thus we have observed that the belief in the *alus* is crucial to the psychobiological functioning of the individual, and to the survival of Ifaluk society and its culture. This analysis thus enables us to understand how an apparently irrational belief continues to survive with such tenacity. As Merton points out: "Seemingly irrational social patterns" may be seen to "perform a function for the group, although this function may be quite remote from the avowed purpose of the behavior."[17]

This interpretation of the Ifaluk malevolent ghosts is not meant to imply that no dysfunctions can be attributed to this belief. We have already indicated the important manifest dysfunctions. The latent dysfunctions are equally severe: the belief serves to drain energy from creative enterprise to that of defense against the *alus*; it serves to preclude investigations of alternative disease theories; it channels much economic activity into non-productive channels; finally, though it resolves many anxieties, it creates a very serious one in its own right—the anxiety created by fear of the *alus* itself.

Notes

1. The field work, won which this paper is based, took place in 1947–1948 as part of the Coordinated Investigation of Micronesian Anthropology, sponsored by the Pacific Science Board of the National Research Council.

2. For a description of Ifaluk culture see Burrows and Spiro (in press).

3. For a description and interpretation of this ethic, see Spiro, 1950b.

4. For a summary of this evidence, see Spiro, 1950b.

5. This analysis consitutes partial confirmation of a hypothesis used in the author's field work, a hypothesis derived from Hallowell (1940), that any society must provide certain socially acceptable outlets for the expression of aggression. After completing the first draft of the paper, the author read Kluckhohn's analysis of Navaho witchcraft (Kluckhohn, 1944) and was struck by the remarkable similarity between Kluckhohn's treatment of witchcraft and his own treatment of ghosts. This paper, therefore, is not to be taken as an original theoretical contribution, but as an independent test of a hypothesis.

6. The *malebush*, during our stay in Ifaluk, included one epileptic child, three subnormal children, one deafmute, one agorophobic adult male, and two schizophrenics. In the treatment of these individuals the people act upon the logic of their belief. Since these individuals are not held to be responsible for their behavior, they are treated with kindness and concern, the only limitations to this kindliness being set by the self-preservation of the group. See Spiro, 1950a.

7. The evidence for this statement, derived from religion, mythology, dreams, art, noninstitutionalized behavior patterns, and projective tests, may be found in Spiro, 1950b.

8. Cf., Dollard, *et al.,* 1939.   9. Dollard, 1938, p. 119.

10. 1944.   11. Burrows, 1952, p. 16.

12. Beaglehole, 1937, p. 320.   13. Spiro, 1950b.

14. Belief in *alus* is not the only institution which could serve this vital function. There are a great number of other institutions which could—and in other cultures do—play the same psychological role that belief in malevolent ghosts serves in Ifaluk. This fact is expressed by the concept of "functional equivalence," which states, in the words of Merton, that "just as the same item may have multiple functions, so may the same function be diversely fulfilled by alternative items. Functional needs are . . . taken to be permissive, rather than determinant of specific social structures." (Merton, 1949, p. 25)

15. That the inhibition of aggression is psychologically disturbing not only follows from the theory of frustration, but is borne out in Ifaluk by empirical observation. To give but one example: After working four days in repairing a canoe house, the men witnessed the collapse of the entire structure. This was a severely frustrating experience for the men, but none indicated his feelings by any overt expression. Later in the afternoon, however, one of the chiefs came to visit, saying he wanted to talk because he felt bad and his "head is very full," a phrase meaning inner turmoil.

16. No immediate causal relationship is implied here, but it is not inconceivable that these two kinds of data could exist in a functional relationship.

17. Merton, 1949, p. 64.

Bibliography

Beaglehole, Ernest, 1937, "Emotional Release on a Polynesian Atoll," *Jr. Abn. and Soc. Psych.,* 32:35–47.

Burrows, Edwin G., 1952, "From Value to Ethos on Ifaluk Atoll," *Southwestern Journal of Anthropology,* 8:13–35.

————, and Melford E. Spiro (in press) *An Atoll Culture: Ethnography of Little Disturbed Ifaluk in the Central Carolines,* Behavior Science Studies, vol. 1, Human Relations Area Files, New Haven.

Dollard, John, 1938. "Fear and Hostility in Social Life," *Social Forces,* 17:15–25.

————, and others, 1939, *Frustration and Aggression.* Yale University Press, New Haven.

Hallowell, A. Irving, 1940, "Aggression in Saulteaux Society, *Psychiatry,* 3:395–407.

Kluckhohn, Clyde, 1944, *Navaho Witchcraft,* Papers of the Peabody Museum, XXII, No. 2.

Merton, Robert, 1949, *Social Theory and Social Structure,* The Free Press, Glencoe.

Spiro, Melford, 1950a, "A Psychotic Personality in the South Seas," *Psychiatry,* 13:189–204.

————, 1950b, *The Problem of Aggression in a South Sea Culture,* doctoral dissertation, on file in Northwestern University Library.

Part V

SOUTH EAST ASIA—INDIA AND THE MALAY PENINSULA

Introduction

Investigations in areas of the Far East, as in areas of Latin America, indicate that the health profile reflects a relatively high incidence of disease. The existing profile has been attributed partly to the attitude and practices of the people who consider health as an existing average, rather than an ideal to be sought. Consequently, a certain amount of illness is accepted as inevitable. This primitive philosophy is explored more fully by Opler and Khare in recent articles appearing in *Human Organization*.[1, 2] They record the cultural definition of illness in village India and in so doing explain the *tridosha* theory as a theory of disease causation. Other causes of disease, as reported by Opler and Khare, are (1) lack of harmony with the supernatural, (2) activity of ghosts, and (3) displeasure of deities. These factors are reported to be brought into play by violation of moral, economic or religious codes. Generally, according to Opler and Khare, supernaturalism is reported to have major significance in disease causation and treatment; however, the degree to which supernaturalism functions varies within a group and the extent of variation is based on social hierarchy, the particular disease and the extent of formal education.

1. *Morris E. Opler, "The Cultural Definition of Illness in Village India,"* Human Organization, *Vol. 22, No. 1 (Spring 1963), pp. 32–35.*
2. *R. S. Khare, "Folk Medicine in a North Indian Village",* Human Organization, *Vol. 22, No. 1 (Spring 1963), pp. 36–40.*

In general, the investigations selected here relate to village people of India and Malaysia—people whose way of life has not been greatly affected by technological change. Health practices are shown to be based on sociocultural influences— the religious factor outstanding. Reliance upon traditional folk practices, even in the face of available scientific practices, more often has been the rule rather than the exception. The folk ways of these people are reported to parallel the ethnocentricity in any other part of the world. Illness is explained chiefly in terms of supernatural phenomena; therefore, the treatment methods generally reflect supernatural qualities.

The research which follows clearly explains (1) the prevailing concept of disease among the people and (2) the effect of culture and cultural blocks on health attitudes and practices. Also, supernaturalism is contrasted with the germ theory, thus explaining certain particulars which impede efforts toward disease control by use of scientific techniques. Finally, some implications of technological change for folk and scientific medicines are shown.

The research of Jelliffe illustrates the extent to which sociocultural factors influence maternal and child health practices in village India. Cultural blocks to nutrition, according to Jelliffe, show direct relationship to traditional concepts of: (1) prestige and social class food, (2) hot-cold food, (3) rice-feeding ceremony, (4) social status, and (5) mixed-feeding practices. Though some traditional customs have no harmful effects, Jelliffe feels that a prerequisite to overcoming harmful customs is understanding and appreciation of the local domestic culture.

Gould suggests that the interaction of folk and scientific medicine brought about by technological change caused a system of selective pragmatism to be brought into existence in village India. Folk medical practices were reported to be employed when chronic non-incapacitating diseases were indicated, while modern practices were sought when the illness seemed to be critical, acute or of an incapacitating nature.

Other factors influencing the increased choice of scientific medicine were socio-economic status and formal education. Gould concludes that the presence of scientific methods has caused an updating of practices by the folk curers; therefore, public health officials face an even greater challenge of altering values by finding an approach which incorporates technical and interpersonal skills.

Wolff shows the health and disease concepts held by the Malays to have a religio-magic origin similar to the concepts of the village Indians. However, his account of the interaction of modern and traditional medicines reveals a cultural heritage which is loosely structured. Therefore, Western practices seem to fit more easily into Malayan cultural structure. He suggests that scientific practices are accepted because they create no disharmony in the existing cultural structure.

15

Social Culture and Nutrition
Cultural Blocks and Protein Malnutrition in Early Childhood in Rural West Bengal

D. B. Jelliffe

Derrick B. Jelliffe, M.D., is Director of the Caribbean Food and Nutrition Institute, University of the West Indies, Kingston, Jamaica. He was formerly UNICEF Professor of Child Health at Makerere University College Medical School, Kampala, Uganda. Dr. Jelliffe's extended research has been chiefly in the area of maternal and child health (especially nutrition of the mother and child). He is co-author with Dr. John Bennett, and others, of many articles in this area. Outstanding among his latest publications are "Education for Child Health Workers in Developing Regions," Postgraduate Medical Journal, London, *(February 1962); and (editor)* Child Health in the Tropics, *Edward Arnold, London, 1962. "Social Culture and Nutrition" is reprinted with the permission of the author and of The American Academy of Pediatrics from* Pediatrics, *20, 1957, pp. 128–138.*

During recent years, it has become apparent that the culture pattern of any group in any region of the world exerts a profound influence on all aspects of medicine and public health. This is particularly true in the field of maternal and child health, where what may be loosely termed the "domestic culture pattern"—including methods of child rearing, customs and rites during pregnancy and childbirth, beliefs regarding causation of disease and locally accepted food ideologies—has obvious and clear-cut repercussions.

Equally, it has become evident that any and all domestic culture patterns contain customs which are either beneficial or harmful, scientifically rational or otherwise. The present paper is an attempt to outline some of the harmful attitudes, affecting certain aspects of child feeding, held by some Bengali village peasant mothers. At the same time, in order to avoid giving a biased picture, it must be clearly stated that there are also facets of the local domestic culture pattern in rural West Bengal, which appear to be scientifically superior to those employed in like situations in many Western countries, notably some of the methods of child rearing—including a highly permissive attitude towards toilet training and breast feeding—which appear to be related to the very low incidence of behavior problems.

Syndromes of Protein Malnutrition

In rural West Bengal, as all over India, malnutrition plays a dominant role as a cause of ill-health in early childhood amongst the lower socio-economic groups. In particular, various syndromes are seen—usually between the ages of 9 months and 2 years—which can be considered in relation to protein deficiency in the diet.

VARIANTS OF KWASHIORKOR. The clinical picture observed varies from an occasional child showing the full classical West African syndrome,[1, 2] to an equally occasional case with the excess blubbery subcutaneous fat and markedly dyspigmented hair of the so-called "sugar-baby" kwashiorkor as described from the West Indies.[3] More usually, however, the clinical picture seen in West Bengal falls between these two extremes, as has been described elsewhere.[4] According to current hypotheses all these variants of kwashiorkor can be considered as being due to severe protein deficiency in young children who are receiving some, adequate, or even excessive calories from predominantly carbohydrate foods.

NUTRITIONAL MARAMUS. Children showing this type of syndrome comprise the commonest and most important variety of malnutrition in this age group in rural West Bengal, being seen at least fifty times as commonly as variants of kwashiorkor. Clinically the main features are severe wasting, with a low body weight and markedly diminished subcutaneous fat and muscle tissue. Etiologically, they are considered to be due primarily to total caloric undernutrition—or, put alternatively, to a generally low intake of all nutrients, including protein— so that the starved child is not only unable to grow, but also has to "cannibalize" his own body stores of fat and muscle in order to maintain basal needs. As elsewhere, for example in Jamaica,[3] intermediate cases, which are extremely difficult to classify, are seen whose clinical appearance lies between kwashiorkor and nutritional maramus.

NUTRITIONAL GROWTH FAILURE. Although difficult to define in precise scientific terms, children are often seen suffering from what may clinically be loosely termed "nutritional growth failure," in that there is stunting, dwarfing and a low body weight, although the body proportions are relatively normal, including the subcutaneous fat and the musculature, and there are few or no associated stigmata of malnutrition, such as avitaminoses, edema or changes in the hair. In these children it would seem probable that diets are more or less balanced, but low in all constituents, including proteins, so that, although the body's basal needs can be met, growth is markedly retarded—with the result that a child two years of age may show the body weight expected of a healthy nine-month-old infant.

Site of Investigation

The present account is based on experience gained during the past two years in a child welfare center or clinic in rural West Bengal about thirty miles from the city of Calcutta. The mothers attending with their children form a more or less homogeneous group, comprising poor, illiterate Bengali peasant women, mostly wives of *chassis* (cultivators), of the Hindu religion and coming from several adjacent villages.

Although the clinic has been open for some years and excellent work has been done, it seems likely that more often than not the local domestic culture pattern has not been affected greatly, although it must certainly have been modified in minor respects as a result of contact with the clinic, at least as compared with similar, but more remote, rural areas.

Etiology of Protein Malnutrition

The etiology of protein malnutrition in early childhood has recently been summarized by Gopalan[6] (Table I), and, almost always, as in any part of the tropics, several overlapping factors will be found to be operative in every case. This was certainly so in affected children in the present study. Basically, it soon became apparent that in almost all cases poverty or economic inability to purchase costly protein foods, such as animal milk, was the prime etiologic factor, aften associated with repeated attacks of enteritis and intestinal parasitism.

Experience and inquiry has shown that on top of this basic background, there exists an extremely complicated and important network of customs, practices and beliefs in relation to infant feeding and child rearing, which all too often tend to exacerbate the situation of an already protein-deficient child, and, indeed, may not infrequently act as the trigger mechanism for the child's precipitation into frank malnutrition. The adverse facets of the local domestic culture pattern—presumably included by Gopalan in his classification under the heading "due to ignorance, faulty dietary habits and faulty home budgeting"[6]—are here referred to as "cultural blocks"—that is

TABLE I

ETIOLOGY OF PROTEIN MALNUTRITION IN
YOUNG CHILDREN (AFTER GOPALAN[6])

(I) *Diminished protein intake:*
  (i) *Primary:*
    (a) due to poverty and economic inability to afford.
    (b) due to ignorance, faulty dietary habits, faulty home budgeting.
  (ii) *Secondary:*
    (a) anorexia due to infections.
    (b) anorexia due to psychologic factors.
(II) *Diminished absorption and utilization:*
  due to infective or psychological factors.
(III) *Increased requirements:*
  due to infection or infestation.

aspects of the village domestic culture which tend to interfere with, or block, the application of scientific health methods, in this case of infant feeding with special reference to protein intake.

Infant Feeding Practices

In order to appreciate the picture clearly it is necessary to outline the methods usually employed in feeding infants and young children in villages adjacent to the clinic.

Breast feeding is universal, easily initiated and carried on without effort by almost all village mothers.[5] Feeds are given on demand and breast feeding is usually prolonged, most frequently for two years or so, or up to the next pregnancy. For the first six or seven months, human milk forms the principal, most important and often the only food, being supplemented in some cases by *misri* (village-manufactured sugar) water, a little barley or sago water, and, for those who can afford it, a few ounces of diluted cow's milk, from about the third month on. During this period, it is the rule for babies to grow very well.

The next stage of infant feeding is dependent to a large extent upon the performance of the customary, traditional rice-feeding ceremony, which is universally carried out by Bengali villagers. This is the present-day equivalent of an ancient Hindu rite (*annaprasan*), one of the *Samskaras*,[7] known in Bengali as *mukhe bhat* (rice eating). Unless there are reasons for delay, it is carried out at six months of age for a boy and at seven months for a girl. The full ceremony, which entails quite considerable expense, is a social and family function of great moment. The main feature consists of the feeding of the infant by preferably a maternal uncle or by a grandfather. For the last mentioned, the baby is put on the feeder's lap and very small fragments of boiled rice are

TABLE II—SOME ASPECTS OF CHILD FEEDING IN WEST BENGAL VILLAGE
(*Based on House-to-House Visiting of 123 Children Aged from Birth to 2 Years*)

| Type of Diet | Age Groups (months) | | | | | |
| | 0–6 | | | 7–12 | | |
	Total Group	No. Pos.	Percent Pos.	Total Group	No. Pos.	Percent Pos.
Milk from breast	36	36	100	42	42	100
Cow's milk	36	16	44	42	23	55
Sago and/or barley	36	9	25	42	22	52
Semisolids and/or solids	36	0	0	42	20	48

| Type of Diet | Age Groups (months) | | | | | |
| | 13–18 | | | 19–24 | | |
	Total Group	No. Pos.	Percent Pos.	Total Group	No. Pos.	Percent Pos.
Milk from breast	21	21	100	24	17	71
Cow's milk	21	7	33	24	8	33
Sago and/or barley	21	6	28	24	6	25
Semisolids and/or solids	21	18	85	24	24	100

placed in the mouth mixed consecutively with curries containing a bitter food, a sour food, green vegetables and fish. Finally the infant is given a taste of *paish* (rice-cow's milk mixture). During the ceremony relatives give their blessing and presents.

The significance of *mukhe bhat* appears to be primarily as an initiation into orthodox Hindu society. As regards diet, prior to this ceremony, the infant is not permitted to eat *shokri* ("ritually dangerous") foods, that is, those which traditionally must be prepared by someone of the same or superior caste. The types of foods embraced by this term vary greatly from group to group, and even from family to family. Boiled rice, or foods cooked with or in contact with rice, are universally considered to be *shokri* and most, but not all, of the present group of Bengali mothers also included *dhals* (legumes), fish, eggs, meat and, according to some, onions. The complexity and variation are further emphasized by the fact that some people considered all foods boiled with added salt as *shokri*.

From other points of view, *mukhe bhat* may also be regarded as a method of celebrating the successful passing of the dangerous first half year of life, while it may perhaps represent an ancient understanding that foods other than milk are needed nutritionally at this age and subsequently.[8]

Following *mukhe bhat*, it might be supposed that an increasingly mixed diet, including rice, would be automatically introduced. This is unfortunately not the case, and experience of the general clinic has been confirmed by a small-scale house-to-house survey conducted in nearby villages. Amongst the group investigated, *mukhe bhat* was universally being carried out at six or seven months of age, unless delayed for certain reasons. Nevertheless, it was found that, of forty-two children aged between seven and 12 months, only twenty (48 percent) were receiving foods other than human and cow's milk, and sago or barley (Table II).

The findings of the survey broadly re-emphasize that many young children aged from about six to seven months to well into the second year of life continue to be fed by a probably small output of milk from the breast, a little animal milk, sago and barley, *together with very small quantities* of other foods which are often very slowly and reluctantly introduced into the diet, and will usually include *muri* (home puffed rice), boiled green banana, potato, soft-boiled rice, fish soup etc. (Table II).

Theoretical Sources of Protein

In the present context, that is with reference to the prevention of protein malnutrition between the ages of six to nine months, when the baby is usually adequately catered for by an abundant supply of milk from the breast, and two years of age, when the child should be capable of taking most of the adult diet, it is obviously necessary to consider the theoretical sources of protein available to the Bengali village mother, which could be used for feeding her child.

The most important source of animal protein is fortunately almost always available in the form of the probably small, but materially significant, amount of human milk taken by the child in prolonged lactation. With regard to animal milk, in the adjacent villages, both cow's and goat's milk are available, but unless a lactating animal is owned by the joint family concerned, it is unusual for poorer mothers to be able to afford more than between a *chuttack* (2 ounces) and half a *pao* (4 ounces) daily. In addition, as anywhere in India, *bazar* (local market) milk is a dubious commodity, almost always being diluted and adulterated. Goat's milk is used even more rarely as it is more expensive, possibly in view of certain alleged virtues, as will be noted later. Products of cow's milk, such as curd or Indian yoghourt (*dahi*) and acid buttermilk (*lassi*) are equally difficult for mothers to obtain owing to their relatively high cost, and the same applies to dried, usually skimmed, milk powders which can be bought in small quantities in the markets of nearby towns, but once again are often adulterated by the vendors.

In essence, then, it can be said that the Bengali village mother does appear to appreciate the great value of animal milk in the feeding of young children, but is unable to afford more than a very small and inadequate quantity from whatever source.

Other theoretical sources of animal protein, include fish (from the village ponds, *dobas*) , eggs (both fowl and duck) , meat (including goat, mutton, chicken and beef) and certain pond shellfish, such as *googli* (fresh water mussels) . In almost all cases these are expensive and beyond the reach of the very slender purse of most village mothers, except in small amounts and occasionally; while, as will be realized, many of these items are made unavailable to the child because of various cultural blocks to be discussed later.

In the same way as with the adult Indian peasant, it is clear that a large part of the protein intake will have to be derived from vegetble sources, including especially the various *dhals* (legumes) and rice—the former having a relatively high content of protein, whereas, although the latter only contains some 8 percent, the amount of this foodstuff eaten by the older child and adult accounts for a high percentage of the total protein intake. In addition, the young child's intake of essential amino acids is very much dependent on the introduction of a really mixed, if mainly vegetarian, diet after the sixth month of life.

Cultural Blocks to Protein Intake

In rural West Bengal, protein malnutrition in young children undoubtedly occurs primarily as a result of poverty and economic inability to buy expensive animal protein foods, especially milk, associated in many cases with poor absorption and increased metabolic demands as a result of recurrent enteritis and intestinal parasitism. However, in addition, certain aspects of the local domestic culture pattern, either singly

or in combination, frequently act as "conditioning" or precipitating factors, forming cultural blocks between the child
and the theoretically available sources of protein. The importance of this aspect of malnutrition has been emphasized
by the fact that investigation of forty unselected, consecutive
children in this age group attending the clinic with various
forms of protein malnutrition showed that, while all appeared
to be primarily associated with poverty, at the same time all
the whole group had one, or usually several, cultural blocks
which had interfered still further with the children's pre-
carious protein equilibrium.

The examples quoted below are mainly those which have
been repeatedly found and thus probably have real practical
importance. However, it has not been possible to calculate
precisely how many village mothers were practicing a particular nutritionally disadvantageous custom. This would, indeed, be difficult to achieve on a statistical basis—the women
attending the clinic are a somewhat selected group, being
mainly of the lowest socio-economic strata and, unfortunately,
sometimes do not attend until their children are already sick
or obviously malnourished. Certainly there is great variation
between different groups and families; while even in village
life, the domestic culture pattern is changing spontaneously
under the pressure of modern technology, as exemplified by
better communications, wider circulation of newspapers, the
spread of advertising, and so on.

Delay in Rice-feeding Ceremony

In most instances *mukhe bhat* is carried out uneventfully
at six months of age for male babies and at seven months for
females. Although theoretically other foods not classified as
shokri can be given beforehand, in actual practice mothers
usually rely mainly on milk from the breast, sometimes combined with a very small quantity of cow's milk and sago or
barley. If the ceremony is carried out at the usual time, this
type of infant feeding caused no obvious nutritional difficulty

—the baby of this age probably being better nourished than at any other subsequent stage in the whole of his life.

Obviously if *mukhe bhat* is delayed, it will mean that the motther will be absolutely unwilling to give *shokri* foods—rice, and, according to some, *dhal*, fish, eggs, meat, onion—so that various cultural factors which may retard this function are extremely relevant. Enquiries have shown that the following may sometimes be responsible: inability to afford the necessary financial outlay for the ceremony, illness of the child, lack of an auspicious day or a very propitious day sometime in the near future, or if all the family are not present. For example, one baby born to refugees from East Pakistan had *mukhe bhat* delayed until the grandmother also arrived; while from the point of view of auspicious days, one infant's rice-feeding ceremony was retarded by almost two months because of a forthcoming especially auspicious time during the *Jugernath puja,* a particular religious celebration, held in a nearby town.

In cases when *mukhe bhat* is delayed, it will be necessary to try to persuade mothers to have this performed as soon as possible, while, at the same time, advising the introduction of selected non-*shokri* foods, such as mashed banana—either ripe and raw, or green and boiled, mashed potato and certain rice preparations, such as *muri* (home-puffed rice), which is not regarded as "rice" (*bhat*) and hence is not considered as a *shokri* food.

Failure to Introduce Mixed Feeding in the Second Six Months of Life

After the rice-feeding ceremony has been completed, it might be expected that the infant's diet would be progressively widened to include all the softer and apparently more digestible or masticable items of the adult dietary in increasing quantity and range, presented initially in the form of pastes or gruels. Experience, however, shows this not to be so with the majority of mothers attending the clinic (Table II), and it is this question of introducing a mixed diet in the second six months of life which is one of the two main problems of infant feeding in rural West Bengal, being second only to the shortage and high cost of cow's milk.

Investigation as to why mothers do not introduce foods during this period shows a variety of stated reasons. Often the mother will say that no teeth or too few teeth are present, or that she feels that the baby will not be able to digest the foods offered and will get diarrhea, or that the abdomen will swell up. While these appear to be the mothers' main beliefs, it also seems likely that the actual additional trouble of feeding the infant with other than fluids—such as milk, sago and barley gruels—may sometimes cause her to be reluctant to make the attempt.

In a probably very small proportion of more orthodox village mothers, a more subtle cultural deterrent may sometimes be operative, based on the "cleanness" or "uncleanness" of the baby's stools. Thus, if the baby is not having *shokri* foods—if, for example, his diet consists of human milk, cow's milk, sago and barley—the stools are "clean" in the ritual sense, being known as *koka pykana* (baby's stool) ; whereas if the child is having *shokri* foods, including especially rice, the stool (*pykana*) becomes "unclean."[9] In the former case, the mother merely has to clean up the baby after he has defecated, while, in the latter instance, she also has to change her *sari,* and, if the bedclothes are at all soiled, she will have to wash *all* the bedding. It seems, therefore, likely that subconsciously this added nuisance may sometimes tend to increase a mother's reluctance to introduce *shokri* foods. Conversely, in case this factor is operative, it may sometimes be well-advised to suggest the use of non-*shokri* foods initially after *mukhe bat,* as, for example, mashed potato and banana. In this context, it is of interest to observe that *muri* (home-puffed rice) , *chira* (a flat rice preparation) and *chana chattu* (toasted Bengal gram flour) are not considered as *shokri*, although both rice and Bengal gram (*Cicer arietinum*), of which these are preparations, are definitely in this category.

It seems likely that the whole problem of apparent resistance to mixed feeding in the second semester of life is more complicated than is at present apparent and certainly deserves much more detailed combined pediatric and socio-anthropologic study. As an infant feeding problem it is certainly outstanding in that it is widespread, lays the basis for much malnutrition—including the syndromes of protein deficiency—most of which present in the second or third years of life, and, in particular, because it is an aspect of infant feeding which should be improvable by means of health education, based on foodstuffs which are already available to the village mother.

Deviation of Cow's Milk

As in many parts of the world, cow's milk may be sold and the money obtained used to purchase less nutrition, mainly carbohydrate foods, etc., the village cow-owner often being unable to afford to use much of the milk for his own family. A particular local form of deviation of milk is seen in some villages of West Bengal, where cow's milk is rapidly curdled with lactic acid to form what is almost pure milk protein or casein (*chhana*) which is freshly prepared daily and transported to Calcutta, where it is used in the preparation of popular Bengali sweets, such as *shondesh* and *fashagola*.

By contrast, there does not appear to be any milk reserved for senior members of the family (as in some parts of Africa); if milk is available, the young child rightly seems to be given considerable preference.

Failure to Use or Produce Certain Foods

FOOD CLASSIFICATIONS. Available foodstuffs in the village appear to be classified in several apparently independent ways. Of these, the following four methods appear to be most important and all are adhered to by the majority of villagers.

(1) *Niramish* (vegetarian) and amish (nonvegetarian) —the latter group comprising fish, eggs, meat and one type of legume (*musuri dhal, Lens esculenta*), while milk and its products are considered as *niramish*.

(2) *Shokri*—as noted previously, *shokri* foods—rice, *dhals*, fish, meat and onions—are those which have to be prepared for an orthodox Hindu by someone of his own or superior caste, as opposed to other foods which can be eaten without such restriction. From the point of view of infant feeding, as observed earlier, these foods cannot be taken until after *mukhe bhat*.

(3) *Garam* (hot) —*tonda* (cold)—this classification is based on alleged, inherent "heating" or "cooling" properties of foodstuffs, and has no connection with either actual temperature or spiciness. Foods which are *garam* to some degree include eggs, meat, milk, *musuri dhal* (*Lens esculenta*), honey, sugar and cod-liver oil; while foods regarded as being to some extent "cold" include fruit juices, *dahi* (curd or Indian yoghourt), *lassi* (acid buttermilk), rice, green *gram* (*kolai dhal. Phaseolus mungo*), water.

As far as can be judged, this classification seems to be scientifically irrational and stems from the humoral theory of Ayurvedic medicine, in which the body is regarded as being composed of three component principles (*doshas*), namely *kapha* (water), *pitta* (heat) and *vayu* (air). It is, however, deeply rooted in the local domestic culture pattern and widely believed by village mothers. As will be mentioned again later, perhaps its main importance lies in the fact that illnesses are also classified as *garam* or *tonda* and "hot" foods must not be given dnuring a like illness, and vice versa. In addition, *garam* foods must not be used in summer and *tonda* foods must be avoided in the cold weather.

(4) *Ponjica* classification—some foods are also classified in the *ponjica* or almanac. Although this is widely followed, and certain foods are forbidden at specific times of the lunar month, this system does not seem to be very nutritionally harm-

ful, as most of the foods detailed are such vegetables as the gourd, the radish and the drumstick (*Moringa oleisera*).[10]

CULTURAL BLOCKS AND SPECIFIC PROTEIN FOODS. The protein foods available to the child will obviously vary with the range eaten by the adults of the family, and this will be modified by the caste, degree of orthodoxy and economic means of that family. For practical purposes, the Bengali villager can be regarded as lacto-pisco-vegetarian, although the amount of milk and fish taken are usually small. The higher the caste and the greater the degree of orthodoxy the less will be the deviation from this baseline. Fish is the most commonly taken non-milk animal protein food, followed by eggs and, after that, meat, in the form of goat or mutton—beef is *never* eaten, being totally prohibited in all strata of Hindu society.

MILK. There appear to be few cultural blocks which are likely to interfere with a young child receiving milk. However, one important local custom is that of overdiluting milk when this is no longer necessary—as when an infant of ten months is having a mixture of half cow's milk and half water. This may quite often be a measure of economy, but is also commonly seen in the well-to-do and is due to a belief that infants are unable to digest undiluted cow's milk, together with the fear—more especially amongst the urban population—that full strength milk is liable to cause "liver," as the much-dreaded Indian childhood cirrhosis is known locally.

An important practice which is sometimes responsible for the onset of kwashiorkor in West Bengal is related to the classification of milk as a *garam* or hot food. All too frequently an infant, who is barely maintaining nutritional balance, develops an infective diarrhea, which is classified as a *garam* illness. Under these circumstances, milk will be stopped completely and the child probably given only barley water thereafter. This regime may be prolonged and sometimes terminates by the infant developing frank kwashiorkor, which has been called "barley-water disease" hereabouts.

One interesting local belief is that goat's milk is more

digestible and useful in children who tend to have loose stools than is cow's milk. The rationale here does not seem clear, unless some children allegedly benefited may have been cases of diarrhea due to allergy to cow's milk. It is perhaps more likely that it is an unconscious "sympathetic magic" type of attitude—the cow's stools being green and watery, whereas those of the goat are hard and solid. In those who can afford it, the choice between goat's milk and cow's milk would appear to be largely immaterial—however, for the poor mother it is a matter of some moment as goat's milk is twice the price of cow's.

One type of present-day change in the local domestic culture pattern, which is well shown by many mothers of the lower socio-economic group in Calcutta city, is the growing tendency to waste money from their slender purses on highly advertised, patented, powdered carbohydrate-milk foods. This is seen as yet to a very limited extent in rural areas, but already one notes this type of product occasionally given to infants by village mothers in almost homeopathic doses, when their money could be much better spent on milk.

FISH. According to Wellin and Muchapiñya, foods may be classified in the minds of men according to different systems—one of which may be related to prestige and social class.[11] Two interesting cultural blocks of this type appear to be of occasional significance with regard to fish in the Bengal village. Two forms of fresh-water fish are available—from the river and from the village ponds (dobas) . The latter are particularly useful as, probably because of their lower oxygen needs, they can be kept in a water-filled dekchi (saucepan) remaining alive for over a week, if the water is changed, and, thereby, acting as a sort of poor man's deep-freeze. Of the pond fish available, the one most preferred for invalids and young children is the singi (saccobranchus fossilis) , and analyses carried out in Bengal have indeed shown this to be an excellent source of protein and to be very low in fat. However, it is expensive and, as an alternative, another type of pond fish known as soal (Opice-

phalus striatus) seems of nearly as good a composition and is about half the price. Attempts to suggest the use of this fish quite frequently meet with lack of enthusiasm, mothers saying that, as well as having a worse flavor and being more difficult to cook, it is "snakelike" and, anyway, a food of lower sorts of people. Similarly, *googli* (fresh water mussels), a minor additional source of protein, are classified as a low-class type of food.

EGGS. Apart from the fact that the more orthodox will not eat eggs at all, it is of great interest to note that chicken's eggs are not readily available in the average village in West Bengal, as the Hindu does not keep fowls, but ducks; whereas with the Muslim villager it is the other way round. The Hindus' failure to keep chickens is perhaps related to these birds' habit of entering village houses and therefore defiling the kitchen which is kept rigidly and ritually "clean" and apart. Another story sometimes heard in explanation is that once, when the Lord Krishna approached the castle of the demon Kongsha for a surprise attack at night, the latter was awakened and warned by the noise of a disturbed flock of chickens—so that since then fowls have not been kept by Hindus.

Of more seriousness is the fact that eggs are regarded as being extremely *garam* or hot; which means that they will not be given during warm weather or if the child is suffering from an illness classified as *garam*.

General Dietary Restriction in Illness

CLASSIFICATION OF ILLNESS. Village mothers in rural West Bengal have their own ideas of the etiology of disease and the following may at different times be thought to be responsible: (1) evil spirits; (2) divine intervention; (3) evil eye (*nazar*); (4) effect of climate (i.e., physical cold or heat).

DIETARY RESTRICTION. While it is difficult to be precise, it seems that in all illnesses—and the village child suffers from an almost uninterrupted procession of them—the mother will tend to restrict the diet and also modify it to suit the *garam-tonda* classification of the particular complaint, as well as employing other forms of treatment according to her ideas as to etiology. As has been observed before, the mother will at best be reluctant to introduce other foods into the young child's diet and, as a result of further dietary restriction applied during a succession of minor illnesses, nutritional marasmus is very likely to develop from resultant chronic or intermittent underfeeding.

Conclusion

The present account is both fragmentary and incomplete, but it is felt that it shows the importance, in the absence of assistance from a trained socio-anthropologist, of making an attempt, however amateurish, to discover the impact of the local domestic culture pattern on whatever aspect of health is under consideration, in this case on the genesis of protein malnutrition in young children.

It is obviously necessary to have as complete an understanding of such local attitudes and practices as possible, both in order to understand and appreciate the mothers' difficulties, and to be able to attempt to overcome harmful customs by means of persuasion, demonstration or modification and integration.[12] Preliminary socio-anthropological surveys of this type will always facilitate the introduction of new public health measures.

Finally, it must be noted that this paper has necessarily been concerned with cultural blocks, or practices which were felt to be harmful with regard to protein nutrition in the young child. It will be realized that equally there are aspects of the local domestic culture which are beneficial in this context in the West Bengal village, as, for example, the practice of prolonged breast feeding.

Summary

Examples of malnutrition related to protein deficiency, including kwashiorkor, nutritional marasmus and "nutritional growth failure," are commonly seen in early childhood in rural West Bengal. While this was mainly due to poverty, and especially the economic inability to buy animal protein foods, together with repeated attacks of enteritis and constant intestinal parasitism, in addition, it was found that certain aspects of the local domestic culture pattern acted as "cultural blocks" between the child and the theoretically available sources of protein. Results of a survey of local methods of infant feeding are summarized and some of the important cultural blocks outlined, including delays in the traditional rice-feeding ceremony, reasons for unwillingness to introduce mixed feedings in the second 6 months of life, failure to use or produce certain foods (with especial relation to the four types of food classification found in the village), general dietary restriction during illness and specific blocks with regard to individual sources of protein. The importance of having health measures based on an understanding of the local domestic culture pattern is emphasized.

Acknowledgments

In a study such as this, it is sometimes difficult for an outsider to perceive the real meaning or purpose of a particular attitude, custom or method, and the author is most grateful to his colleagues at the All-India Institute of Hygiene and Public Health, Calcutta for their advice and constructive criticism, and especially to Doctors J. Deb, Probodh Chandra Sen and Nurgez Sethna.

References

1. Williams, C. D.: Kwashiorkor: A nutritional disease of children associated with a maize diet. Lancet, 2:1151, 1935.

2. Jelliffe, D. B.: Clinical notes on Kwashiorkor in western Nigeria. J. Trop. Med., 56:104, 1953.

3. Jelliffe, D. B., Bras, G., and Stuart, K. L.: Kwashiorkor and marasmus in Jamaican infants. West Indian M. J., 3:43, 1954.

4. Mukherjee, K. L., and Jelliffe, D. B.: Clinical observations on kwashiorkor in Calcutta. J. Trop. Pediat., 1:61, 1955.

5. Jelliffe, D. B.: Breast feeding in technically developing regions, with especial relation to West Bengal. *Courrier,* 6:191, 1956.

6. Gopalan, C.: Kwashiorkor in Uganda and Coonoor. J. Trop. Pediat., 1:206, 1955.

7. The *Samskaras* are ancient *Vedic* rites that mark the transition from one age or period of life to another.

8. This may or may not be so. There is a great tendency for culturally conscious health workers in any part of the world, to apply what may be termed a "golden age" interpretation to all ancient customs. While it seems certain that many of these were indeed empirically based on what are presently understood as scientifically sound principles, many would also appear to be dogmatic and irrational. In addition, it seems equally true that quite often customs beneficial in quite different social settings thousands of years previously may no longer be so today—or, alternatively, may have become so modified that only the husk of the ceremonial is adhered to, without the beneficial substance of the practice being carried out. Nutritionally, the present-day observation of *mukhe bhat* may be a case in point.

9. Among many mothers, this attitude does not prevail and the young child's stool is regarded as "clean" until he is aged about five years irrespective of diet.

10. Dr. Probodh Chandra Sen (personal communication) comments on this classification as follows: "There are elaborate rules prohibiting consumption of various articles of diet on certain days of the lunar month. For example, if (i) *patol* (*Trichosanthas dioica*) is eaten on the third day of the moon, the consumer will have the misfortune of increasing the number of his enemies; (ii) radish on the fourth would mean the loss of wealth; (iii) coconut on the eighth day would make the consumer a dunce; (iv) beans on the eleventh day would lead to sinful acts; (v) gourd and allied vegetables on the thirteenth day might result in the loss of one's son, and so on. The restrictions are minutely recorded in the Hindu calendar and one wonders what could be the reason for such restrictions. They may have been designed as an attempt to assure stable conditions of food supply by regulating the distribution of edible fruits and vegetables."

11. Wellin, E., and Muchapiñya, A. G.: Child-feeding and food ideology in a Peruvian village. Report prepared by the ICA Anthropology project. WHO Mimeographed Document (MH/AS/160.154), 1953.

12. Jelliffe, D. B.: Cultural variation and the practical pediatrician. *J. Pediat.,* 49:661, 1956.

16

Modern Medicine and Folk Cognition in Rural India

by Harold A. Gould

Harold a Gould, Ph.D., is Professor of Anthropology, University of Pittsburgh. He was a National Science Foundation Fellow, Lucknow, India, 1959–60; National Institute of Mental Health Fellow, (1960–62); and an Andrew W. Mellon Fellow, Pittsburgh, 1962–63. His major interests encompass the areas of peasant society, urban society, social organization, and social change in India. He holds membership in several sociocultural organizations, including the Association for Asian Studies and the Royal Anthropological Society of Great Britain and Ireland. His "Modern Medicine and Folk Cognition in Rural India" is reprinted with the permission of the author of The Society for Applied Anthropology from Human Organization, *Vol. 24, No. 3, Fall, 1965, pp. 201–208.*

In an earlier paper dealing with the impact of technological change on the medical practices of some villagers in North India, I conceptualized a distinction between chronic nonincapacitating dysfunctions and critical incapacitating dysfunctions. By chronic nonincapacitating dysfunction were meant,

> conditions manifesting drawn-out periods of suffering, sometimes cyclical in character, usually not fatal (or fatal by slow degrees), and only partially debilitating (enabling the sufferer to maintain a semblance of his daily routine).[1]

Critical incapacitating dysfunctions were marked by

316

the opposite inventory of symptoms: that is, maladies involving sudden and often violent onset, and rather complete debilitation with reference to some aspects of the individual's routine.

Since scientific medicine had proved popular with the villagers only with respect to the critical incapacitating dysfunctions, I concluded that,

a competition between folk and scientific medicine has been occurring in Sherupur [pseudonym for the village studied] through which each has come to serve a distinct class of ailments within a general range of culturally perceived maladies.[2]

The basic insight, then, which led to this way of interpreting the place which scientific medical practices had come to occupy in this peasant community was that victims of illness only turned to doctors of modern medicine when they were desperate and when to their way of thinking the help the doctor could render was demonstrably quicker and/or more effective than indigenous approaches. The other side of this was that for some kinds of illness scientific procedures were either dubiously effective or nonexistent and that in these instances peasants unabashedly used and recognized as superior indigenous, nonscientific therapeutic systems and their underlying conceptualizations. The villagers were, in short, pragmatists who resorted to whatever systems of medicine were available and seemed valuable to them.

Medical Practices and Cognitive Processes

Intervening years have not altered the conviction that at the level of therapeutic practices this dichotomous characteristic of contemporary medicine in Sherupur is a real and viable feature of its social life, nor that a kind of rustic pragmatism is a root mechanism which facilitates such a dichotomy. However, an opportunity to do three additional years of field work in India between 1959 and 1962, some of which time was spent revisiting Sherupur, has helped make it clear that a number of modifications and refinements in my original contribution are necessary.

Perhaps the main deficiency in my original essay was the failure to recognize the important relationship obtaining between medical practices and cognitive orientation. It was indeed true that the people of Sherupur exercised a rustic pragmatism whereby some diseases were more readily treated by scientific than by folk therapies; however, further field work made it equally clear that the acceptance of modern medical help for critical incapacitating dysfunctions involved no concomitant conversion to scientific thoughtways concerning the causation and etiology of diseases. The germ theory was just as much a mystery in Sherupur in 1961 as it had been in 1954 or in the centuries prior to the advent of European rule. When I attempted to explain the germ theory to one of Sherupur's more informed citizens in 1961, I realized that the language itself is so undeveloped in this domain of experience that the task was semantically hopeless. In Hindustani, one could only depict germs as tiny insects, an imagery which certainly failed to convey the reality to a listener who knew no English and was unschooled in any science whatsoever.

The Personal Equation and Therapy

Another factor which received inadequate attention in my initial study was the role which the personal relationship plays in the peasant community. To the peasant, trustworthy relationships are personal relationships between individuals who by virtue of caste, kinship, and community ties share common values and are consequently bound together within a system of mutually enforceable obligations. This is one of the great gaps separating modern medical practitioners in India from their potential peasant clienteles. The former are rarely able, because rarely inclined, to establish the kind of rapport that would win acceptance of *themselves* in the villages; yet without this acceptance there is little hope of gaining much acceptance there of what they represent professionally. What Parsons[3] has called the "functionally specific" relationship, where personal considerations are held in abeyance, remains incomprehensible and, therefore, suspect to a peasant because it is structurally alien to him. Speaking of another north Indian village in this connection, Marriott has said:

> The people of Kishan Garhi thus recognize three great social realms—that of kinship and family, which is an area controlled by limitless demands and mutual trust; that of the village and caste, which is an area in part controlled by particular obligations and formal respect; and that of the outside world, of government and market place, which is an area controllable only by money and power—things which the villager scarcely possesses.[4]

Disease Etiologies and Therapeutic Approach

Still another factor that proved to be important was the complexity of disease etiologies. One may not simply attach a name to a malady and, on this basis, assign it a single place in a neat classificatory scheme. Illnesses strike people who are different from one another both organically and psychologically; they strike persons who are members of particular sociocultural systems, each with its particular cognitive world. The same disease, scientifically defined, may strike an ultraconservative person who rigidly adheres to indigenous medicine at all costs or a liberal-minded person who as uncritically turns to a modern medical practitioner. It may strike a person with a strong constitution, on the one hand, or a person with a weak one, on the other, with the result that it may constitute a chronic nonincapacitating dysfunction to the one and a critical incapacitating dysfunction to the other. A given illness may fall within the ambit of what is defined in a culture as the realm of divine ordination and may, therefore, be singled out for special supernatural treatment. In short, what a disease *is* will be inevitably conditioned by a very complicated set of factors which must be conceptually disentangled as carefully as possible by the observer.

In order to illustrate these and other points, let us turn now to data obtained during my latest visits to Sherupur. Tables 1 and 2 summarize some aspects of therapeutic activities in the village which may serve as a point of departure for the discussion to follow.

Experience made it plain this time that only when allowance was made for my presence in Sherupur could a comprehensive inventory of sickness and medical therapy be compiled. The total amount of time I spent in this community of 750 people was approximately ten months spread at intervals over a three-year period. During these interludes of residence, I myself entered actively into the cognitive world and the action pattern system of the population through the roles I came to play in the treatment of the sick. The tables reveal the consequences of this. Where choices of therapy were made independently, which usually meant when I was absent from the village, the pattern was about the same as was indicated in my earlier article; especially is this the case if we ignore smallpox which, although a critical incapacitating dysfunction, is a special problem, as will be shown later. But where I was a factor in therapeutic-choice situations, a radical departure from the former pattern occurred.

The primary variable accounting for this difference was, of course, the personal relationship per se. The kind of person I was, with the kind of powers and resources at my disposal, became an aspect of the structure of village medicine in Sherupur. Once I had become accepted and trusted in Sherupur, even people suffering from critical incapacitating dysfunctions who sought relief through scientific medical procedures nevertheless preferred to use me as an intermediary between themselves and scientific medicine rather than directly approach its professional practitioners. Part of the reason for this was that

TABLE 1—"Disease Situations" in Relation to Form of Therapy Received by People in Sherupur

Type of Illness	Independently Chosen		Personal Tie with Anthropologist	
	Indigenous Therapy	Scientific Therapy	Accepts Med. from Anthro.	Induced by Anthro. See Doctor
Chronic Nonincapacitating Dysfunctions				
Chronic Asthma	1	—	—	—
Mild Fever, Cough, Cold	8	—	8	—
Old Age Aches and Pains	4	—	1	—
"Weakness" (Ambulatory)	6	—	—	—
Early or Chronic TB	2	—	—	—
Stomach and Bowel Disorder	9	—	6	—
Sprains, Cuts, Bruises	3	—	2	—
Cutaneous Infections	6	—	3	—
Uterine Discharge	1	—	1	—
Anemia	—	—	2	2
	(40)	(—)	(23)	(2)
Critical Incapacitating Dysfunctions				
Asthmatic Complications	—	1	—	—
Severe TB	—	1	—	—
Severe Dysentery	—	—	2	1
Cholera	—	1	—	—
Smallpox	6	—	1	—
Embedded Testicles	—	1	—	—
Ulcerous Cutaneous Infections	—	—	9	—
Severe Sprains, Cuts, Bruises	—	—	2	—
Severe Foreskin Infection	—	—	2	1
Eye Infections	—	—	23	—
Multiple Insect Bites	—	—	1	—
Rheumatic Filaria	—	—	1	1
	(6)	(4)	(41)	(3)
Total	46	4	64	5

TABLE 2—DEGREE OF RESORT TO VARIOUS CATEGORIES OF THERAPY
IN RELATION TO THE DISTINCTION BETWEEN CHRONIC
NONINCAPACITATING AND CRITICAL INCAPACITATING
DYSFUNCTIONS (IN PERCENTAGES)

	Independently Chosen		Personal Tie with Anthropologist	
Type of Illness	Indigenous Therapy	Scientific Therapy	Accepts Med. from Anthro.	Induced by Anthro. See Doctor
Chronic Nonincapacitating Dysfunctions	Percent 62	Percent —	Percent 35	Percent 3
Critical Incapacitating Dysfunctions	11	7	76	6

I was there in Sherupur whereas doctors were at least a mile
and a half distant. But this is only part of the story because,
as my reputation spread, people began coming to me from
other villages that were sometimes closer to a hospital or clinic
than to my residence. It should be noted here that I had received some training as a medic during World War II. This
proved useful not only in coping with certain kinds of illness,
but also in making me aware of the necessity for never attempting to treat any malady personally which I suspected to
be outside my competence. In such instances I would take the
sufferer to a doctor or else consult with a doctor on the person's behalf. Throughout my stay in the community I maintained close working relationships with doctors who were personal friends as well as ones who were associated with various
state and central government health schemes. In short, I tried
to recognize my personal limitations in the field of medicine
and to operate strictly within them. This careful delineation
of the role I was prepared to play in Sherupur seems to have
helped me to quickly gain the villagers' confidence. They knew
what to expect from me, what they could *depend* upon in case
of trouble.

Certainly one of the most striking facts which emerged from the tabulations is that in one-third of all the recorded instances of chronic nonincapacitating dysfunctions, victims accepted medicines from me, an avowed advocate of scientific therapy. This is the most important manifestation of all of the preference for personal relationships. For it is doubtful whether my scientific medicines helped any of these cases any more than did indigenous remedies, and I believe the villagers were themselves fairly well aware of this. Their main reason for approaching me for such maladies was a mixture of the mystical and the honorific. It was their way of saying that they accepted me as an esteemed member of the community, on a par with other esteemed members of the community, who was expected to give aid and comfort in times of crisis; who was expected to provide reassurance through words and deeds because I possessed certain half-understood powers capable of bringing about good results. As Carstairs[5] has pointed out, it is important in village medicine that there be someone at hand who vitally matters, who can proclaim that things will have a favorable outcome. That, in Sherupur, persons like this are indeed valued in the areas of sickness is attested not only by the general results in the tables but also by incidents such as the following, which occurred frequently. After a number of people had received help from me, a woman summoned me and requested that I purchase a glass bangle for her infant daughter and place it myself on the child's wrist. She believed this would ward off illness in the future after I had departed from Sherupur. The diffuse powers I represented in this woman's eyes must be made to linger on after my departure.

What was said previously about problems of disease diagnosis also stands out in the tables. One cannot merely determine that a subject suffers from, say, asthma and then inflexibly conclude that, in terms of treatment, it is a case which can be assigned to the category of chronic nonincapacitating dysfunctions. Asthma may be mild or severe, or it may be mild at times and severe at other times in the same individual.

It may alternate within very circumscribed limits of severity for years and then change its pattern profoundly, as when a heart complication develops. Just such a case as this in Sherupur was Badari, a member of a cultivator and dairying caste known as Ahir. He had served in World War II as a private soldier and afterwards had returned to the village and resumed farming. He developed an asthmatic condition which he treated with indigenous remedies despite the fact that his condition had been diagnosed by an army doctor. For years he continued this therapeutic pattern until eventually complications from an enlarged heart began to seriously incapacitate him. When this happened, Badari went to a doctor for further diagnosis and treatment. Ultimately he died from the heart condition.

From the standpoint of folk cognitive structure, this Ahir had not suffered from one malady, but two. One was a chronic ailment best handled by folk medicine, the other was a critical ailment best handled by scientific medicine as understood by the peasant. Some rather vague continuity was perceived between the two phases of Badari's illness, to be sure; that is, people said that one thing had more or less led to the other. Essentially, however, it was held that there had been two disease situations, each calling for a therapeutic approach that was valid for its appropriate domain. True, the latter of the two therapies had failed, but this was not seen as being a result of the prior failure of the former.

Looking now at the critical incapacitating dysfunctions, it is clear that the most frequent complaints in this category were eye infections and skin diseases involving painful ulceration or scabbing. One reason why I was so often approached for these disorders is that penicillin eye ointment and both penicillin and sulfa-based skin ointments achieved in most cases truly dramatic results, probably due to the fact that the villagers had acquired no prior tolerances for these drugs. Again, however, this must be seen in conjunction with the personal relationship. For, once learning of the power of penicillin and sulfa, they could have easily and cheaply purchased these drugs on their own. But it was important that I be the agent of dispensation; my person was somehow intertwined with the medicines. This was not simply because they could obtain free medicines from me either, because some who could pay willingly did so when I asked them to. In other words, my medicines and I had become integral parts of certain disease situations. In this sense, the acceptance of scientific medicines from me, and from doctors too for that matter, resulted in no material changes in basic folk cognitive structure. These experiences were filtered through the screen of this cognitive system and converted into meanings which did no violence to it. One therefore wonders whether it is correct to say that the villagers accepted modern technology or that they converted modern medical technology into folk medicine. One wonders, furthermore, whether more can be expected as long as the peasant social system survives intact to maintain the fabric of folk culture.

Primitive Medicine in the Folk Setting

Smallpox illustrates the degree to which still essentially primitive cognitive orientations may remain an integral part of the folk orientation to some diseases. Smallpox is quite obviously a critical incapacitating dysfunction in every sense of the word. It is a great killer that is deeply feared by the peasantry. Yet this illness is deemed an entirely religious matter. It is thought that a goddess named Bhagoti Mai (also called Sitala Mai and Sitala Mata) causes smallpox and that the only way to expunge her influence is by performing religious rituals. If an individual household is struck by the disease, a senior member will place an offering of water contained in a clay cup before a *Nīm* tree. One *Nīm* tree is enshrined as the abode of *Bhagoti Mai* in Sherupur but a worshipper may not necessarily place his offering before that particular tree. In individual cases, different *Nīm* trees are

employed which suggests that it is the tree's symbolic importance as a source of curative power (many remedies are prepared from its bark and leaves) that is decisive. If the disease
reaches epidemic proportions, however, a Brahman priest is
engaged to perform more elaborate rituals at the site of the
Bhagoti Mai shrine.

It is almost impossible to get peasants to accept vaccination
to prevent smallpox or to accept any medicines once they have
contracted it. Modern medicines have very little effect, as a
matter of fact, once a person contracts smallpox. Consequently
the modern medical practitioner is not able to counter the
powerful religious aversions to treatment with a powerful cure
of his own. This may help to make smallpox one of the last
serious diseases to be brought under control by public health
programs in India.

A Case of Smallpox in Sherupur

A case in which I was deeply involved will illustrate many of
the problems connected with smallpox and, at the same time,
will afford insight into a number of the other questions that
have been raised throughout this discussion, especially pertaining to cognitive orientation and acceptance of change.

During early 1961, the ten-year-old son of a very poor, illiterate low-caste family with whom I had been close friends for
many years contracted a bad cough. His parents consulted me
and I consulted a doctor in their behalf. It was decided that a
course of sulfa drugs and aspirin would adequately deal with
the condition. It seemed to be only a bad cold. Shortly after
initiating this therapy I left the village for several days. When
I returned friends informed me that Bakara Ram (the boy's
name) had grown gravely ill in my absence and the parents
were extremely worried. The parents, however, had not summoned me upon my return so I rushed at once to their small
dwelling at the edge of Sherupur.

When I reached the place, the door was closed and some

of the other young children of the household were sitting disconsolately about in the front compound. When I asked where the parents were, the children were evasive. Finally, I learned from them that their mother had shut herself up inside the house with Balaka Ram and had left word for me that my assistance was not required. I knocked on the door, however, and when there was no response I pushed it open and entered. Lying on a stringed cot and covered by a blanket I found Balaka Ram and his mother. It was clear that the child was desperately ill. His fever was very high and he was weak and incoherent. His mother, however, kept insisting that everything was all right and that my help was not needed. This agitated me greatly so I went to search for Balaka Ram's father who, I thought, as head of the household would be more reasonable.

It was only after locating Balaka Ram's father that I learned what the trouble was. They believed he was suffering from smallpox and that all one could do under the circumstances was make the boy abstain from eating and perform religious rites. I insisted that a doctor be summoned at once and Balaka Ram's father finally reluctantly agreed, largely because my status and our friendship made it impossible for him flatly to refuse.

By the time I returned with a doctor, the boy's father had been joined by his wife, his two adult sisters and his aged mother. The mother had been abandoned many years ago by her husband and had been the family's head ever since. She was very strong-willed, energetic, aggressive, and outspoken. In the interim this old matriarch had clearly assumed control of her family and was now leading the group that barred the entry of the doctor and me into the house where Balaka Ram lay. The argument that ensued centered around the issue of whether the doctor should be allowed to intervene in an illness that called for religious measures alone. The women became frenzied and shouted and wailed that to permit injections, or even an examination, would further anger Bhagoti Mai and then she would kill Balaka Ram for certain.

After much effort, I convinced the old matriarch and her daughters and daughter-in-law that they could safely permit an examination of Balaka Ram by the doctor provided he promised to administer no medicines of any kind. The doctor made his examination and concluded that this was not a case of smallpox but of pneumonia and bronchitis made worse by the fast which the child had been compelled to endure. But by now the doctor had become extremely truculent over the reception he had received at the hands of people whom he deemed social inferiors and ignorant savages. He had called the grandmother an old hag and had berated the whole family for their blind superstition which prevented them from getting the help required to save this boy's life. After the examination and some further refusal by Balaka Ram's domestic group to accept modern medicine, the doctor departed in anger from Sherupur and vowed to have no further dealings with the case.

Once the doctor had departed, I continued talking to the old woman and the rest of the family. At one point, after Balaka Ram's grandmother repeated her conviction that this was an exclusively supernatural matter, I countered by asking her how she could be so certain that God works only in one narrow way. Here I was quite consciously attempting to awaken in her rustic mind some of the implications of Hindu pantheism. Is it not true, I asked her, that God is to be found in everything and that he acts in many different ways? He lives in the earth, does he not, and in the *Nīm* tree, and in animals, and even in the walls of this house. May he not also live in the doctor and work through his medicines? Could she be sure this might not be so, I asked. Would it not be wise to do the religious rites and then also let the doctor and me help through medicines?

To my amazement, the old woman suddenly burst into tears, knelt down and touched my feet and commenced telling me with great emotion that she was just an ignorant old woman who tried to do her best. She thanked me for what I was trying to do and agreed to let the doctor's medicines be tried. Meanwhile the rituals would be performed. I was delighted, of course, because I knew that Balaka Ram did not have smallpox and would undoubtedly recover now. It seemed to me unimportant whether modern medicine or Bhagoti Mai got the credit so long as the boy survived.

The doctor refused to return to Sherupur, as he had vowed he would never do, but he was willing to perscribe the appropriate medicines, mainly pentid-sulfa tablets, cough medicine, and proper diet. We decided to attempt no hypodermics because of the religious fears concerning them, for it had to be remembered that Balaka Ram's family still believed him to be suffering from smallpox. In time the boy recovered completely and it was doubtless one of the few times, if not the first time, in the history of Sherupur that anyone had accepted modern medical therapy for what was believed to have been a case of smallpox.

Some Observations on the Smallpox Case

In this incident, then, many different things stand out. First, the villagers' conceptualization of the causes and cure of smallpox are firmly rooted in the typical primitive cognitive orientation, where, as Simmons[6] says,

> medical beliefs and practices seem to be well integrated with the religion and morality of the group and play a prominent role among the mechanisms of social control.

Others, similarly rooted, include snake bite, evil eye and bewitchment. Bhagoti Mai strikes because moral transgression has occurred; religious rites and fasting alone can correct this condition. The rituals performed have been assimilated into the corpus of Hinduism, but the cognitive foundations remain aboriginal— *viz*, disease is intermeshed with the supernatural and with social control. Recall that in the direct encounter between scientific and primitive world views which my intervention in Balaka Ram's case engendered, refusal to accept modern medical aid was based upon the belief that Bhagoti Mai would be made angrier and would inflict more severe misfortune on the household. At the same time, this encounter revealed how under ordinary conditions a scrupulous differentiation is made and maintained between the spheres of competence of the various medicines employed in the villages. Violation of these functional boundaries, particularly where the extreme poles of scientific and supernatural world views are brought into direct conflict, can generate severe anxiety and extremely volatile reactions.

Second, the power of the personal relationship has been demonstrated through two of its consequences in this case. On the one hand, its strength was sufficient, where combined with great perseverance and appropriate status, to facilitate partial overriding of the most powerful religious sanctions against the use of scientific medicine. On the other hand, in its absence, the professional relationship exercised by itself proved to be utterly inoperable. The doctor whom I had summoned wished to be accepted on the basis of his professional proclivities alone. In essence, he demanded of these villagers an immediate and uncompromising conversion to the ideologies of modern science and modern social structure with disastrous results for the goals which his professional training had equipped him to achieve. Villagers do not understand or trust the professional relationship because they are not in any meaningful sense members of the culture in which the sanctions and premises underlying such a relationship form integral aspects of the socialization process.

It seems to me that observations of this kind have vast overtones for efforts nowadays being directed at helping and changing the so-called underdeveloped peoples of the world. For one question naturally arises if there is any general validity to what has been said here. How can one design institutions and train personnel able to bring to the peasantry and the aboriginal the innumerable material advantages which flow from modern technology, whose very nature requires the professional type (and here I refer to a whole person and not just a technical skill) , in a manner which enables the agents of this new technology to simultaneously establish the deep personal ties with those to be benefited which they alone trust. At least this is the problem as long as the peasantry persists as a structural phenomenon towards whom the members of the modern world feel they have a mission. At the point where technological change dissolved the peasantry, of course, the problem would no longer have any meaning because then there would be a single world view in which disease and medical therapy enjoyed the same sets of premises among all categories of the population and in which social interaction was keyed to mutually intelligible roles set in compatible social institutions.

A third point is the strength of the pragmatic impulse. The old woman, once her religious resistance had been modified, rather automatically moved to the position that henceforth *both* religious rites *and* scientific medicine would be utilized in dealing with Balaka Ram's illness. There was no notion on her part that one thing must be rejected in behalf of the other. The underlying dictum always seems to be: Try anything that is available and culturally legitimate.

Fourth, we must reiterate that in folk medicine, just as in scientific medicine, there are always problems about correct diagnosis. The canons employed by peasants for identifying illness are not invariably successful even with respect to purely indigenous maladies. With smallpox, villagers believe that the stool reveals by its texture and color the presence of the disease. In Balaka Ram's case, this was the main symptomatological tenet of his kins' adamant refusal to accept the doctor's conclusion that the child was suffering from pneumonia and not smallpox. Linked with their mistaken interpretation of symptoms was the general mood of the community, however. Smallpox was fairly rife in Sherupur at the time and there was no doubt a consequent tendency to believe that any illness whose symptoms remotely resembled those believed to be associated with smallpox was indeed an instance of Bhagoti Mai's wrath. The point is, at any rate, that peasants can be objectively wrong in determinations made about the nature and cause of sickness as defined by their own extranaturalistic and supernaturalistic premises. Partly this is because these premises include no basis for the articulation of critical mechanisms such as ideally, at least, are the essence of the scientific method. But failure of diagnosis also occurs in the domain of folk medicine for a reason that is common to scientific medicine as well, *viz*, the complexity of disease etiologies. Declares Nurge:

> Diseases do not exist as categories which can be identified, named and brought for treatment according to the classification . . . especially to the layman, symptoms are confusing, are interpreted naively, and are subject to frequent reinterpretation. A particular malaise is not quickly and accurately identified by either a villager or anthropologist.[7]

Yet in this very ambiguity inherent in symptomatology may also lie one of the strengths of both folk and primitive medicine. From an objective standpoint, wrong diagnoses are undoubtedly being made constantly in folk and primitive sociocultural settings. Disease classifications ordinarily aid this tendency by their vagueness; they will subsume under the heading of a particular named malady, on the basis of superficially understood symptoms, a multitude of objectively distinct diseases ranging in severity from the easily curable to the incurable. Take the illness called fever (*bookhār*) in Sherupur; it can cover everything from a slight case of flu to pneumonia and worse. You take medicines for fever and it can be pointed out that most people recover after taking the appropriate indigenous medicines. Some die of fever, of course, but the number are few compared to those who recover, which means to the peasant that in most cases the medicine he employs is efficacious. In other words, indigenous medicines have a wide mark to shoot at which virtually guarantees the appearance of success no matter what their chemical composition. It is well known that the same logic operates in the modern world with respect to the sale of remedies for headaches, colds, neuralgia, etc.

Some Action Implications

Conclusions that might be useful for public health workers and programs are difficult to draw because so much remains unknown or at most half-understood about primitive and folk world views when they encounter modern technology and the sociocultural systems that accompany it. One thing seems clear, however. Mechanisms like rustic pragmatism are often valuable as pathways for the acceptance of many modern health *practices*, but transformations in *thoughtways* concerning sickness and debilitation should not be expected to accompany such acceptance readily or indeed, in many instances, ever. This, at least, must be regarded as axiomatic as long as technological change and economic development do not proceed far enough to achieve the *structural elimination* of peasantries and primitives.

The reactions to the incursion of scientific health procedures can be remarkable sometimes at both the general and the specific levels. What Simmons[8] characterizes as "defensive reactions" to modern medical technology are very striking. In essence the more modern medicine becomes entrenched in, say, the domain of critical incapacitating dysfunctions, the more indigenous practitioners stabilize their control over the treatment of chronic non-incapacitating dysfunctions. The latter even adopt the paraphernalia of modern medicine in order to intensify their psychological impact on their patients. There is one in Sherupur who administers many of his indigenous compounds with a hypodermic syringe and his business has boomed since he began doing this. In Simmon's words:

The explicit delimitation of the domain of popular medicine by the people is in part a defensive reaction to their acculturation experience. The illnesses placed in the domain and defined as inaccessible to the ministrations of modern medicine represent precisely those popular medical beliefs that have been ignored or attacked most consistently by the representatives of modern medicine with whom the people have come in contact, beliefs which the former in no case have taken seriously.[9]

The routinized impersonality so intrinsically a component of the professional role probably intensifies this defensive reaction. For it stems as much from fear and misunderstanding of the *persons* who possess professional medical skills as from the content of these skills. Often I found peasants wanting very much to receive modern medical treatment but avoiding doing so because it necessitated their attending an outpatient clinic or being admitted to a hospital. It is hard to describe the aversion the peasants feel to the institutional structures in which modern medicine is presented to them and into which they are compelled to enter if they are to be treated. For them the *social experience* is the crucial variable, the very aspect which from the standpoint of the ideology of modern social interaction is not supposed to be allowed to stand in the way of maintaining good health. But the peasant sees hospitals and clinics as places where he will be compelled to wait endless hours in congested anterooms, castigated and mocked by officious attendants, and finally examined and treated by a doctor who will show no personal interest in him whatsoever. This is the main reason why people in Sherupur preferred to get medicines from me and to be seen by doctors whom I personally brought into the village for the purpose, for here medicine was being integrated into patterns of social interaction which they understood and which did not drain from them every ounce of their self-respect as the price for being benefited by what the modern world has to offer. Carstairs has given a delightful illustration of the difference one's approach to villagers can make:

Another method, adopted in the early years of this century by the chief health officer of Jodhpur State, turned upon a judicious use of showmanship. This doctor, an Irishman and a famous athlete, included in his retinue one of those emaciated beggars, blind and pockmarked, who are still all too common a sight in India. When he came to a village he would summon everyone with his stentorian voice. "Take a look at him," he would bellow, "that is what Mataji [the Goddess of Smallpox] does for you! And now look at this: this is what vaccination does for you!" He would then strip to the waist and display not only his vaccination scars but also his muscular torso. The demonstration was convincing.

In contrast . . . I witnessed a conspicuously less successful technique. The public vaccinator came to pay his annual visit of a few days. He was a supercilious young man from Udaipur city . . . and he regarded villagers as an inferior and stupid lot . . . During his four-day stay . . . the task degenerated into a hunt. I would see a herd of children and young mothers come bolting out of an alleyway with hilarity and panic mingled in their shrieks, while the vaccinator pursued them, brandishing the weapons of his trade.[10]

Rapid modernization of non-modern thoughtways respecting sickness and its treatment is going to require, it seems to me, a series of gradual culture changes that cut both ways. That is, changes must be made in the professional role which reflect awareness of the nature of primitive and peasant cognitive and social structure. Without them efforts to achieve any fundamental shifts by peasants and primitives toward values that the modern world cherishes appear doomed. The challenge is to find ways of creating an institutionalized approach to public health in the underdeveloped societies which incorporates *into a single role* the technical qualifications conferred by professional training and the interpersonal skills needed for dealing with primitives and peasants in their own institutional terms which successful anthropological training confers.

References

1. Harold A. Gould, "The Implications of Technological Change for Folk and Scientific Medicine," *American Anthropologist*, LIX, 507–516.

2. *Ibid.*

3. Talcott Parsons, *The Social System*, The Free Press, Glencoe, Ill., 1952.

4. McKim Marriott, "Western Medicine in a Village of North India," Benjamin Paul (ed.) , *Health, Culture and Community*, Russell Sage Foundation, New York, 1955.

5. G. Morris Carstairs, "Medicine and Faith in Rajasthan" in Benjamin Paul, ed., *Health, Culture and Community*, Russell Sage Foundation, New York, 1955.

6. Ozzie Simmons, "Popular and Modern Medicine in Mestizo Communities of Coastal Peru and Chile" in Dorrian C. Apple (ed.), *Sociological Studies of Health and Sickness*, McGraw-Hill, New York, 1960.

7. Ethel Nurge, "Etiology of Illness in Guinhangdan," *Proceedings of Rip Van Winkle Clinic*, IX, no. 4 (1958), 16–36.

8. Simmons, *op. cit.*

9. *Ibid.*, 81–82.

10. Carstairs, p. 108.

17

Modern Medicine and Traditional Culture: Confrontation on the Malay Peninsula[1]

by Robert J. Wolff

Robert J. Wolff, Ph.D., is Associate Professor, School of Public Health, University of Hawaii. Previously, he was Associate Clinical Professor of Social Psychology, Hooper Foundation Medical Center, San Francisco; Project Psychologist (follow-up study), State Department Public Welfare, Minnesota (1957–61); and Psychologist, Government Suriname, South America (1953–55). His publications include "Population Description," Vox Guanae and "Meaning of Food", Tropical and Geographical Medicine, (1965). His article "Modern Medicine and Traditional Culture" is reprinted with the permission of the author and of The Society for Applied Anthropology from Human Organization, Vol. 24, No. 4, Winter 1965, pp. 339–345.

It has become commonplace to say that the world today is characterized by change. Naturally, people in previous ages have also had to adapt to changed circumstances, but the changes today seem more violent—there are more changes per unit of time.

That is not all, however. Today's changes are not merely technological improvements, they are very basic reorientations.

Some years ago an irate Frenchman coined the term "cocacolanization" to describe the attempt to replace native wines with Coca Cola. The real issue, of course, was not whether the taste of one drink was preferable to the taste of another, but whether one way of life would replace another. As wine is a symbol of a certain way of life, so too is Coca Cola—of a very different kind of life.

Where in France the difference between the old and the new, between *Kultur* and mass culture, were real enough then (and seem to be a problem even now), the differences elsewhere between the traditional way of life and the new were truly staggering. It is no exaggeration to say that the change-over to a new way of life, to new values, to new ideas, is a revolution on a scale perhaps never equalled in the world's history.

Barbara Ward Jackson, in a recent book,[2] lucidly describes this revolution. She points to the sudden and almost universal spread of a number of important *ideas* which are changing the world. The idea that all men are equal or at least should have equal opportunities in education, in business, in development, is revolutionary and new in almost all areas of the world. Or, the idea that we can and should improve our material, physical well-being in this world rather than wait for compensatory improvement in the next, is revolutionary and new in the history of the world. And the idea that science and technology can and should be applied to the solution of immediate problems of this world rather than to the mystical truths of the universe, is new and revolutionary to many ancient cultures.

Medical Services as Agents of Change

Modern medicine has been in the vanguard of this revolution. The application of science to problems of everyday living and health, and the idea that the benefits of modern medicine should be made available to everyone, have been instrumental in causing an unprecedented increase in the number of living human beings in this world, and, often, in improving the health of the people.

It may seem strange to us Westerners, who initiated this revolution (and have made it such an apparent success), that others did not actually *demand* the benefits of modern medicine, or modern economics, or modern political systems. Most people did not ask for change. As colonizers, not so very long ago, we imposed our medical science, as we imposed our kind of economics, and as we imposed our kind of government.

Today, however, the revolution of new ideas, which we originally introduced, has led to the establishment of nations with civil services, medical services, and other manifestations of the modern state. It is these services that now bring the changes in their own nations, with or without assistance from outside. Even though the innovations may be carried out by natives, the ideas behind the technological changes are still foreign importations.

Modern medical practices are being introduced by probably all Medical Services in all developing nations. But modern medicine is not only scientific medicine, as contrasted to traditional medicine, it is above all Western medicine. It is important to consider that there might be a difference between the ease with which the tools and the skills of Western medicine are adopted and accepted, and the difficulty of understanding and accepting the ideas underlying the technology of medicine.

It is relatively easy to accept antibiotics, or modern diagnostic tools, or even modern diets—it is difficult to understand or accept the *ideas* that have resulted in the continuing development of antibiotics, diagnostic tools, or diets. It is difficult to accept for many peoples the idea of causality in health and disease, which we Westerners take for granted because it is so much part of our culture to think in terms of cause and effect; it is difficult for others to understand the idea, which we Westerners now take so much for granted, that we should apply all our scientific efforts to the alleviation of pain and to the prolongation of life; and it is difficult for some, to understand that the benefits of modern medical science should be equally available to all, regardless of social class or social importance.

Malaya and Malay Culture

I should like to present a few of the problems inherent in the introduction of Western medical practice as they are manifest in Malaya.[3] Malaya is perhaps not untypical of the developing countries, although it is considerably wealthier than many such nations. Malaya today is going through a period of change, even revolution, on many fronts. Concerted attempts are being made to lift Malaya from a traditional society to a modern nation. Politically, economically, and medically, new tools and skills are being introduced almost daily.

In some ways, Malaya is also unique perhaps, in that within a relatively small territory a number of populations live side by side, each with its own unique culture, and each with its own standards of material civilization. If one counts the island of Singapore in with the total population of the peninsula, there is no majority: both Malays and Chinese form about 40 percent of the total population. There is a minority of Indians, about 11 percent of the total, and a number of smaller minorities, including what is loosely called aborigines. The Malays dominate the country politically, the Chinese economically. The former consider themselves the original population and think of the Chinese and Indians as guests in their country. Actually, a large proportion of the Malay population has immigrated from Indonesia only one or two generations ago—no accurate figures are available, but it is estimated that in parts of the west coast up to 40 percent of Malays immigrated less than two generations ago. At the same time, there is a sizable group of Chinese in Malaya who can trace their ancestors back several hundred years.

Historically, Malaya has always been a crossroads. There have been waves of migrations passing through Malaya; some of the aborigines are probably descendants of people who moved through Malaya a thousand or more years ago. There have also been cultural invasions. Even today there are very evident remnants of Hindu, Buddhist, Arabic (Muslim), and, of course, Western influences.

The observable differences between Chinese and Malay cultures are great, and they are exaggerated possibly by the fact that almost all city dwellers are Chinese, whereas almost all Malays live in the rural areas. This means, among other things, that the Chinese, being more urbanized, also seem more Western in many ways; the Malays, being more rural, seem more traditional.

The Malays, although they live on the land and use the fruits of the land, do not farm intensively. Only a small proportion of them grow rice commercially, and the rice grown in Malaya is not sufficient for the country's needs—although probably the majority of Malays grow some rice for home consumption. Rice-growing, however, is more a traditional pursuit, a cultural heritage, than a commercial proposition (much as folk dancing might be a cultural heritage to another people). Many Malays own rubber trees, which they either tap themselves or rent out to Chinese. Malays do not grow vegetables, either commercially or for their own consumption. They own fruit trees, but rarely make an attempt to improve yield or otherwise farm more intensively. Despite the fact that the Malays have a long tradition of rural living, their pattern of agriculture seems more like gathering of jungle products than growing.

The Malays appear to live a very leisurely life: they are not poor, although they may not have much ready cash. Their houses are simply built, but generally airy, cool, and comfortable. Their diet is monotonous, but not because they do not have access to more variety in foodstuffs: it is the traditional way of living.

In contrast, the Chinese generally live in crowded quarters, with less comfort, less space. Their way of life seems very unleisurely. Their diet is simple but varied, and probably more adequate nutritionally than the Malay diet. The unit of Chinese society is the family, not the village.

It would be tempting to say that the unit of Malay society is the village, but this would be a simplification distorting reality. It would be more accurate to say that there is no real unit of society among Malays, that possibly the small nuclear family, in a very vague sort of way is their unit of society. What binds Malay society, however, is Malay culture, Malay customs and traditions.

For hundreds of years Malays in this peninsula have been subjected to foreign influences. Long before the invasion of Europeans, there were Indian outposts. Even today the influence of Hindu culture is readily visible: the language contains many words of Sanskrit origin, Malay shadow plays continue to show the stories of the Ramayana, many of the titles and traditions connected with royalty are Indian. Later, other Indians brought Islam, and today Malaya is by constitution an Islamic nation: by law, all Malays are Muslim. Islam plays a predominant role in the daily life of all Malays. But, as any Malay will point out, this is *Malayan* Islam, not Egyptian Islam. What this means is that Islam too is incorporated into the Malay culture.

Perhaps as a consequence of these varied historical influences, Malay culture is a mixture of elements that to an outsider often seem to blend very poorly.

Malays are strict monotheistic Muslims, but at the same time they implicitly believe in a host of spirits, demons, devils and gods, many of them of pre-Hindu origin. Malay society in the villages is strictly egalitarian, or democratic: no man is more than another—and yet, at the same time Malay society in a larger sense is feudal, with various classes of royalty considered almost as castes. To an outsider it seems that this astonishing variety of seemingly contradictory beliefs cannot possibly fit into a meaningful whole. There seems no unity, no strong central idea in this conglomeration. For the Malay this is no problem.

One of the items of furniture sometimes found in a wealthier Malay home is a small cupboard, usually with a glass door (if it is named at all it is usually called an *almeira*, a Portuguese word). On its shelves is a fantastic array of odds and ends: often a collection of those small sample bottles of liqueur,[4] some dolls, some ash trays and cigarette lighters, some objects made locally out of straw or bamboo, maybe some knitted doilies. The items usually are not arranged in any particular way. They are generally gifts, not retained because of any economic or esthetic value, but only because they were gifts. The total impression is very unartistic!

Perhaps Malay culture is like that: it is the cupboard in which are stored all the gifts from other cultures, not arranged in any particular way. There is no connection between the items on one shelf and those on the next—or even any linkage among the items on a shelf. But they are all the possessions of one person.

How does one live with such a collection of gifts? As with the cupboard—cautiously. One is careful not to upset the delicate lack of arrangement. A new gift can always be fitted in, but slowly, cautiously, for fear of upsetting the little china cat on the left or the shell-bird on the right.

Unifying Principles of Malay Culture

Any culture, of course, is the current collection of inherited, acquired, and stolen bric-à-brac accumulated over a long period of time. But must there not be some method to the madness of collecting? It would seem that for a culture to be viable it must have some underlying principles of collection: some items are rejected because they are not practical, some because they do not fit in with the rest of the items. Anthropological and historical literature is a record of the many principles of selection applied by different peoples at different times. The Malay cultural heritage collection is held together by two principles, mutually dependent. One is that the whole collection is valuable not for any intrinsic worth, but because it is peculiarly Malay: some of it is old, and so has value as antiquity; some of it is unique—no one else has it. But it is the totality of the collection that makes it really valuable, because it is Malay. The second principle is the central concept of what might best be termed harmony. The world itself is perceived as in many ways incomprehensible, consisting of often conflicting facts. But somehow there is harmony in a live-and-let-live sense. People too are different, and they are expected to be. Yet they must learn to live harmoniously. And by harmonious is meant *gentle:* one's actions must be such that they do not cause hurt or embarrassment.

There are two words in Malay that describe this dimension: *halus* and *kasar. Kasar* is coarse, or rough of texture, but it also means large, crude, overbearing, vulgar, boisterous, loud, rude and inconsiderate. *Halus*, in contrast, means smooth, soft, gentle, cultured and refined, small, delicate—and also polite, noble, tender. It even has the connotation of finely chiseled features and smooth skin. Malays are supposed to be *halus*, others are often *kasar*—especially Chinese and Europeans.

No one can escape, I think, the charm of a Malay village. Even a short visit casts the quiet spell of peaceful surroundings and friendly people. At almost any time of day one can find people sitting around, playing with small children, talking, or just daydreaming. Conversation is low-keyed: a man will need considerable provocation to raise his voice, and a woman who raises hers will be looked upon with amused tolerance. No one ever yells or screams at the top of his voice.

The content of conversation too is mild. One expresses an opinion very tentatively in Malay company. No one will contradict, there is always the softly murmured assent from listeners. Disagreement is expressed through stating an opinion rather independently of previously expressed sentiments. This gives Malay conversation a curious tone: the gentle unemotionality may give an impression of vagueness, of uninvolved talk about the weather, whereas actually, important issues may be in discussion. The differences in idea or opinion are always played down, agreement is stressed. And two completely diametrical notions will be expressed as just two side-by-side statements. In extreme cases, disagreement may be expressed by changing the subject or withdrawing from the conversation altogether. This is, of course, a generalization and it would be most unfair to attempt to characterize the totality of a culture by the kind of conversation evidenced. Nevertheless, this is certainly the model of the culture—it is what social intercourse *should* be.

The same model applies to society. Many contradictory elements are apparent in the structure of Malay society, but the contradiction is ignored. Each village or *kampong* has a village chief who is both appointed and elected, although the process is never as crude as actually appointing or electing. The elders of the *kampong* will discuss among themselves who would be most suitable for the position, if there is a vacancy. Occasionally it may be the son of a previous village chief, because hereditary virtues are one of the considerations discussed. A village chief need not be wealthy, although that too may be a consideration: his position entails a certain amount of responsibility and it helps to have some means. He must be a respected member of the community, but, equally important, the sort of person who can handle himself properly outside his own community. Very possibly the district chief will sit in on at least some of these conferences and he will learn much about the feelings of the elders. He will rarely, however, go so far as to actually ask for the name of a candidate. In the end, the district chief will appoint someone he knows the elders have "elected." If the elders are reasonably agreed, it is a smooth, refined process. If, for whatever reason, one or more of the elders disagrees (this, of course, would never be referred to openly), the process of appointing will be put off, sometimes for years. There is seldom, if ever, a formal meeting of the district chief with the elders of a village to discuss the appointment of a new village chief. Once all parties are agreed through informal discussions, however, the appointment is made officially.

The village chief has little formal authority. His role is not to rule the villagers—they rule themselves, through adhering to the customs of their culture, especially the rules governing human relationships. The village chief will rarely, if ever, be called upon to mediate a dispute. Such a dispute—over land or land use—will be taken to a court or to the district officer, a government servant. All the elders may be asked to mediate a dispute over property. The *imam,* the religious leader, may be asked to intervene in marital disputes. The *bomoh* (medicine man, or shaman) may be asked to arbitrate disputes over customs. And, of course, it is almost a disgrace to get into a dispute in the first place—and a disgrace, or at least an embarrassment (which is the same thing) to both parties.

The village chief is the "face" of the village—the façade it carries to confront the outside. That is why one of the most important qualities of a village chief is the skill of talking. He must be able to speak properly. This means not only that he speak good Malay, but above all that he be fluent in the proper uses of all the phrases, figures of speech, and addresses which are part of the language. He must say what others expect him to say; he must be well versed in the elaborate double-talk of the cultured Malay. Yet he must know how to communicate when it is necessary—no mean task. The village chief has prestige, but not much more than other elders. He has influence, but not much more than the *imam,* the *bomoh,* or any of a number of other individuals. He is not expected to display qualities of leadership—no one is. Nor is he expected to influence opinion, even less, action—no one is. In a sense he is a figurehead, but it would be unthinkable to treat him as such. It would be considered very rude to march into a *kampong* to do a survey, or to administer to the sick, or to talk to any of the villagers, without first stating one's business to the village chief. He will be most gracious, invite one to his village, offer his support. But it should be understood that his support is a formal phrase, he cannot guarantee the cooperation of the villagers.

The role and function of the village chief is but one example of the informal but traditional nature of the structure of Malay society. It is a society which provides remarkably few restraints —or rewards—for its inhabitants: any individual is free to believe what he wants, to act as he wants. The only restriction, and it is a severe one, is that never is one individual to embarrass another. To act aggressively is embarrassing, but it is equally embarrassing to act in such a way that one forces another to be aggressive! The nature of this restraint, however, is cultural rather than social. It is not society, through any channels of authority or law, which enforces good behavior: it is the culture as a whole—the value of being a Malay. The only punishment is ostracism, the only reward is being accepted.

It is perhaps not surprising that in this culture Western medicine and modern medical practices have been accepted in unlikely ways. Malay culture certainly allows for change, for introduction of new practices. It has incorporated many new practices and customs in the past and continues to do so today. However, these new practices must be introduced gently, softly, gradually. And it is the new practices per se that are incorporated, not a new way of looking at things or organizing facts. In the cupboard of cultural bric-à-brac, new customs can always be fitted in, but the system does not allow for the rearrangement of the shelves.

Malay concepts of disease, of treatment, of life and death, are as varied as their culture. Disease is caused by bad spirits— and the spirits are bad either because one has not properly propitiated them or because some evil person has manipulated them. But disease is also caused by wind (perhaps a Chinese concept?) , and by bad living: if one is not *halus,* it is possible to become violently ill. Disease is also given by God, either as punishment or as a test.

The treatment of disease is, of course, related to these varying concepts of cause: a disease caused by spirits must be treated by manipulating these spirits. Or a disease may be treated by internal or external application of herbs. Or, a disease must be suffered. It is not at all unusual to find Malays who treat a disease with all these methods at once. A *bomoh* may be called to exorcise the spirits, but he will, for good measure, prescribe herbs too. He may even use modern Western drugs if he is a modern *bomoh*. If any or all of these treatments fail, it is obviously the will of God, and the patient and those around him must accept this fact.

Hence it is not surprising that some modern medical practices are readily acceptable. Almost everybody now knows that aspirin brings down a fever and that quinine helps alleviate an attack of malaria (although most people also know that chloroquine is better because it actually cures the disease). Most, too, know or have heard that injections cure yaws, and know and accept that certain pills give a mother back her strength after delivery. Today in Malaya the Malays will readily accept modern drugs and they know the efficacy of injections. They will consult a doctor (either after having consulted a *bomoh* or at the same time) when they expect the doctor to prescribe pills or injections. They have not accepted surgery, however, saying that it is an injunction from the Kor'an not to cut or in any way mutilate the body. Their real fear, notwithstanding, seems to be not of the cutting itself but rather that part of the body may be removed.

Very generally the Malays have accepted government-trained midwives, yet rarely to the exclusion of *kampong*-trained ones. It is recognized that the former may be more skilled than the latter, but nevertheless there is seldom an attempt to substitute one for the other.

During a recent outbreak of para-cholera, the chief of a village assured me that all the people had had immunizations. A brief investigation showed that perhaps two-thirds of the villagers had indeed been immunized, some of them because they believed in the efficacy of this procedure, most of them because the immunizations were given free. The ones who were not immunized all gave reasons: they were busy at the time, they were asleep when the truck came to the village, they forgot about it, although they planned to get the injection, etc. In this same village a large ceremony was staged also, beginning with prayers in the Mosque and ending with a torchlight parade to scare away the evil spirits. Most houses at this time sported a charm outside the main entrance to remind the cholera spirits that the necessary precautionary steps had already been performed. Almost *all* villagers, too, expressed the conviction that cholera was certainly a scourge from God Himself and that there was little one could do to guard against it.

This, I believe, is an essential element of the Malay attitude towards Western medicine: if a procedure can be fitted into the conglomeration of existing facts, customs, practices and beliefs, it is accepted—but on a footing of equality with previously held beliefs. The pills and potions handed out by a Western clinic do not *replace* native herbs or traditional medical practices. On the contrary, they are included in the repertoire of the *bomoh*.

Points of Friction

Westerners often seem dogmatic to the Malays for this reason: to us a thing is, at least theoretically, either true or false. If it is false we reject it completely; if it is true we accept it completely. This, to the Malays, is a very strange, almost unnatural way of thinking. One old man told me when we were discussing this: "Truth cannot be held in the hand—it is something you may see, or rather, guess at—but do not touch it, or put it into words, because it will evaporate." There are two words in Malay which mean truth: *kebenaran*, which contains the root *benar*, meaning real or authentic but also correct; and *hakekat*, an Arabic word having the connotation of essence but also nature. Both words also are used for justice. There is no word for *truth*, however, that has an opposite *falsehood*.

In view of this orientation to reality as something to be

circumscribed at best, never pinned down—a point of view which makes it difficult to accept any kind of manipulation of the external world as well—it is interesting to examine again the incidents occurring in the village during the cholera epidemic. The inoculation campaign was, of course, preventive, as were the prayers and charms. But it was clear from the number of preventive measures taken that no one believed very much in the efficacy of any of these measures. I am convinced that the people who had availed themselves of three kinds of prevention did not feel any safer than those who had only taken out one kind of insurance—nor did they necessarily feel any safer than those who had not done anything at all.

The radio and newspapers at that time stressed not only the importance of getting "pab-injects," but also cautioned against eating raw vegetables or drinking unboiled water. During this period the cooking and eating habits of Malays in the village did not change: they still used unboiled water at times (although they might use boiled water if it was convenient to do so).

The Chinese, on the other hand, seemed to take precautionary measures more seriously—because they "believed." It was the Chinese who clamored for mass inoculations and who apparently religiously boiled all their water. It was the Chinese, too, who said frequently: "I do not have to worry any more, I have had my injection." The Chinese took the advice of the government because they believed in the efficacy of these Western medical measures—the Malays availed themselves of the inoculations (when they were brought to their doorsteps) because authority said they should. Since a sufficient number of individuals went along with what the government said, everybody acted properly—no feelings were hurt, no one was ambarrassed.

The Government Medical Service was satisfied because millions of cholera inoculations were dispensed. They were satisfied especially because apparently the Chinese appeared to accept not only the inoculations, but the idea behind these preventive measures provided by modern medical science. The Malays, on the other hand, although they accepted the inoculations readily enough (free, and delivered to the villages), did not seem to want to substitute Western preventive measures for their own, nor did they seem particularly impressed with the efficacy of this new method.

There are other indications that the Malays may accept new methods, but do not seem inclined to make a choice between the old and the new. The government is providing excellent training for midwives, yet it is doubtful that these government-trained midwives are at present replacing traditional midwives, perhaps euphemistically referred to as *Kampong*-trained. Government-trained midwives are accepted, their training is appreciated, but the attitude of many women seems to be that this is no reason to prefer them over other midwives. Partly perhaps because to choose might embarrass, partly also because it is a very basic value of Malay culture to accept almost anything without attempting to favor one thing or another, because that would destroy the delicate harmony of the whole.

The government also has started a very ambitious program of providing rural health clinics; these are well staffed and well equipped, and yet not always fully utilized. In one village a number of women told me that they no longer went to the clinic—"because the nurses talk rough."

It is, of course, not unusual for people to make medical decisions on nonmedical grounds. We might also choose a physician for his bedside manner, and if he would "talk rough" we might very well consider finding another doctor. Yet there seems to be a difference. We may stop going to a certain doctor because he talks rough, but more than likely we would immediately try to find another whom we considered at least as well qualified medically. We would not go without a doctor altogether. The alternative to these Malay women, however, was not to go to any clinic at all.

Another Perspective

Such behavior seems to us, and to Western-trained Malayans, hopelessly illogical. Nevertheless it is perfectly logical, of course, in the context of another culture. The idea of gentle harmony binding together often incomprehensible or even contradictory facts, as it underlies Malay culture, is apparently a very workable one. It means that individuals may well have an open mind, may try and use new techniques, but it also means that one should be very careful not to substitute one for another.

At one time I thought that there might be a pattern to the preference of Malay women in using the services of a *Kampong*-trained midwife, a government-trained midwife, or, in the city, even the maternity hospital. There seemed to be a large number of women who had their first child in the hospital, if they lived in the city—until it was learned that the delivery of a first child was free, the delivery of subsequent children had to be paid for in the hospital. I thought that perhaps there was a predominance of women in the rural areas who had had their first delivery assisted by a *Kampong*-trained midwife, but subsequent deliveries with the help of a government-trained midwife—until I found that the government-trained midwife had only recently arrived in this village and had not been available earlier. A survey of recent deliveries when women could make a choice showed that no choice was actually made. In fact, the determining factor seemed to be whether the *Kampong*-trained or the government-trained midwife discovered the pregnancy first. The mother had no preference, or, at least, was careful not to express any preference.

This seemingly uncritical acceptance of anything new, provided it can be incorporated on an equal footing with the old, is typical of contemporary Malay culture, and probably has been typical of Malay culture in the past. Perhaps this is why the Malays today seem to have accepted Western medical practices—as they have accepted Chinese medicinal herbs, and Indian Ayurvedic medical practices—without having accepted Western *medicine:* they have accepted the technology but not the ideas behind it.

Another illustration of this is the Malays' attitude towards hospitals and hospitalization. The importance of hospitals has been very difficult to communicate. The idea of a hospital as a preferred place of treatment is foreign to the Malays, as it is foreign to many peoples. There is no precedent in Malay attitudes toward disease and treatment for this kind of isolation. All health statistics show that even if one controls for proximity of hospitals, distribution of population, and availability of other medical facilities, the percentage of Malays admitted to hospitals, either on an in-patient or an out-patient basis, is significantly less than comparable percentages for the other population groups.

The assumptions underlying the establishment of hospitals are ideas, and as such, much more difficult, if not impossible, to incorporate in the culture than practices or pills. Unfortunately these assumptions (ideas) are rarely considered when educating people to the benefits of a better system of medical treatment. The establishment of hospitals is based upon the idea that certain diseases are contagious and thus patients should be isolated; or that proper care can be given only by properly trained technicians in a properly prepared environment; or that the most efficient treatment proceeds not only from a first diagnosis but from a continuing evaluation of the patient's state of health, best determined by laboratory tests. These assumptions or theories form the very basis of Western medicine.

Conclusions

For really good medical services to be established anywhere, it is necessary to acquaint the people not only with more modern tools, more efficient techniques, but with a new and acceptable way of thinking about disease, about causation of disease, about treatment of disease.

To the Malay, however, there is no need to assume a single theory to explain the causality of disease—disease, like any other phenomenon of the natural world, is many-faceted and essentially incomprehensible in the sense that no single theory will cover all known facts perfectly. Where we are satisfied with a theory and accept a number of exceptions to the rules we make in accordance with that theory (until we adopt a new theory), the Malay is satisfied in regarding *all* the facts without the need for any sort of theory to explain all, or even many, of these facts.

Doubtless it is not accidental that there are very few Malay doctors and nurses, since to become a good Western-trained doctor or nurse requires the relinquishing of a basic cultural orientation and the acceptance of *one* explanation of existing facts. Surely it is rather *kasar* to put oneself so squarely in one immutable position, and it is certainly *kasar* to assume a position of opposition or disagreement with any and all of the many other positions others may choose to assume.

It would seem, then, that the introduction of Western medical services to the Malays is difficult not just because there is a conflict of cultures—it is perhaps doubly difficult because the elements of our Western medical subculture are bound together in a meaningful, causal, logical sequence, whereas Malay culture does not recognize any such kind of order, except the order he perceives in the world around him, an order which is the harmony between not necessarily related phenomena.

The conflict between the culture of the Malays and the culture of modern medicine—or, modern medicine as one facet of Western culture—exists under the surface only, where ideas and values underlying the cultures seem incompatible; the fruits of modern medicine, the pills and potions and even injections, are freely accepted. Perhaps this is not an exception, but rather the rule in the world today. Few people in the world will reject nylon, automobiles, antibiotics, and Coca Cola—but many reject the principles of Western government, production and consumption, medical science, principles which have made possible the development of these "miraculous" fruits of our Western civilization.

It is easy to enjoy the fruits of an alien civilization, but very difficult to change one's own civilization to produce similar fruits. Perhaps the Malays will demonstrate the possibility of the Malayanization of Western cultural elements, rather than the Westernization of Malay culture.

It may well be that Malay society is fortunate in having a culture which can absorb elements of foreign cultures so relatively painlessly. As one village chief told me, "One should never fight progress: the fighting may kill you, as progress may kill you; we accept anything, and then find that it does not change our lives much after all."

References

1. This article is based on material collected during 1962–1964 in the Malay Peninsula, and supported by USPHS Research Grant GM 11329 (ICMRT); it is a much modified version of a paper read at the ICMRT Advisory Committee meeting, NIH, Bethesda, Md., November, 1963.

2. Barbara Ward (Jackson) : *The Rich Nations and the Poor Nations,* W. W. Norton, 1962.

3. Malaya, in this article, refers to the Malayan Peninsula—I am not here speaking of the new poltical unit of Malaysia.

4. Islam forbids the use of alcohol.

Part VI

THE MIDDLE EAST AND AFRICA

Introduction

The research that follows indicates that conservatism, fatalism, and improvidence are factors that decidedly affect health attitudes and values of the Middle Eastern and African populations represented. Yet, certain other differences in basic concepts of health and disease between these populations tend to characterize them as almost antipodal and unique in their own right.

In the Middle East, Darity reports the existence of two basic concepts relative to preventive and curative medicine—belief in animism (spirits) and belief in animatism (impersonal powers, evil eye). These concepts are reported to be especially prevalent among the rural populace and the loss advanced, economically and educationally.

Though poverty is a deterrent to progress, Darity found an interrelatedness of cultural change in education and in other aspects of life. He noted a growing awareness of, and an increasing interest in, nationalism, world prestige, and Western educational practices; therefore, he concludes that any new venture in health and medicine will more likely be accepted if presented in a manner that purports the enhancement of the national image. Shiloh's Middle East research[1] corroborates the findings of Darity and others in the assertion that acceptance and integration of many Western medical practices are occurring among Middle Easterners not because the underly-

1. *Ailon Shiloh, "Middle East Culture and Health,"* The Health Education Journal *16, no. 4 (1958), pp. 232–342.*

ing rationale is understood but because of a desire of self and/or national enhancement.

In Africa, as elsewhere, numerous symptoms of medicine and health practices are reported to exist. Though the degree of complexity of the cultural symptoms varies, each medical system is found to operate according to the dictates of a specific framework of cultural behavior. The selections which follow offer a general description of some typical systems of African popular medicine, some socio-cultural practices affecting health behavior, and some prevailing attitudes toward both "primitive" and "modern" practices.

Gelfand declares that in some areas of Africa, especially Central Africa, the witch doctor (Nganga) holds a secure and respected place in society. Also, he suggests that in these areas the general concept of disease causation is spiritual; therefore, treatment is spiritually inclined—chiefly methods of exorcism or propitiation of spirits are employed. Other agents of disease existing in Africa, according to Gelfand, are witches (usually women) who are believed to have the capacity to inflict illness at will.

In a general way, Shiloh's study of leprosy among the Hausa of Northern Nigeria concurs with the research with other cultures regarding the interaction of scientific (Western) and folk systems of medical and health practices. In his examination of the dynamics occurring from the interaction of the Hausa and Western systems of medicine, Shiloh reported the increased acceptance of the new to be due to (1) increased use of native personnel in the program, and (2) having personnel take the services to the recipients rather than requiring recipients to travel long distances to clinics.[2]

An investigation of an Ibadan population, recorded by Maclean, revealed that a majority (up to 90 percent) of the individuals had resorted to native curing practices, even

2. Shiloh, "A Case Study of Disease and Culture in Action: Leprosy Among the Hausa of Northern Nigeria," Human Organization 24, no. 2 (Summer 1965), pp. 140–47.

though they were familiar with scientific medicine and could secure treatment with relative ease. Maclean further implies that increased utilization of Western health services might be expected with increased education of the recipient population to the values of Western medicine and of the dispensing personnel in regard to traditional health philosophy.[3]

Gerlach contends that numerous socio-cultural factors influence the diet of the North East Coastal Bantu and he offers the results of efforts to reduce *kwashiorkor* (protein malnutrition) as support for his contentions. The Bantu, according to Gerlach, considers *kwashiorkor* to be caused by broken taboos; therefore, increased protein production brought about by improved agricultural methods has not effected protein consumption. He concludes that experts might expect to alter the *kwashiorkor* profile only when they have understood the existing concept of *chirwa* (something forbidden), and have devised ways to alter basic attitudes and habits.

---

3. Catherine MacLean, "Hospitals or Healers? An Attitude Survey in Abadan," Human Organization 25, no. 2 (Summer 1966), pp. 131–39.

18

Some Sociocultural Factors in the Administration of
Technical Assistance and Training in Health

William A. Darity

William A. Darity, Ph.D., is Professor of Public Health, University
of Massachusetts, Amherst. Among his outstanding achievements
have been the following: Public Health Educator in areas of North
Carolina and Virginia; W H O Consultant, Un Relief and Work
Agency; W H O Professor in Health Education, American Univer-
sity, Beirut; W H O short-term Consultant and Director of Program
Development, North Carolina Fund. His research activities have
included the areas of community health and family planning. His
publications include: "Some Consideration in Developing Family
Planning Service," Public Health Reports, *(August 1967); co-author,*
"Some Implications of Pregnancy on Campus," Journal of the
American College Health Association, *(February 1968). His article*
"Some Sociocultural Factors in the Administration of Technical
Assistance and Training in Health" is reprinted with permission of
the author and of The Society for Applied Anthropology from
Human Organization, *Vol. 24, No. 1 (Spring 1965), pp. 78–82.*

Introduction

Cultural change in the Middle East has been very rapid in
the last fifty years, especially since World War I. These changes
are probably most evident with regard to the expansion of
Western educational programs which have had a profound
effect on the various social relationships as they exist at community and family levels. They have had an effect on the

prevailing values and practices of the Middle East. This article discusses some of the author's observations on the interrelationships of these changes and certain considerations which should be given to them by those concerned with the administration and practical application of technical assistance, especially in the administration of health services and the training of health personnel.

Some General Observations

The achievement of a certain educational level is probably one of the most prized attainments in the Middle East. Among the middle class, the possession of high educational attainment has more value if it is received through, or based on, Western educational philosophy and practices. It is even more prized if carried out in a Western language, say English or French. The ability to read, write, and speak a foreign language is itself a status symbol and places its possessor on the inside with foreigners. Such people are usually an asset at a cocktail party, and the newly arrived foreign technician feels comforted to find that among "these foreigners" there are some who do not seem foreign, who "speak *our* language, dress like *us,* and act like *us.*" What the foreign technician should recognize is that this Westernized Middle Easterner does not really think completely "like us." His thoughts and rationalizations are intermingled with the experiences which he has undergone during a lifetime. This fact becomes more evident when it is realized that the change to Western educational practices is rather new among the Middle Eastern countries. It is, in fact, such a recent import that conservatism, fatalism, and improvidence in the rural areas still survive to a high degree. Elementary schools are increasing in the rural areas but at a very slow rate considering the population increase.[1] Nevertheless, the desire for education is one of the forces which has become, more or less, a cultural pattern among the people of the Middle East. However, this quest for education, this increasing interest in the learned man, is hampered by a multitude of social problems, particularly poverty and all the factors normally associated with it. In this connection, Himadeh says:

> The major social problem in the Arab countries of the Middle East is poverty, with its normal concomitants of malnutrition, poor housing, bad sanitation, and disease. It is also the chief social problem in the more developed countries, but there are differences in degree, extent, and permanence. Poverty in the Arab countries is so extreme that it often endangers physical subsistence; it embraces a very large proportion of the population; and for the most part it is chronic, not temporary or cyclical as it is in the more advanced countries.[2]

It has been observed that even the low-income people of the Middle East have desires for education, since they view education as a means of solving their many problems, although it is the middle class and the nobility who have the most opportunity really to enjoy the benefits of education. Huxley observed this while discussing a proposed UNESCO-sponsored conference with the late King Abdullah. The fact that the conference was being held in the Middle East, Huxley believed, provided a great opportunity for the countries of the region to demonstrate their keen interest in education as well as their international goodwill.[3] Huxley continues by saying of King Abdullah:

> However he seemed much less interested in this than in the general point the UNESCO represented world education, science, and culture. This clearly appealed to this traditional Arab respect for learning and learned men.[4]

The same respect for the education of women was not exhibited by the King. Huxley says that when mention of women was made, King Abdullah pointed out that they were a necessary evil.[5]

These contrasting attitudes on education for women and

education in general as held by King Abdullah cannot be considered to be representative of the attitude of all Arabs, but the problem is related to perception of women's roles. Women are conceived of as the makers of the home and the persons to bear children, functions for which it is thought a high degree of education is not important. There are many women who are receiving higher educational degrees in the Middle East, but although they are getting these degrees, the general concept of family has not changed noticeably. In all walks of life, there is strong parental control over the actions and decisions of children. This is evident in the selection of marital partners, which is almost solely the function of the parents. Sometimes these marriages are arranged at an early age, and usually a cousin is preferred. Such an arrangement proves to be less expensive for both sides of the family since a dowry must be paid.[6] This procedure does not permit the Western practice of courtship. However, on the campus of the American University of Beirut, Lebanon, I observed many of the students carrying out the same practices of courtship and friendship that are evident in the United States and Europe. As an outsider, I assumed that these students had fully accepted the concept of these practices. However, in addressing them in normal American terms such as, "Was that your girl friend with whom I saw you talking?" I always encountered a negative, and sometimes an apparently indignant, reply. In this connection, I carried out a study to discover the effect of the American educational institution on ideas and practices concerning courtship and marriage. I interviewed 123 male university students from the Middle Eastern countries each of whom had a continuous friendship with one girl, as evidenced by taking her to dances, walking with her on the campus, and having a sandwich with her at a snack bar. These students were asked the question: "Do you want to select your own marital partner?" There were 85 (or 70 percent) who said "yes"; nineteen (or 15 percent) who said "no"; and 15 percent who said they did not know. When they were asked whether they had a special girl friend, 50 percent replied in the affirmative, 30 percent in the negative, and 20 percent did not reply. However, when they were asked whether they believed in courtship, 87 percent replied in the negative, and later, 90 percent said they did not think it was wrong for parents to select their marital partners.[7]

The results of these interviews indicated that the Middle Eastern male wants the best of two different cultures. He has a strong feeling for the Western method of mate selection but on the other hand an ambivalent feeling where parental control is concerned. This is one of the types of situation of which the foreign technician should be aware. It precludes the possibility of carrying on the same type of relationship that one would with a Westerner. The general appropriateness of asking about one's wife, sister, or daughter may not be recognized. Yet, the Middle Easterner, realizing that it is a Western custom, may do so, and the Westerner should not assume that it indicates a complete meeting of sociocultural views. Some of the ways in which these factors may have an effect on health services and practices will now be discussed.

Some Sociocultural Factors Affecting Health Services

Health in most societies is considered a valued asset when the individual is sick. Yet, when there is no evidence of sickness, it is difficult to interest the individual or group in taking preventive measures. However, in the Middle East, there is a constant awareness of the encroachment of the evil spirit which brings an illness. This may be in the form of the evil eye or the evil soul (or breath), which are two of the supernatural powers that play an important part in the etiology of disease.[8] Hamady says:

> The belief in the evil eye is strong and widespread among Arab people. In their view, its bad influence spares nothing, for rarely can anyone escape the injury that it is able to inflict. It is considered a frequent cause of misfortunes,

such as sickness, death, or bad luck. There are many popular sayings that mark its fatal effects: "It empties the houses and fills the tombs," "It is to the evil eye that belongs two-thirds of the graveyards."[9]

To the Western technician these ideas may seem to be superficial, but they are a part of a culture. They cause not only the rural people to wear amulets to ward off evil spirits but highly sophisticated urban middle-class professional groups as well. It is not unusual to see a baby of middle-class highly Westernized parents wearing a blue amulet attached to the clothes or the hair. The technician who believes that these practices can be overcome in a short period of time among rural nonsophisticated groups must first examine the practices of the highly sophisticated groups. It is in the framework of such practices and beliefs that health programs must be developed and health services organized. Powers and Darity point out that:

> Health . . . procedures used in the more developed countries must be so radically changed in their adaption to countries of the Middle East that one often has difficulty in finding any similarity to common practices. The procedures must be organized not only to overcome certain traditions, but also must be adapted to fit into the cultural patterns in a manner acceptable to a major segment of the population. Examples of these traditions which have deep cultural significance are: (1) a patient with measles placed in a dark room covered with red clothing will be cured; (2) illness is due to the evil eye and can be cured by burning incense with prayers.[10]

Considering the facts that the isolation of measles in a dark room is not bad practice and that red clothing may be helpful in the progress of the case, both may be highly significant to the mental welfare of the patient and his family.[11]

The authors ask:

> Would it not be better to add to the use of incense and

prayers modern concepts of treatment, rather than the impossible attempt to change, within any reasonable period of time, these age old beliefs?[12]

Another common practice to which the Western medical technician will have to become accustomed is that of dressing boys like girls until they are five years of age. In many circles this is highly criticized, and I had a Western-trained psychologist tell me it would cause the boys to adopt feminine traits. Although not in a position to deny this statement, I questioned its validity, pointing out that if all boys in a village are dressed like girls up to the age of five, this would have little or no effect on them since there is no other frame of reference. Hamady explains this practice as follows:

Male children are highly prized in Arab society. One reason for dressing them as girls till the age of five is to keep the evil eyes from focusing on them; and from the moment they are born many protective means are used to annihilate the harmful effects of such eyes on them.[13]

Health officials in the Middle East are concerned with the possible effects of such attitudes towards boys and the higher rate of infant mortality among girls. For the Westerner to accept at face value the premise that boys are more desirable than girls, without considering all factors involved, would be a mistake. One factor is that, traditionally, men have been considered to be the breadwinners and to be responsible for the parents in old age. As women become better educated and more financially self-sufficient, they will be able to share more in these responsibilities. Health personnel, in encouraging better health care for infant girls, should stress the contribution that the girls can make to the parents in their old age. Without this consideration of the future (the Middle Easterner is future-oriented as far as children are concerned), no amount of health services will bring the incidence of infant mortality among girls down to the same level as it is for boys.

Reactions to disease and health in the Middle East are intermingled with various patterns of values, superstitions, and attitudes, and the foreign technicians will have to work within the framework of them. The basic approach will have to be the acceptance of these patterns as the starting point of the organization of services.[14]

Some Sociocultural Factors Related to the Training of Health Personnel

Although those persons who undergo training in the countries of the Middle East have had better than average educational opportunities and wider contacts, it cannot be overemphasized that they come from less educated cultural backgrounds. Even though they have been able consciously to dispense with a good many of their traditional beliefs, they are still vulnerable to them.[15] The major problem in their training is that in many cases they may become more critical of traditional practices and beliefs than the Western technician who tries to learn what they are and to adapt to them. It has been observed that many of the native health workers have a tendency to appear to be ashamed of their traditional past, to lack patience with lower-income groups; and to deny or ridicule certain expressions and superstitions which may be brought out in a clinical situation. For example, mothers are encouraged to deliver their babies in clinics. One of the traditional practices at childbirth is described as follows by Granqvist:

> When she has given birth a mother steps three times over the threshold and back, she and the child. Another woman carries the child if she is too weak. This is for fear of harm, or fear that she will not have any more children.[16]

Student nurses in a clinic refused to let one mother step across the threshold and ridiculed the practice. During most of her confinement, the mother was extremely unhappy, moody, and untalkative. Then suddenly one day, her attitude changed. It was discovered that during the night, without any assistance from the nurse, she had got up and made her three steps across the threshold. This satisfied her and relieved her anxieties. Students of public health should thus be taught to work within the framework of these practices and not to work against them. It would have been better for the mother to have made the three steps back and forth with the assistance of the nurse immediately after birth. This would also have made her more appreciative of the services of the clinic and definitely would have encouraged her to urge other mothers to attend.

In addition to trying to get the students of the Middle East to accept their own countrymen as they are and develop health programs on this basis, the foreign technician who is concerned with health training will also have to face the problem of nationalism. This nationalism is a search for a native national character which will blend well with the customs, and utilize the technical skills, of the West. This search dates back as early as 1914.[17] However, to fit a program of modern health services into this developing nationalistic feeling is difficult. The person who is carrying out health training, if a Western-trained national, is always under suspicion of trying to undermine either the progress or the customs of the country. Therefore, as often as possible, all frames of reference should be in terms of the country itself or the region in general. Sources very close to the region, as well as teaching examples, should be used. Those in the health professions usually represent the highest intellectually trained group. They are in many cases concerned with economic and social modernization of their countries as well as health improvement. Staley points out the following:

> Factors in the demand for economic modernization in under-developed countries, other than the desire to overcome poverty include:
> 1. The desire of new, self conscious nationalism to attain

or preserve independence, and to be free of foreign political or economic dominance, real or imagined.

2. The desire for the means of national defense and security. In some cases there may be an unavowed or latent desire for expansion at the expense of neighbors.

3. The desire for national and personal respect, status, prestige, and importance in the world, which experience shows not to be readily accorded to "backward" weak countries or citizens.[18]

Therefore, to relate health training only to the alleviation of poverty and the various diseased conditions which have emanated from or through poverty will not always sufficiently stimulate the desire to solve health problems. In the Middle East, almost everyone is concerned with some aspect of the political development of his country, and it is within this framework that health training must begin. It will be impossible not to recognize the important factor of nationalism and its unavoidable connection with training in the health professions.

The question we now raise is how can health problems be solved when all Middle Easterners are concerned with prestigious jobs? Middle Easterners like jobs that will require the wearing of a coat and tie, or the white jacket associated with the laboratory. The day-to-day hard core job of reaching people in the villages with an idea towards improving sanitation, housing, water supplies, and the like, requires someone who is not a white-collar worker. This is the work of the sanitarian or the nurse who can get out into the local community and who has the skills to communicate in something other than a patronizing manner. The factor of prestigious work in the Middle East, regardless of the limitations of salary such jobs often bring, is one of the overriding characteristics which the foreign technician will face. For example, the American student who wants a university education will wait on tables, do construction work, or any number of other chores during the summer and during the school year in order to earn money to pay for his education. Such is not the case in the Middle East. Even when jobs have been made available to assist students, if they are not white-collar jobs, most of the students will not accept them. In one of the countries of the Middle East, I was approached by some students concerning work they might do in order to attend the university. Arrangement was made for them to work with a construction company, helping a foreman at a site. Out of the group of six, only one accepted the job. The other five informed me that they were looking for office work, this despite the fact, also, that the construction work paid considerably more than the office jobs they desired. Some four years later, I happened to see three of these people again. The student who had accepted the construction job was then entering graduate school, while the others were working as clerks for a very minimal salary. They both expressed the wish that they had gone on to the university, but qualified it with statements to the effect, that, "We just couldn't accept that type of work."

This type of attitude, coupled with pride, nationalism, and some of the representative customs I have mentioned, poses an immense problem for the recruitment and training of health personnel to work in the rural areas of the Middle East. The foreign technician must search for a new approach. Recruitment from the local areas and training in large cities eliminates, to a great degree, the development of a health technician who will be satisfied to go back to the rural area to work. Training in the rural areas eliminates the possibility of the high level technical proficiency required if the problems in the rural areas are to be salved.

Where do we go from here? How can the foreign technician, within this changing Middle East, contribute to constructive work in the field of health and other social welfare endeavors? How can the differences in practices between the two cultures be made less? How can an appreciation for the tradition of work with the hands be developed and how can this be dignified so that more health practitioners can be trained for work in rural areas? How can the overriding problems of fatalism and conservatism, on one hand, and nationalism on the other, come to a meeting ground? The foreign technician who is either concerned with advising and assisting in the development of services or with the training of health personnel, must consider all of these questions prior to embarking on a course of action that will yield beneficial results. Without these considerations he will be doomed to failure from the beginning and may in fact do more harm than good.

Summary

Cultural changes in the Middle East have been very rapid in the last fifty years. Western educational procedures have become more and more accepted as a model. However, various practices of the West have created ambivalence among some students exposed to American educational systems. Therefore, it is impossible to accept the Middle Easterner who speaks a Western language and knows well many of the Western customs, as being a fully Western-oriented individual.

Likewise, in the organization of health services and the training of health personnel, careful consideration should be given to the influence of superstitions such as the evil eye, ritual practices during childbirth, practices in the treatment of diseases, as well as prevailing feelings of fatalism, conservatism, and nationalism. The major problem may be posed in this question: "How can the Western-oriented technician, who is concerned with helping countries solve problems of poverty, develop schemes which will take into consideration all of these factors?" Huxley raises the same question, from the political point of view, when he says:

> Regional politics operate under the shadow of oil and the rivalry of great power blocs, so that development is constantly being distorted by pressures from without and resentful reactions from within. Can the relation between the great powers, with their resources of capital and techni-

cal experience, on the one hand, and the countries of the Middle East on the other, be converted from the primarily exploitative activities of the Western world in the past . . . into one of mutually advantageous and complementary participation in a common enterprise? That is the over-riding question for the Middle East.[19]

References

1. Sa'id B. Himadeh, "The Arab Middle East" in Phillips Ruopp, *Approaches to Community Development*, W. Van Hoeve, Ltd., The Hague and Bandung, 1953, p. 286.

2. *Ibid.*, p. 283.

3. Julian Huxley, *From an Antique Land*, Max Parrish, London, 1954, p. 112.

4. *Ibid.*, p. 112.

5. *Ibid.*, p. 112.

6. Florence M. Fitch, *The Daughter of Abd Salam: The Story of a Peasant Woman of Palestine*, Bruce Humphries, Inc., Boston, 1934, pp. 19–20.

7. This study was carried out in the spring of 1958 as a means of trying to understand how better to counsel students from the Middle East.

8. Hilma Grandqvist, *Child Problems Among the Arabs*, Soderstrom and Co., Helsingfors, 1950, p. 236.

9. Sania Hamady, *Temperament and Character of the Arabs*, Twayne Publishers, New York, 1960, p. 171.

10. Leland E. Powers and William A. Darity, "In the Middle East Training Begins Where People Are," *Health Educators at Work* 9 (May, 1958), 14–19; 15.

11. *Ibid.*, 15.

12. *Ibid.*, 15.

13. Sania Hamady, p. 236.

14. Powers and Darity, 16.

15. *Ibid.*, 15.

16. Hilma Granqvist, *Birth and Childhood Among the Arabs*, Soderstrom & Co., Helsingfors, 1947, p. 87.

17. Washington Platt, *National Character in Action: Intelligence Factors in Foreign Relations*, Rutgers University Press, New Brunswick, 1961, pp. 150–151.

18. Eugene Staley, *The Future of Underdeveloped Countries*, Frederick A. Praeger, New York, (rev. ed.), 1961, pp. 21–22.

19. Huxley, p. 113.

19

Meet The Nganga

Michael Gelfand

Michael Gelfand, M.D., is Professor of Medicine, University College of Medicine, Rhodesia, Salisbury. Among his latest publications are: African Background: The Traditional Culture of the Shona-Speaking People, *Verry, 1965;* Africa's Religion: The Spirit of Nerjajena, *Verry, 1966; and* Medicine and Custom in Africa, *Williams and Wilkins, 1964. "Meet the Nganga" is reprinted with permission of the author and of Abbott Laboratories from* Abbottempo, *Vol. 2, no. 2 (May 15, 1964), pp. 30–34.*

All readers of novels about Africa have heard about the witch doctor, or nganga, yet few have any conception of what sort of person he is, or what he does. This is hardly surprising, for the only way to understand his procedures is to talk to him as well as attending his consultations.

Anyone who takes the trouble to meet a nganga in the flesh will soon discover that he is not the frightening monster of fiction, but that he is respected by his people, who place implicit faith both in his opinions and in his remedies.

Despite the many outward changes taking place today with the emergence of independent African States, the witch doctor still retains a secure place in the social structure of the people.

His services are much sought after, and his advice is much needed by the masses, who possess an infinite faith in his magic.

The nganga, like the Western physician, obviously believes that sickness has a cause but, instead of attributing it to the invasion of an organ by a virus or bacterium, he holds that it has a spiritual causation.

It follows, therefore, that if a spirit is responsible, the first line of treatment must be to find out what has upset the particular spirit and, secondly, what the spirit requires to be propitiated. For instance, the offended spirit may demand that a beast be sacrificed and that some of its meat be roasted and offered to it while the rest can be enjoyed by members of the family.

The most important spirit in a family unit is that from a dead grandparent or parent. First in importance comes the spirit of the grandfather, then that of the grandmother and so on. Any neglect of a rite or religious practice may offend one of these spirits. If, for example, the dead person is not buried in the correct manner, the spirits are upset.

In the complicated marriage formalities, any omission of part of the dowry would anger the spirits concerned. When a daughter marries, the son-in-law must present his mother-in-law with a cow, but should he neglect to do this, the departed grandmother is sure to inflict punishment on the guilty individual.

As a rule Africans love their parents and accord them the highest regard and respect. "Honor thy parents" is ingrained in the Africans' philosophy. It must be extremely rare for an African to display any unkindness towards his parents; no matter how bad a parent may be in ordinary life, his children respect his memory.

Hence in African society the elderly are shown every consideration, and their dependents never fail to make the family elders comfortable and to share their food with them.

The other equally important cause of sickness or death is that which results from the evil machinations of a witch. A strong belief exists throughout Africa that there are people (mostly women) who are endowed with evil which is passed on from parent to child.

The witch can inflict death or sickness on any individual she selects. Any person who crosses her path, who excites her jealousy or who is boastful is likely to be attacked. The witch is envious of success, riches or good fortune in the broadest sense. She therefore attacks people she knows, but not the stranger.

Illnesses inflicted by the witch may be of any kind, but more often they are sudden, severe, mysterious and often painful. An unexpected death is apt to be linked in the minds of the African with witchcraft. The poison of the witch is so severe that death follows quickly but, if it has not had sufficient time to act, the individual is spared from death.

One of the chief duties of the nganga, therefore, is to discover the witch and to prescribe a method of treatment which clears the evil from the body.

A popular form of exorcism is simply to suck out the evil cause from the patient's body. Africans go miles in search of a nganga with a reputation for "sucking out" the sickness. When this specialist is sought the usual complaints are rheumatism, arthritis or a painful disorder of locomotion.

The nganga applies his mouth to the painful part and sucks vigorously for a minute or two, after which he generally spits out a form of foreign material from his mouth, such as a piece of bone, and promptly displays it in the palm of his hand to the patient.

Another popular method is for the nganga to take a goat and go with the patient to a crossroad where the nganga, after giving the animal some medicine by mouth, proclaims aloud that the evil spirit should leave the person and enter the animal; after that it is chased away, taking the evil away with it.

So far, I have tried to show that the nganga is a diagnostician in that he endeavors primarily to discover the cause of the illness.

In itself, this may suffice to cure the patient, provided the effect on the individual has not been marked; but the nganga does appreciate that the damage already caused by the spirit can be removed by administering a medicine which will complete the cure.

This herbalistic function of the nganga probably originates from the early Egyptians who, some 4,000 years ago, were among the first people apparently to recognize that many cures for man's diseases were to be found in nature—in the plant and animal kingdoms.

So there has developed over the years a very extensive herbal pharmacopeia employed by nganga. Hundreds of different herbs (also parts of animals, insects or reptiles) are carefully collected and regularly employed. Nor are these remedies used haphazardly because many of them are known to the nganga, who have learned by trial and error, through the centuries, which plants can be given with safety.

In most parts of Central Africa the nganga is, theoretically, either a diviner or a herbalist, with a clear division of duties. But I have found a great overlap of function.

Should the patient be intent on knowing the cause of the sickness he consults a diviner, but should he prefer medicine he finds a herbalist.

Divining procedures vary greatly throughout tropical Africa but most of the techniques are based on the principles of a game of dice in which the nganga throws his divining set, observing how the "dice" lie on the ground after being cast in the air. There are a variety of falls or combinations, each with its own meaning.

In Mashonaland the set of *hakata* comprises four flat rectangular pieces of wood carved from a tree whose wood is specially hard. Any man with a gift for carving prepares a set which he sells to the nganga. On one side of each wooden piece a special design is cut and as a set consists of four *hakata* it follows that there are sixteen different combinations which can result when the lot is cast. Each combination has its own meaning.

Before he is allowed to divine, the nganga must carry out

a ritual which enables the set to "see clearly." One practice is to leave the unused set overnight at the ashpit of a village. But even though this is done the nganga must never omit to spit a special mixture on the *hakata* on each occasion he begins to divine.

As the nganga divines he chants, calling on the spiritual world to tell him what is troubling the patient. He first asks whether it is one of the spirits (*vadzimu*) of the family. If the combination confirms his questions he chants again, asking which spirit is angered.

Is it the grandfather? If this is the reason for the illness, the nganga divines again, asking what it wants in order to be propitiated; perhaps a blanket or a goat. Should his *hakata* fail to prove that a *mudzimu*—spirit of a departed relative who during his lifetime practiced as a nganga—is responsible for the illness, the nganga might easily chant once more, asking if the illness is due to natural causes, in which event there is nothing one can do about it except to prescribe a herb in order to alleviate the symptoms.

In Mashonaland, one of the most responsible duties of the diviner is to provide the reason for an individual's death. No matter how many nganga a person may have consulted during his illness, once he passes on his family must consult a reliable diviner in all instances, for death is not natural except perhaps in old age.

It is all important to know whether the offended spirits are appeased, or if witchcraft is still operating against the person and his family.

Since the nganga owes his skill to a spiritual endowment, it follows that his training or qualifying procedures are bound up with the spiritual world. It is true that apprenticeship to a practicing nganga plays a part.

In Mashonaland, which I know best, apprenticeship to a nganga may last for weeks or months, but almost without fail the main emphasis is possession of the selected individual by a *mudzimu*.

Thus, on the death of the father, his spirit might sooner or later elect to enter a relative, when the spirit reveals itself in sickness. The young initiate complains of various symptoms. Often enough he becomes mentally confused but he may be troubled with pains, cough, weakness and so on.

Not knowing the nature of the trouble he tries different remedies, but all fail until he goes to the right diviner, who discovers that the spirit of the father desires the relative to follow in his footsteps and agree to practice as he once did.

The African knows that it is useless to protest—he accepts willingly and gladly. Having done so, he starts to dream regularly about remedies or divining procedures.

In others, there is no preliminary illness but the initiate begins to dream. In his dream he sees his father, as a nganga before him, instructing him how to manage different complaints or how he should divine.

Some continue to dream in this way after they are in practice whereas others dream only when they encounter a specially difficult case.

The members of his family already are aware that he will soon be a proper nganga. But before he can practice he must hold a ritual ceremony attended by a number of nganga and his relatives and close friends.

Beer is brewed for the occasion and, during the ceremony, the spirit of his dead father enters and possesses him. In this state the spirit speaks through him aloud, explaining to the gathering that he is the medium for the healing spirit, that he is able to treat disease or divine, as the case may be, and that as long as he remembers to respect the spirit he will be able to continue to help the people.

With this public ceremony behind him the young nganga is ready to be entrusted with the care of any patient who wishes to consult him.

Every nganga charges a fee. There is no free service and the public is quite willing to pay for his help. The nganga has to earn a living just like any other tribesman. He works in the fields and tends his cattle, when he is not otherwise engaged in private practice.

The Africans believe that for any service rendered there should be some payment, however small. A nganga has few bad debts. Rarely does a patient fail to pay him.

The herbalist is paid on cure. As to when a cure is deemed to have been effected is largely left to the judgment of the sick person's family. The amount of the fee varies greatly from a very little to as much as 30 dollars, depending on the skill of the nganga.

But this payment for cure is not the only charge; there is also a small fee for the medicine which the nganga has had to find.

Further, if the nganga has to go a long way to the patient's house he is entitled to a small payment to cover travelling expenses and to food when he arrives at the patient's village.

The fee for divining, however, differs from that given to a herbalist on cure. It is handed over before the nganga starts to divine.

In my experience the ethics practiced by the nganga are good. I have never heard any nganga say anything disparaging about his colleagues, and this is all the more significant because I have been on intimate terms with many of the Mashonaland nganga.

Speaking generally, nganga do admit that there are nganga who practice evil and they are to be likened to witches, but they do not approve of running down their colleagues. They argue that should any nganga criticize his colleagues, this will at once show him up as a man of poor quality.

There may be other reasons for nganga not displaying signs of professional jealousy. One potent explanation is that nganga work on their own and contact one with another hardly ever takes place in the professional sphere of treatment.

Each nganga proudly guards his remedies and knowledge, for, should he divulge them to other nganga, there is a distinct risk that he will upset the spirit of his dead father.

Another reason for good relations among nganga is that they all possess a piece of land and are thus assured of a basic living.

Throughout Africa the nganga continues to take a big part in treating the diseases of his people, but the scientific principles of Western medicine are not known to him. He does not follow the principles of anatomy and physiology and their applied science of pathology.

Moreover, much of his treatment lacks value and scientific appraisal. On the other hand, it is possible that a number of his herbal remedies may well have a specific value in disease.

There exist already a number of outstanding examples, such as quinine and curare, which have proved of inestimable value to mankind.

It is more than likely that one or more specific remedies exist in the pharmacopoeia of the nganga.

In the psychological field, however, the nganga may play a useful role in his society, as he often discovers, through direct questioning, what his patient's problems are.

The patient goes into minute detail about his disappointments in life, his failures and what is threatening him—and perhaps precipitating an acute anxiety state.

Here, then, we see the nganga at his best, for he may now prove of greater help than the physician or psychiatrist because of his more intimate appreciation of the customs and ritual practices of his people.

There is, therefore, good reason in Africa for not opposing the practice of the nganga, even though we realize that, because of his limited diagnostic abilities, organic disease is recognized late and much suffering results among the tribal patients.

20

Socio-Cultural Factors Affecting the Diet of the Northeast Coastal Bantu[1]

by Luther P. Gerlach

Luther P. Gerlach, Ph. D., is Associate Professor of Anthropology, University of Minnesota, Minneapolis. To a considerable extent, his research reflects interest in peoples of the less advanced areas of the world, especially Asian and African underpriviledged groups. Among his publications are: "Nutrition in its Sociocultural Matrix: Food Getting and Using Along the East African Coast," Ecology and Economic Development, *Institute of International Studies, University of California, (1965); and (co-author), "Five Factors Crucial to the Growth and Spread of a Modern Religious Movement,"* Journal of Science for Study of Religion *(Spring 1968). His article "Socio-Cultural Factors Affecting the Diet of the Northeast Coastal Bantu" is reprinted with the permission of the American Dietetic Association from their* Journal, *Vol. 45, November 1964, pp. 420–424.*

The diet of any people depends on their patterns of and capabilities in food production, distribution, preparation, acceptance, and consumption. In turn, these patterns are dependent on a host of socio-cultural and environmental factors. Those concerned with the problem of improving nutrition among any group of people must thus deal with a complex of dynamically interrelated variables, both to determine the existence and cause of nutritional deficiencies and to implement appropriate remedial measures. On one hand, they must attend to the technologic and economic factors necessary to produce and distribute foods, appreciating that since these factors are functionally related to social, political, magico-religious, and attitudinal as well as environmental factors, technical and economic change is, in a sense, both the cause and effect of pervasive socio-cultural change. On the other hand, they must be prepared to cope with the complex of interlocking attitudes and practices which prevent a people from (a) utilizing adequately the foods which their technology and economy make available to them and (b) understanding and eliminating the causes of malnutrition.

Scholars such as Malinowski,[2] Firth,[3, 4] Richards,[6, 7] Mead,[8, 9] Read,[10] and Herskovits[11] have long commented on this need functionally to relate patterns of food use to their socio-cultural context. Similarly, experts of the Food and Agriculture organization and the World Health Organization (FAO and WHO) have declared that the "existing system of beliefs and ideas" of a people must be taken into account in order to change their eating habits.[12, 13] Unfortunately, programs designed to help people improve their technology, economy, and diet may still be implemented without such "contextualization." This was true of development projects for the Digo, Duruma, and related Bantu-speaking peoples of the Kenya and Tanganyika coast, sometimes referred to as the Nyika group of tribes, amongst whom I conducted anthropological research from 1958 to 1960.

I should like now to analyze Nyika patterns of food production, distribution, and utilization, relating them to important socio-cultural factors and indicating how failure to understand these patterns and the factors which affect them prevented authorities from improving the Nyika diet. I shall pay special attention to the Digo and Duruma tribes.[14-18]

Food Production Practices

The Nyika vary in their mode of livelihood. The Digo are primarily agriculturalists, specializing in maize, cassava, bananas, and coconuts. Most Duruma and Giriama are chiefly pastoralists, with large herds of cattle, sheep, and goats. The Shirazi and certain Digo who live within a few miles of the Indian Ocean are mainly ocean fishermen. A number of younger men and a few women from all of the tribes now work for wages on large Indian- or European-owned plantations or in such cities as Mombasa in Kenya or Tanga in Tanganyika. A growing number of young men are becoming full- or part-time traders in foods, livestock, trinkets, and notions. Such differences in occupation and livelihood are in part the functions of differences in physical environment and in part of differences in attitudes about what constitutes proper work and the good life.

Motivation to work and to produce food relates to various key social and cultural factors. For example, many of the older Digo feels that hard physical work is demeaning, probably because this is the work that their slaves performed until slavery was ended some forty years ago. The Duruma, who apparently did not have so pervasive a slave system as did the Arabicized Digo, tend in general to have a higher regard for manual labor and often are hired by the Digo to work for them. Many younger Digo, who tend to have less concern than their elders about the slave system of the past, also indicate a greater willingness to labor with their hands.

It is even more important to note that most of the coastal people share the feeling that it is often not worth while to work hard and diligently in order to achieve individual success. For one, they believe, that success is partly a function of impersonal supernatural forces, of the will of God and of fate. These forces do not always reward hard work with success. For another, if a coastal African is successful, he will be greatly envied by his neighbors and kinsmen, who also then fear that he may use his growing wealth to increase his power and to extend his influence and control over resources at their expense. His wife will probably also fear that he will now have enough wealth to be able to afford either another wife or a mistress and that this will be disadvantageous to her. A prosperous individual is typically called on to share his wealth with his kinsmen and wives, either by direct gifts or by financing ceremonials and rituals in which food and other goods are distributed. Those who clearly refuse to share their wealth will in turn be denied financial or other aid if they ever require it. Furthermore, they will perhaps be accused of being witches who became prosperous not by hard work but by cheating and stealing from others, often using black magic.

Such patterns and pressures tend to militate against individual striving and also to prevent individuals from saving profits and personally amassing capital for reinvestment. On the other hand, this system of sharing does facilitate food distribution and prevents a division of society into opposing groups of well-fed "haves" and hungry "have nots." In effect, prosperous individuals invest in their kin groups and thus obtain a host of social, economic, and political rewards. By helping others a clever person can benefit by extending his sphere of influence and obligating others to aid him.

A small but apparently growing number of Digo and Duruma entrepreneurs are learning how to manipulate this system of sharing so that they obtain more aid and support than they give and are able to become successful businessmen in the developing market-exchange economy of the Kenya and Tanganyika coast. Certainly, one thing a coastal African should do to protect his assets and his reputation is to appear poor, hungry, and needy—not only to his neighbors and relatives but also to government officials and tax collectors. This misleads those interested in measuring local economic development and food consumption. They may well calculate that a people are poverty-stricken and close to starvation when they are in fact living rather well.

Agricultural Practices

Certainly an important factor in food production is technology. The food production technology of the Nyika peoples

is probably not as inefficient as many Americans and Europeans like to believe. The Nyika practice slash-and-burn agriculture and shifting cultivation. After their gardens are exhausted by four to seven years of cultivation, they allow them
to lie fallow. They clear a new field of trees and other large
growth by girdling and by fire; and they clear a field of grass
and light growth by cutting this at the roots. Firing often
burns larger areas than will be cultivated, destroys valuable
forest, and may become hot enough to damage the soil. The
Nyika attempt to clear an area for cultivation immediately
before the rains fall, but on occasion the rains come late or
fail entirely and the burned fields become a wasteland of
baked mud or dust. If it rains adequately, however, crops
grow well in the newly prepared soil, fertilized by the ashes
of the burnt growth. Furthermore, as some local administrators and agricultural officers indicated, the fire clears the area
of rodents, insects, rusts, and other diseases harbored in the
soil.

If a field is covered only by grass and other light growth, they
will often not burn this growth but rather chop it off at the
roots, using their favorite agricultural implement, the all-purpose short-handled hoe.[19] Then, instead of raking off this
grass as American or European farmers usually do, they allow
it to remain on the ground, where it serves as a cover from the
sun, protecting the soil, seed, and plant, and eventually rots,
becoming fertilizer. Nyika weed their crops only once or twice
and again do not rake the weeds from the field but instead
allow them to cover the soil. They do not plant their crops in
neat and orderly rows, but since they do not use machines to
plow, plant, or harvest, they have no real need for such order.
They also do not pull weaker seedlings and plants from their
fields, because they do not feel that this will actually assist
the stronger crops to grow.

The Digo, whom we observed in the location known as
Lungalunga, obtained good harvests using these methods.
The Digo teacher in the local government primary school had

his students grow crops using European methods which he had learned in teachers' college. His students used long-handled hoes in the American and English manner, although most found them awkward to handle and some cut their toes as a result. They raked the land clear of weeds and grass, and the hot sun baked the exposed soil, killing most of the improved maize seedlings given by the government. Interestingly, the teacher's wife grew maize and other crops in a smaller adjoining field, using traditional methods. When I asked the teacher about this, he smiled and said in effect, "Well, women don't like to try new methods and, after all, we must get enough to eat." Indeed, she had a much larger harvest than did her husband and his students.

The government has a large experimental agricultural station near Mombasa and often invites Nyika peoples to see demonstrations of new and improved methods and seeds. The Nyika are not as slow to accept innovations as some of the government people believed, but they were not always as certain that the government station adequately demonstrated that European and American techniques were superior to Nyika ways.

Livestock Production

The Duruma and Giriama, who manifest the typical East African cattle complex and desire to have as many cattle and goats as possible, have adopted many aspects of western animal husbandry technology, and veterinary medicine.[20, 21] Cattle and goats provide the chief source of food and income for most of these people. They are the most important form of inheritable wealth and investment and are used to pay bride wealth and blood debt and to provide food for rituals and ceremony. Men rise to power and influence by giving cattle and goats to kinsmen and friends to herd and milk.

The Duruma and Giriama have been quite pleased to see their herds multiply rapidly as a result of Western technique and medicine, but they have not been willing to keep the size of their herds to that which their land can carry. In respect to their use of cattle, a few scrawny cows are worth much more to them than one fine animal. As a result, the introduction of Western medicine and other technology has led to extremely serious overgrazing in this and other areas of Africa, and large areas of formerly rich grassland are rapidly becoming eroded wasteland and useless thorn desert. Clearly, rather sweeping socio-cultural change must accompany technologic change in this instance if this technologic change is not to have adverse consequences and lead in time to reduced rather than expanded food production.

Problems of Irrigation

There are yet other cases where a number of socio-cultural factors in effect prevent the Nyika from accepting a technologic change which would increase food production. For example, the people of Lungalunga in Kenya know well how to irrigate their fields by channeling water from the neighboring Umba River and that irrigation will enable them to increase their rice productions. They now grow "dry" rice in swamps filled mostly by rain water, although they are quite aware that the Arabs, Shirazi, and Digo of Vanga, less than fifteen miles away, grow much more rice per acre by irrigation from the Umba. Unlike the people of Vanga, the Lungalungans do not have the social, political, or economic organization necessary to implement irrigation agriculture. The Lungalungans are afraid that they will quarrel with kinsmen and neighbors over land rights and water rights if they irrigate and that they will not have the production organization—the organization for work—required to assure that they work together where necessary instead of against each other.

Because of past Arab control of Vanga, the Vangans have a different land-tenure system and different production organization and are therefore able to irrigate. (Interestingly enough, recent conflict between Africans and Arabs has weakened the social and political supports for irrigation agriculture and rice production has declined.) All of this indicates that it is important to study the socio-cultural factors which relate to production organization since such organization is as important to food production as technology. Certainly, the key to the production of more food among the Nyika is not simply more and better Western technology.

Factors Influencing Food Production

In any event, production is not enough to give people the food they need. Distribution is just as vital, and distribution clearly relates to all manner of economic as well as noneconomic factors. Food is distributed partly by patterns of extensive gift exchange and reciprocal aid, partly by the practice of sharing in feasts at frequent rituals and curing ceremonies, and partly by patterns of trading and marketing.[15] While the latter method is increasing in importance, the other forms of distribution are not to be ignored. The three methods together assure that the agriculturalists get fish and meat and milk, that the cattle herders get fruit and vegetables and fish, that the fishermen in turn obtain the products of garden and pasture, and that the wage laborer can buy what he needs.

Unfortunately, attempts by the United Nations Educational, Scientific, and Cultural Organization (UNESCO) and governments to improve production and distribution have actually had the reverse effect in some instances. For example, the establishment along the coast of a governmental program in which Indian merchants and government cooperated to purchase, process, and market local milk inadvertently caused the cattle herders to sell more milk than they could part with, increased African enmity towards the Indian merchants and government agents who handled the milk program, and injured the rapidly developing business of the African trader in milk, vegetables, and fish by raising the cost of milk and controlling the milk supply.

This program, known as the Mariakani Milk Scheme, has

been lauded by local and international authorities and by representatives of the International Bank for Reconstruction and Development (IBRD).[22] Its major defects appear only when it is studied in the context of developing African trade and conflict between Africans and the Indian merchants who are their patrons and creditors. It would seem more desirable to stimulate the development of the Nyika entrepreneurs, since they have the capacity to market available foods, to stimulate or increase demand for new or traditional products, and to contribute to widespread and basic economic development and political stability.

Acceptance and Consumption of Food

Finally, it must be emphasized that even if technologic, economic, and other changes do cause more food of different types to be made available to the coastal Africans, this does not then necessarily mean that these foods will be used and the diet improved. Habits of food preparation and consumption are hard to change. The coastal Africans, like many other peoples throughout the world, may well reject new and better foods in favor of more traditional foods, or they may continue to cook their food in such a way that much of its nutritional value is lost. For example, many coastal Africans still regard fresh fish as bad for their health and will eat only dried fish, such as shark from South Arabia.[17] Digo, Duruma, and other coastal fish traders peddling fresh fish on bicycle are doing their best to change this attitude, and since about 1959 they have stimulated many women to demand that their husbands purchase fresh fish at least three times a week.[14, 15]

These traders characteristically market fish, meat, and vegetables, and governmental interference in the milk trade is hurting their overall trade in all of their wares. Furthermore, the distribution of free powdered milk in this area has, in many cases, backfired because of local habits of food preparation and use.

Nyika women have been slow to believe that this substance was really milk which could supplement or replace milk from their breasts for their children. Also, they have frequently mixed this powdered milk with unboiled, contaminated water and have fed it to their infants, causing illness and perhaps death. The Nyika, like many other Africans, believe that the only proper food, especially for infants and ill adults, is a starchy, protein-deficient porridge or gruel made from corn, millet, cassava meal, or rice.[7] Only this can properly be termed "food" (*chakuria* in Digo, *chakula* in Swahili). Only this is emotionally satisfying; only this "fills the belly" and makes one feel as if he has really eaten well. Meat, fish, eggs, animal milk, and the like are all regarded not as "food" but as "sauce" or "dressing" (*chitoweo*). The Nyika are convinced that while healthy adults can eat such *chitoweo* with relative impunity, children under about three or four years of age must be protected and should be restricted to a diet of mother's milk and *chakuria*. Those who are sick, no matter how old, should also be limited to a diet of *chakuria*.

We found it possible to encourage some women of one Digo location to mix their maize (corn) meal with chicken eggs, milk, and sugar (all available locally at low price) and to feed the resulting *chakuria*—like pudding—to their infants. Presumably, it would be possible to cause this innovation to spread throughout the coastal area, and it might be truly beneficial if enough were eaten. Presently, however, most infants do not obtain protein other than that in the customary *chakuria* and in mother's milk, and few mothers are able to provide adequate milk for the required period.

Malnutrition—Kwashiorkor

Protein malnutrition, or kwashiorkor, is hence not uncommon among infants and some adults in the coastal area, but when a local African sees a person suffering from what Western observers conceptualize as inadequate nutrition, the Africans feel instead that this person is suffering because he or his parents broke important sexual taboos. The term *chirwa,* which is the passive form of the verb *kuchira,* meaning in effect "to do something forbidden," is used to identify those suffering from these violated prohibitions.

The major taboos, violation of which leads to *chirwa,* are sexual intercourse between husband and wife during the period before a child born to them is old enough to be weaned (three to four years of age) and adultery by either parent during this period or during the period of gestation of this child. If a new child is conceived before its sibling has reached the desired age for weaning, it is said that the new child will "steal the strength" of the former. While few Nyika are willing to abstain from sexual intercourse for the required period, they do make every attempt to prevent conception. If conception does occur or if there is other evidence that the taboos have been violated, the close relatives of the endangered former child may well accuse the guilty parent or parents of trying to kill this child.

Western observers have most incorrectly translated the term *chirwa* as "rickets" or "protein malnutrition," but it most certainly does not mean that to the Africans. When Western medical authorities ask, as they do, to see those suffering from *chirwa,* they are usually shown no one since the Nyika hate to admit publicly that they have broken the sexual taboos and that they have a child with *chirwa.* When the Western officials argue that the Nyika should feed their children more "food" (*chakuria*) to counter *chirwa,* they are regarded by the Africans as quite foolish, if not presumptuous. First of all, the Nyika feel that they do give their children more than enough *chakuria;* second, they know quite well that one does not remedy broken taboos by eating more *chakuria.* They believe that only traditional Nyika methods administered by Nyika specialists can be employed to deal with *chirwa.*

Not even the best intentioned technical expert, nutritionist, aid administrator, or Peace Corps volunteer can effectively counter protein malnutrition in this area of Africa unless he understands the concept of *chirwa* and unless he can also change some fundamental attitudes and food habits so that available protein foods can be eaten by children and those who are ill. But even here, it must be noted that seemingly desirable change may perhaps have some undesirable consequences. Destruction of the concept of *chirwa* as a retribution for "out of season" intercourse, combined with improved health and diet, may well lead to such an increase in births and in longevity of life that malnutrition then does become clearly a result of too little food for too many people rather than primarily a result of inadequate use of increasingly available food.

In conclusion, it is seen that diet is dependent on a complex web of intertwining social, economic, political, magico-religious, technologic, attitudinal, and environmental factors. These factors influence food production, distribution, acceptance, and consumption. Those who wish to improve diet must, therefore, study *all* aspects of the food-getting and -using complex in its socio-cultural and environmental matrix and implement programs of change and development accordingly. Authorities who fail to do this may actually cause harm to a people's food supply and diet while attempting to help them.

References

1. Presented at a Symposium on Cultural Influences and Diet presented jointly by the American Antropological Association and The American Dietetic Association at the annual meeting of the American Association for the Advancement of Science in Cleveland, on December 28, 1963.

2. Malinowski, B., "The primitive economics of the Trobriand Islanders." *Econ. J. 31:* 1, 1921.

3. *Ibid., Coral Gardens and Their Magic. A Study of the Methods of Tilling the Soil and of Agricultural Rites in the Trobriand Islands.* Vol. 1, *The Description of Gardening.* New York: American Book Co., 1935.

4. Firth, R. W., *Primitive Economics of the New Zealand Maori.* New York: E. P. Dutton & Co., 1929.

5. *Ibid., Human Types: An Introduction to Social Anthropology.* Rev. ed. New York. Barnes & Noble, Inc., 1957.

6. Richards, A. I., *Hunger and Work in a Savage Tribe: A Functional Study of Nutrition among the Southern Bantu.* London: Routledge & Kegan Paul, Ltd., 1932.

7. *Ibid., Land, Labour and Diet in Northern Rhodesia: An Economic Study of the Bemba Tribe.* London: Oxford Univ. Press, 1939.

8. Comm. on Food Habits, "The Problem of Changing Food Habits." *Natl. Acad. Sci.—Natl. Research Council Bull. No. 108,* 1943; reprinted 1964.

9. Mead, M., "Cultural patterning of nutritionally relevant behavior." *J. Am. Dietet. A.* 25: 677, 1949.

10. Read, M., *Sociological and Psychological Bases for Food Habits.* Proc. 2nd Intl. Congress of Dietetics, Rome, 1956.

11. Herskovits, M. J., *The Economic Life of Primitive Peoples.* New York: Alfred A. Knopf, Inc., 1940.

12. Joint FAO/WHO Expert Committee on Nutrition, Fourth Report. WHO Tech. Rep. Ser. 97, July 1955.

13. Drogat, N., *The Challenge of Hunger.* London: Newman Press, 1962.

14. Gerlach, L. P.: "Economy and protein malnutrition among Digo." *Proc. Minn. Acad. Sci.* 29: 1, 1961.

15. *Ibid.,* "Traders on bicycle: A study of entrepreneurship and culture change among the Digo and Duruma of Kenya." *Sociologus* 13:32, 1963.

16. *Ibid.,* "Nyika." *Encyclopaedia Britanica.*

17. Murdock, G. P., *Africa: Its Peoples and Their Culture History.* New York: McGraw-Hill Book Co., Inc., 1959.

18. Prins, A. H. J., *The Coastal Tribes of the North-Eastern Bantu: Pokomo, Nyika and Teita.* London: Intl. African Inst., 1961.

19. Stamp, L. D., Africa. *A Study in Tropical Development.* London: Chapman & Hall, Ltd., 1953.

20. Herskovits, M. J., "The cattle complex in East Africa." *Amer. Anthropologist* 28: 230, 1926.

21. Schneider, H. K., "The subsistence role of cattle among the Pakot and in East Africa." *Amer. Anthropologist* 59: 278, 1957.

22. Intl. Bank for Reconstruction & Development, *The Economic Development of Tanganyika.* Baltimore: Johns Hopkins Press, 1961, p. 170.

Part VII

WHAT'S PAST IS PROLOGUE

Introduction

Primitive is defined as original or primary. From the cultural anthropologist's point of view, primitive health measures might well be considered a basis for scientific medicine and justifiably so when considered in the light of twentieth-century research in primitive medicine. In general, this research asserts that various types of primitive or folk medicine have world wide existence, though the extent of usage seems to vary inversely with the technological and economic advancement of the culture. Further, each type of primitive medicine is reportedly conditioned by and adapted to the culture in which it is found to be operative.

Ackernecht's research is of particular interest in that it suggests an interrelatedness of primitive and scientific medicines. He suggests that one should show tolerance for primitive medicine in this statement: "But our medicine is not the medicine nor our religion the religion, and there is not one medicine but numerous and quite different medicines in the different parts of the world and in the past, present and future."[1] He suggests that primitive medicine has served a purpose and has persisted through the ages because of its (1) psychotherapeutic characteristic, (2) social interrelations, and (3) satisfaction of a basic craving in humanity, a metaphysical need. He offers further support for his suggestion as follows:

1. *Erwin H. Ackernecht, "Problems of Primitive Medicine,"* Bulletin of the History of Medicine *11 (1942), p. 503.*

> Because magic gives the mystical unity which we feel so important, this deep satisfaction by metaphysical participation, it could be repressed, condemned to a hidden and almost unconscious existence (like ratio lives in primitive mentality) but it could not die, it still lives and acts.[2]

In his brilliant description of the psychotherapeutic aspects of primitive medicine, Ari Kiev[3], not unlike Ackernecht, found that primitive medicine, like modern psychotherapy, has therapeutic effect in that it mobilizes the patient's hope for relief. Also, he suggests that primitive medical systems reveal differences that seem directly related to the degree of economic and technological development; and, with increased complexity of a society, the folk curer's methods show a greater parallelism to Western psychiatry, which often ascribes the patient's illness to interpersonal and intrapsychic conflicts.

The research that follows lends credence to the foregone contentions. It explains that folk medicine, like any other human endeavor is (1) a social activity, (2) has psychotherapeutic value, (3) is present to some extent in all cultures, (4) might be expected to change as scientific knowledge is gained and (5) serves as prologue to scientific medical practices.

Saunders and Hewes express the idea that folk medical practices embody a religious characteristic and persist in all cultures, including our own. They contend that folk and scientific medicines pervade each other to the extent that a constant two-way interchange is set up, and that those in our culture who share folk medical tradition are more often than not receptive to scientific medicine. Among the less advanced people, according to Saunders and Hewes, *cultural lag* inhibits objective consideration of illness causation; therefore, through understanding and tolerance, physicians might use many folk concepts in ways advantageous to the patients.

---

2. Ibid., *pp. 516–17.*
3. *Ari Kiev, "The Psychotherapeutic Aspects of Primitive Medicine,"* Human Organization *21, no. 1 (Spring 1962), p. 25–29.*

Erasmus' research implies that a parallel exists between folk beliefs and scientific knowledge; likewise, progress from folk concepts to science is directly related to acquired economic status. He offers the idea that folk beliefs evince inductive inferences based on reported observations; and, in this respect folk beliefs bear semblance to scientific medicine.

Thus primitive and ritualistic ways have been accorded a place in the evolution of culture, our own among the rest. Taking an introspective look at American culture, Horace Minor depicts the *Nacirema* (Americans) as a ritualistic people in spite of (or because of) technological advancement. He implies that *Nacirema* customs result from social interaction and the development of values and attitudes acceptable to the group—a civilized way that has evolved from less complicated (primitive) habits and customs. Malinowsky further re-emphasized the worth of primitiveness and recounts civilization's evolvement from primitive ways when he wrote:

Looking from far and above, from our high places of safety in the developed civilization, it is easy to see all the crudity and irrelevance of magic. But without its power and guidance early man could not have mastered his practical difficulties as he has done, nor could man have advanced to the higher stages of civilization.[5]

Finally, the whole concept of primitiveness as the forebear of technological advancement might be amply summarized in the statement by Shakespeare: "What's past is prologue."[6]

---

4. *Horace Minor, "Body Rituals Among the Nacirema,"* American Anthropologist *58, no. 3 (June 1965), pp. 603–7.*
5. *Bronislaw Malinowsky,* Magic, Science and Religion. *Glencoe: The Free Press, 1948, p. 70.*
6. The Tempest *2. 1. 253.*

21

Folk Medicine and Medical Practice

by Lyle Saunders and Gordon W. Hewes

Lyle Saunders, M.D., is Professor of Medicine and Public Health, University of Colorado Medical School, Denver. He is the author of Cultural Differences and Medical Care, Russell Sage, 1954.

Gordon W. Hewes, Ph.D., is Professor of Anthropology at the University of Colorado, Boulder. He was a Fulbright Lecturer in Keio and Tokyo (1955–56), and Lima (1960). His chief concern, as reflected in his research and writings, is culture history, psychoethnology, and cultural geography, especially of Africa and Asia. He holds membership in the American Ethnological Society, Association of Ethnic Geography, Association of Asian Studies, and the Japanese Ethnological Society.

"Folk Medicine and Medical Practice" is reprinted with the permission of the authors and of the Association of American Medical Colleges from The Journal of Medical Education, *Vol. 28, no. 9 (September 1953), pp. 43–46.*

The practice of medicine, in whatever form it may take, is a social activity. Inevitably it involves interaction between two or more socially conditioned human beings. Invariably it takes place within a social system which defines the roles the participants may take, specifies the kinds of behavior appropriate to those roles, and provides the sets of values and orientations in terms of which the actors are motivated.[1]

In the practice of medicine, as in any other area of human behavior, the outcome of any interactive situation is a function of the attitudes, values, cognitions and expectations both or all the participants bring to the situation and of what all expect to get out of it. Thus, in the relationship between a doctor and a patient, what goes on in the interaction, what satisfactions each derive from the relationship and what other relationship situations eventuate are determined not only by what the doctor brings to the relationship, but also what the patient brings.

The patient is not, as is sometimes supposed, a passive, uninformed, completely receptive partner in the relationship, but an active participant with his own notions about what is wrong with him and what could or should be done about it. He also has his own ideas of how far he will go in accepting the advice and direction given by the doctor. It is the patient who makes the first diagnosis and the first assessment of the relative severity of his condition. It is the patient or some member of his family who initiates contact with the doctor; frequently only after alternative procedures have been considered or tried. Thus, the first reference point for the identification of an illness, the first steps toward cure or relief and possibly a good deal of the subsequent activity with respect to the illness are likely to derive from that body of belief and practice which we know as folk medicine.

The term folk medicine is popularly thought of as referring mainly to the esoteric and bizarre health practices of ancient or primitive peoples. But the concept is equally applicable to that vast body of belief in our own culture, lying partly within and partly outside the field of scientific medicine that is available to and used by laymen and "marginal professionals" in the diagnosis and treatment of ailments.

It is a truism that all cultures have among their elements and patterns a body of beliefs and practices centering in the recognition and treatment of illness. In our culture there are two interrelated sets of such beliefs and practices: scientific medicine—that which, by the methods of science, is systematically developed, disseminated and practiced by "legitimate professionals" in medical schools, laboratories, clinics, and hospitals

—and folk medicine—that which, informally developed and disseminated, is more or less the common property of everybody in the culture. The two cannot be sharply differentiated, since many elements are common to both.[2] What probably distinguishes them is the emphasis in scientific medicine on understanding cause and effect relationships in illness and recovery and the relative lack of such an emphasis in folk medicine.

It is easy to see that scientific medical practices do not even begin to encompass the entire range of beliefs and practices dealing with illness and curing within our culture. There are, for example, aside from qualified physicians at least fifty different kinds of persons from whom one may seek medical advice or treatment. A person may consult somebody (a druggist, an electrotherapist, a naturopath), may visit an institution (a shrine, a hot spring, a gymnasium, a Turkish bath), may change his residence, may purchase and use an appliance (a sun lamp, an elastic stocking, a hot-water bottle, an exercising machine), may seek relief in drugs (Hadacol, Lydia Pinkham's Vegetable Compound, Carter's Liver Pills), may change his diet (more or fewer vegetables, nuts, gravies, starches, fruits), may choose a household remedy (bicarbonate of soda, salt, vinegar, oil of cloves), may follow a procedure (sun-bathing, cold baths, eye exercises, prayer), or may turn to the written word (a home medical book, a newspaper, a copy of *Reader's Digest*) for information and advice. All of these and innumerable other choices may fall outside the field of scientific medicine and can be made without any contact with a licensed physician.

Folk Beliefs

Although there is vast literature on folk medicine, there has been relatively little attention given to it and little use made of available information by professionally trained medical personnel. Folk medicine, when it is considered at all, is likely to be thought of as a curious survival, having about the same relation to medical science that alchemy has to chemistry. Medical personnel seldom have any systematic knowledge of the folk medicine of their own or other cultures, and no sharp awareness of the extent to which folk medical ideas and practices permeate our culture and influence behavior with respect to illness.

Except when the physician lives and works in a cultural environment radically different from his own, he is not likely to realize the extent to which the folk medical beliefs of his patients modify their responses to their symptoms and to his therapeutic procedures. It is perhaps with patients who differ from the physician only in subcultural orientation (i.e., patients who are members of a social class different from that of the physician or of a different ethnic group partially sharing his culture) that the "blind spot" of the physician with respect to the folk medical beliefs of his patients may most seriously interfere with the establishment of an effective therapeutic relationship. Here the difference in medical knowledge and attitudes may lead to suspicion, hostility and distrust of the doctor, who may not understand the necessity of being asked apparently irrelevant questions; the need for elaborate and time-consuming laboratory procedures, the delay in establishing a definitive diagnosis and instituting treatment. The doctor feels impatient, annoyed and impeded when the patient fails to follow his advice or to cooperate in the treatment process.

The folk medical beliefs of patients inevitably influence their relations with physicians. When the doctor does not recognize the existence of such beliefs and persists in seeing them as evidence of ignorance or superstition, the influence is likely to be an adverse one. When the doctor is aware of folk beliefs and sensitive to the meaning they may have for patients, the beliefs can be used by him in attaining the ends he seeks in the relationship. Recognition and understanding by the physician of folk medical beliefs and practices does not mean that such beliefs and practices must be accepted as scientifically valid. It is only necessary to recognize that they exist, that they can influence the outcome of therapy in many cases, and that they can sometimes be used to the advantage of the patient.

Medical Viewpoint

The prevalent attitude of many practitioners of medicine toward folk medicine—when its existence is recognized at all—is frequently one of attack by such direct means as exposure or ridicule or by resort to "educational" measures designed to eliminate what is considered to be mainly medical ignorance. Such an approach is likely to be less harmful to the persistence of folk medical beliefs than it is to the quality of the relationship between the physician and his patient, and is more effective in driving patients deeper into a dependence on folk medicine than drawing them into the folds of the enlightened followers of science.

Rather than being mere ignorance or a random collection of superstitious notions, folk medical beliefs constitute a fairly well-organized and reasonably consistent theory of medicine. Rooted in time and tested by the experience of many generations, they are tenaciously held.[3] Success in treatment is taken as proof of their validity; failure is rationalized or ignored.

In many respects, folk medical beliefs are similar to religious beliefs and are almost as impervious to rational argument, demonstration of their error, ridicule or other forms of direct attack. The fact that a large proportion of the people who share the folk medical traditions of our culture are also receptive to scientific medicine is no indication that the older beliefs are being rapidly supplanted by the new, but rather the new is constantly fitted and adjusted to the old. Traditional beliefs are given up very slowly and many persist almost indefinitely, along with the latest in medical advances. Witchcraft, for example, may continue to be regarded as a basic cause of disease even after the role of microorganisms as causative agents is well understood and accepted. Treatment procedures which are frankly magical in nature may be used along with the latest techniques, if not with the physician's knowledge and consent, then without them and in defiance of him.[4]

Scientific knowledge may even reinforce folk beliefs and apparently even confirm them as, for example, when a people who believe disease is caused by animals in the body are shown microorganisms under a microscope or have the germ theory of disease explained to them.[5] The ability of folk medicine to absorb and assimilate new ideas and new practices is almost limitless, and folk medicine in our culture, rather than diminishing under the impact of the scientific point of view, is probably expanding and flourishing as new elements are added at a much faster rate than old ones are dropped.

The differences between scientific medicine and folk medical traditions and practices will continue indefinitely because of the phenomenon of cultural lag and the practical impossibility of a culture in which individuals can be expected to regard themselves and their illnesses and disabilities from a purely objective, rational, scientific point of view. Practitioners of scientific medicine, however, can do much to narrow the gap by becoming aware of the content and meaning of the medical knowledge their patients bring to the patient-physician relationship, by concentrating their educational and other efforts toward the elimination of those folk beliefs and practices clearly recognized as harmful in the light of scientific knowledge, and by using the remainder of them in ways beneficial to individual patients and their families.[6]

In the doctor-patient relationship the primary objective of the doctor much of the time must be to motivate the patient to follow the course of treatment the doctor prescribes. This end probably can be more certainly and more effectively attained if the treatment course is determined by a knowledge of folk as well as of scientific medicine, and is thus the closest desirable approximation to the patient's own ideas of what is good treatment in his particular case.

References

1. In more simple terms: in the practice of medicine, as in all other areas of human behavior, *what* is done, *who* does it, and *why* (i.e., for what reasons) it is done are largely matters of social prescription.

2. There is a constant two-way interchange between the two. Remedies developed by scientific medicine become part of the pharmacopeia of folk medicine (e.g., the use of aspirin to relieve minor aches and pains); others with a long history of folk use are "discovered," analyzed, tested and ultimately used in scientific medicine (e.g., opium, quinine, cocaine).

3. No small part of their appeal is the fact that they do have a good deal of functional value.

4. Many examples of the use of folk remedies by patients undergoing treatment in modern hospitals have been observed.

5. In Denver, there is a widely accepted belief among Spanish-speaking patients that the medicines used in "shots" are nothing more than new forms of old familiar "weeds" that have long been used in popular medicine.

6. See George Foster, editor: "A Cross-Cultural Analysis of a Technical Aid Program." Washington, D. C., Smithsonian Institution, 1951.

22

Changing Folk Beliefs and the Relativity of Empirical Knowledge[1]

Charles John Erasmus

Charles John Erasmus, Ph.D., is Professor of Anthropology, University of California, Santa Barbara. Previously, he was Field Ethnologist, Institute of Social Anthropology, Smithsonian Institute; Applied Anthropologist, Institute of Inter-American Affairs, Columbia, Haiti, Ecuador, and Chile; and Associate Professor of Sociology and Anthropology, North Carolina University. He has been Consultant, Land Tenure Center, University of Wisconsin and has served with the U. S. Agency for International Development, Venezuela. His publications include: Man Takes Control: Cultural Development and American Aid, *University of Minnesota Press (1965); "Upper Limits of Peasantry and Agrarian Reform,"* Ethnology *(1967); "Cultural Change in Northwest Mexico," Vol. III of* Contemporary Change in Traditional Societies *(1967); and "Community Development and the Encogido Syndrome,"* Human Organization *(Spring 1968). His "Changing Folk Beliefs and the Relativity of Empirical Knowledge" is reprinted with the permission of the author and of the* Southwestern Journal of Anthropology *from Vol. 8 (1952), pp. 411–428.*

One of the most fascinating of all the acculturation problems in Latin America today is that resulting from the contact between folk and modern medicine, for here it is possible to study not only the conflict between two systems of knowledge but also the differences between those two polarities we call magic and science. We are generally inclined to think of backward peoples as being more concerned with the supernatural and with magic than ourselves, a circumstance which led Levy-Bruhl, for instance, to consider primitive man to be pre-logical in his thinking. Recently, in his search for an "objective" criterion of progress (which he defines as the "advance to something better"), Kroeber has suggested that the advancement of a culture can be determined by the degree to which it has disengaged itself from reliance on magic and superstition. Retarded peoples, he says, place greater emphasis on phenomena that have only mental or subjective existence and thereby tend to reward certain types of psychotic and neurotic behavior that more advanced groups would consider pathological.[2]

More recently, Tax has said that although primitives reach conclusions through the same logical processes that we do, they reason from premises which differ from ours according to their "content of cultural experience." He therefore proposes a cross-cultural distinction between "knowledge" and "ignorance" by defining knowledge as "any item of information that is derived from the scientific interrelating of sense-perceived phenomena" and which accumulates through increased intercultural contacts, literacy, improved technology, increased division of labor, and the greater secularization of society. Furthermore, he equates "rational thinking" with "knowledge of the world of nature and of man" provided by the "scientific method" while "irrational thinking" he equates with "ignorance," the state in which mankind began.[3] Pointing out that "experimental verification" at best yields only "a statement of probability based on a correlation," Rowe accuses Tax of setting up universal cultural values on an ethnocentric basis, of assuming "absolute truth" and of suggesting a unilinear evolution of knowledge whose furthest development to date is represented by our own culture.[4]

To what extent can we truthfully say that backward peoples think differently from ourselves, that their knowledge and beliefs are less empirical, that a transition from magic to science represents progress or that an evolutionary concept of knowledge must be unilinear and ethnocentric? In the pages which follow we shall endeavor to throw more light on these questions through a study of folk vs. modern medicine in Ecuador. Special attention will be given to situations where folk practices and beliefs are being challenged by their modern counterparts, for the type of acceptances and resistances we encounter in these situations can help us to evaluate whatever differences may exist between folk and modern thought.

Our study will be divided into three sections. The first will present a summary sketch of the relevant data on folk medical beliefs and practices collected in the poorer districts of Quito. Although our material on the subject from the towns of Tulcán and Esmeraldas was in general very similar to that from Quito, it is not included in this section in order to avoid the geographical comparisons that would be necessary. Field methods used for the collection of this data included interviewing, observation of the curing procedures of folk practitioners, and a statistical study of the sale of remedial herbs in the central public market of Quito. Secondly, we shall describe special situations of change in Quito, Tulcán and Esmeraldas. Methods here included interviewing, small public opinion surveys, and the testing of school children, nursing students, and nurses' aides. The final section will be devoted to a theoretical analysis of our data in relation to the questions we have asked.

Folk Medicine

Beginning with the folk concepts of disease etiology, we may consider first those illnesses attributed to contagion, although the folk concept of contagion is different from the modern one. The major folk explanation is concerned with the fear of bad body humor. This is most commonly described as due to lack of personal cleanliness. It is a substance which exudes with perspiration, and if one does not bathe frequently it may re-enter the pores and infect the blood. Not only is it a source of auto-infection, but it may also be passed between persons. Thus it may cause such ailments as skin diseases, infected wounds, and syphilis. Close contact, sexual relations, or seats still warm from a previous occupant are means by which it may pass from one individual to another.

Next we may consider those folk illnesses attributed to "mechanical" etiologies. By mechanical we refer to such things as temperature change, harmful foods, fatigue, and body blows. Of all the mechanical causes those concerning temperature are probably the most important for the folk. Exposure to cold air when overheated is considered very dangerous, and being caught in a thunder shower when working in the fields or drinking cold water when perspiring are other variants. Symptoms may include dysentery, menstrual and postnatal cramps, pneumonia, urinary difficulties, rheumatism, measles, partial paralysis, and malaria. Body heat may cause skin diseases, and heat generated in the body by coughing may lead to angina. Certain foods are dangerous by reason of their "heaviness," "sourness," "acidity," or inherent "coldness." Some foods stick to the stomach and others lead to an overabundance of body bile which is related to liver trouble. Any cooked food which is left to stand acquires a quality of coldness which is especially feared. Fatigue from hard work and insufficient food leads to "liver" and "kidney" ailments as well as skin infections and "inflamed uterus." Body blows can cause meningitis and tumors. Diarrhea with fever is said invariably to accompany the process of teething. For some informants, diarrhea at this age is simply a kind of "natural" consequence. Others give a psychological explanation. They say that because the child is irritated he develops "anger" sickness.

There are several illnesses that the folk ascribe to psychological causes. Among these is anger sickness due to quarrels, jealousy, etc. This may result in such symptoms as vomiting, diarrhea, fever, inability to walk, depression, "fits," and "palpitation of the stomach." An unfilled desire such as a sexual desire, a food craving of a pregnant woman, or the desire of a small child to possess a toy or candy may result in a variety of maladies. "Fits," syphilis, and urinary difficulties are examples. Sadness due to a personal loss (loss of a loved one, money, property, etc.) may also cause "fits" as well as palpitation of the heart, fever, lack of appetite, severe headaches, loss of consciousness, etc.

Among the supernatural ailments fright and malevolent air are the two most frequent causes and the victims are predominantly children. The stimulus for a fright may be anything as natural as a sudden fall or as supernatural as an encounter with a ghost or a spirit. For many individuals there seems to be a definite feeling that the fright produces soul-loss. Malevolent air may be contracted by a small child if he is taken to a cemetery, too close to a corpse, to solitary places in the mountains, down into mountain canyons, or is exposed to a rainbow or night air. Another prevalent childhood illness, especially among pretty children, is that due to evil eye, the malevolent glance of certain adults who have "electrical" or "strong" eyes. For adults witchcraft is the primary supernatural cause of illness. The methods of the witch include magical poisoning of the victim's food and imitative magic using dolls to represent the victim. Symptoms of all ailments having supernatural etiologies are so generalized that they could point to almost any malady in a modern classification. However, among those listed for children, informants always included fever, vomiting, and diarrhea.

The pains frequently experienced by women after parturition are also attributed to supernatural causes, for they are considered likely to occur if the placenta is discarded in such a way that it comes in contact with water or cold air or is eaten by dogs. The placenta should be buried in a dry, safe place such as the ground beneath the kitchen hearth.

Folk preventive measures may be classified as either mechanical or supernatural. The "contagious" diseases are prevented by such mechanical means as bathing and by avoiding warm seats. The "mechanical" illnesses can be prevented by avoiding sudden changes of temperature, by regularly taking cathartics to keep the stomach clean, etc. Psychological illnesses are considered almost impossible to prevent since they are brought on by circumstances which the individual cannot control or readily avoid. Supernatural ailments may be prevented by both mechanical and supernatural means. Avoidance of those situations in which a child is susceptible to supernatural infections could be considered mechanical. But since avoidance is not always possible, the supernatural means of prevention predominate. Wearing certain objects on one's person is the most common type of preventive measure. The beak of a parrot or the wool of a llama will protect against witchcraft. A rosary around the neck of a child will guard it against malevolent air while crossing a canyon. Steel rings protect their wearers against both malevolent air and witchcraft, while a red ribbon will protect a child against the evil eye.

Very often diagnosis is made by reflecting over preceding events. Was the sick person recently exposed to a sudden change of temperature? Did he enter a canyon where there might have been spirits? Did he make an enemy who might have had him bewitched? Professional curers diagnose largely by magical means such as measurement of the patient with red ribbons (Esmeraldas), cracking the patient's back, or throwing corn grains in the embers of a fire. Some of these magical methods of diagnosis are curative as well.

The predominating type of folk remedy consists of herbal solutions and broths, the cathartics being the most popular of all. Calmative herbal broths employed for stopping diarrhea and vomiting as well as sudorific herbal broths are, like the cathartics, usually taken orally while others are administered in the form of enemas and vaginal douches. Among the external remedies, herbal poultices are very often used. On the supernatural side, cupping may be employed to extract malevolent air. But the most popular remedy for ailments with supernatural etiologies is that of "cleaning" the patient with special plants, eggs, or guinea pigs. The "cleaning" process consists of slowly rubbing the remedy over the patient's body until the illness is drawn into it. Religion also plays an important part in curing in the form of vows to saints or praying "Our Father" and Credos in magical sets of three, etc.

In a sense, every adult is a medical specialist. The folk share a common knowledge concerning the diagnosis, classification, and treatment of symptoms and are most likely to consult a curer only when their own household remedies fail. If a supernatural cause is suspected, however, only the curer is considered capable of properly administering the "cleaning" treatment.

An attempt was made to gauge the incidence of folk illnesses and the extent to which folk remedies are used by observing purchases of herbs for a period of several days at the central public market in Quito. These remedies were sought for practically every kind of malady imaginable, but a few illnesses had a considerably higher incidence than others. The six illnesses of highest incidence were malevolent air (nearly all children), "cough" (children), fright sickness (children), menstrual difficulties (mostly cases of retarded flow, and the cathartics purchased may well have abortive effects), urinary difficulties (mostly adults with symptoms of blood and pain), and bewitchment (all adults). If the period at which the investigation was made is representative of yearly conditions, at least 180,000 purchases are made each year in this one market alone, a figure almost as great as that of the population of Quito. One fifth of all the purchases were for supernatural ailments and consisted of herbs with magical "cleaning" properties.

Change and Conflict

Some general knowledge of the modern concept of microbial infection was found to exist in all locales where studies were made. However, even though school children in particular were often capable of giving good explanations of modern concepts of disease etiology, they were also capable of giving just as good explanations of the traditional concepts. To check the impressions obtained from interview material, tests were given to grammar school children in Quito. Their responses showed they knew and adhered closely to the folk beliefs which had previously been uncovered in the personal interviews. On questions concerning the doctor's ability to cure those ailments whose etiologies we have classified as supernatural, the answers were almost unanimously negative. Since doctors do not study these maladies, they do not know the curing techniques appropriate for them. Answers to a question on the nature of the microbe and its dangers indicated some understanding of it. It was defined as a tiny animal that could only be seen with a microscope, that lived in unclean food and water, etc., and was an agent of disease. But the diseases actually associated with the microbe were those with modern names such as tuberculosis, typhoid, and whooping cough. When asked if microbes could be the agents of such ailments as fright sickness, malevolent air, and bewitchment, the responses were again almost entirely negative. If a microbe can be seen only through a microscope, how can it frighten anyone? Such illnesses are caused by spirits, cold winds, and evil persons and are not the results of contagion or infection.

Interview material showed that in general the illnesses with supernatural etiologies are treated by folk specialists, while others such as infected wounds, measles, anger sickness, and skin infections are treated at home. However, even such folk specialists as curers and professional herbalists will agree that the doctor is the one best qualified to treat such ailments as diphtheria, tuberculosis, venereal disease, and appendicitis. In many cases the informant will admit that he goes to the doctor only when his own remedies or those of the curer have failed. Judging from the symptoms given for many of the folk etiologies, it would seem that even though the folk have more confidence in the doctor as a medical practitioner for many maladies with modern names, they do not always classify their symptoms according to those names until the doctor has been consulted at an advanced stage.

In another set of tests conducted in a Quito grammar school, the children were given a list of twenty-two illnesses and asked to check the ones they would treat at home, those they would have treated by folk curers, and those they would have treated by a doctor. The list included folk and modern illnesses and in no case was there a 100 percent response in favor of any particular means of treatment. Responses in favor of the doctor ranged from 96 percent in the case of tuberculosis to only 2 percent in the case of fright sickness. All the supernatural ailments as well as such maladies as skin infections, infected wounds, and diarrhea fell among those for which more than 50 percent of the subjects would seek a curer or treat at home. For ailments such as bronchitis, typhoid, paralysis, whooping cough, and malaria more than 50 percent preferred the doctor. The same children were also given a list of causes and asked to match them with these illnesses. The most frequently indicated causes of illness was microbes, which gained its weight from those disease on the list bearing modern names. In all, however, it accounted for only 19 percent of the total number of responses. Folk causes were predominantly given for illnesses treated at home or by a curer. The most significant fact was that even in the case of those illnesses for which medical treatment was favored, supernatural causes were in some cases predominant.

From a consideration of our data so far, it would appear that the folk look up to the doctor for his ability to cure serious illnesses for which their own remedies are less likely to be efficacious, independently of whether or not they understand or believe in his explanation of causes. Their acceptance of the doctor rests primarily upon empirical observation and experience. To test this further, we will now compare the results of investigations at Esmeraldas and Tulcán. In the Negro coastal area about Esmeraldas, yaws was a prevalent disease until an extensive campaign of injecting penicillin was inaugurated. Doctors who served in the campaign encountered considerable public resistance at first. By the time of my visit, however, yaws had been pretty well brought under control, and if there ever had been any resistance to the program it was certainly no longer in evidence. Although investigations in Esmeraldas showed a strong adherence to folk medical beliefs and treatment, house-to-house interviews disclosed nothing but praise for the yaws campaign and a complete conviction that yaws was a disease which the doctor alone was capable of curing. This attitude was shared even by local curers. As some informants expressed it, you cannot deny what you see with your own eyes.

The situation in the highland town of Tulcán was somewhat different. A water purification system had just been installed and house-to-house visits revealed that while the folk were very much in favor of the purified water, their reasons had nothing to do with disease prevention. Previously they had had to let their water stand in buckets until the dirt settled; now it was possible to use it directly from the public taps. For the most part, however, they did not believe that the former water had caused them any harm. Interviews with informants and a native curer disclosed that the symptoms of intestinal infection were being attributed to malevolent air and fright sickness and were being treated by magical means.

The data from Esmeraldas and Tulcán give further indication that the acceptance of the doctor is based primarily on empirical knowledge and observation. The campaign at Esmeraldas was curative with spectacular and observable results. At Tulcán, on the other hand, the program was one of preventive medicine based on modern concepts of disease etiology that were not as easy to grasp on a purely empirical basis. Perhaps a noticeable change in the incidence of certain syndromes at Tulcán will lead the folk to an empirical judgment in favor of modern preventive medicine. But it seems just as likely that their failure to grasp the modern concepts of disease etiology will result in the contamination of food and water through other means, thus preventing any noticeable change in the incidence of syndromes.

Let us now turn back to Quito and the new charity maternity hospital, Isidro Ayora, where attendance runs as high as 60 percent of the total number of Quito births. On interviewing mothers concerning the hospital it was found that some profound changes were transpiring in their beliefs. Such hospital practices as flushing placentas down the drain and requiring patients to leave in five days (according to tradition a mother should remain in bed for fifteen and in the house for forty) were causes for alarm, but all women who had attended the hospital stated that their fears were evidently groundless since no ill effects had resulted. Arguments overheard between mothers who had attended the hospital and mothers who had not indicated that those who have attended are "selling" the hospital to others and arguing against their own former folk beliefs. The fact that all services at the hospital are free and that many mothers are recommending it seem to be the primary motivating factors for attendance in the case of young mothers going for the first time.

However, not all goes smoothly at the new maternity hospital. Because the modern concepts of medicine are not understood, many of the preventive measures find little acceptance. Once inside the hospital, mothers for the most part refuse to be bathed after parturition, to eat certain foods which they consider harmful, or to go without their postnatal laxative. Those hospital practices in conflict with their beliefs but over which they have no control are effecting changes in those same beliefs on an empirical basis. Those beliefs in conflict with hospital practice that the mothers can control by fits of crying or threats to leave are persisting and disrupting the hospital routine.

As far as tradition is concerned, we may say that the folk beliefs in themselves are offering no resistance to modern medical practices in so far as those practices may be judged

by the folk on an empirical basis. Preventive medicine, however, is being resisted because its comprehension is largely at
a theoretical level that does not readily lend itself to empirical
observation. Let us now consider the effect produced on
the folk beliefs by higher education and special theoretical
training.

A test on medical beliefs was given to fifty-five nurses' aides
at the maternity hospital Isidro Ayora and an equal number
of student nurses at the national school of nursing. While the
nurses' aides had had only grammar-school education, the
student nurses were all high-school graduates.

By comparing, first, the responses of the nurses' aides (who
had had little additional theoretical training) with interview
material and the tests of grammar-school children, it is possible
to make come estimate of the extent to which hospital life has
affected their beliefs. In doing so we find that the only clear
distinction pertains to the more supernatural ideas. Causes
such as witchcraft and improper disposal of the placenta, preventive measures such as red ribbons and religious medals,
and such treatments as "cleaning" and praying were no longer
important to them. However, while beginning nursing students, with the advantage of a high-school education, were
much more inclined to affirm their disbelief on these questions,
many of the nurses' aides refused to answer them. Third-year
nurses showed the most remarkable change, for over 75 percent
stated disbelief. Third-year nurses also distinguished themselves from all the rest by a 45 to 61 percent greater frequency
of stated disbelief concerning postnatal food taboos, "natural"
diarrhea as an accompaniment of teething, fright sickness,
malevolent air, and sickness due to desire. The most persistent
beliefs among all groups were those concerning anger and sadness, body humors, body biles, temperature changes, and the
preventive and curative use of laxatives. (Among the better
educated groups very innocent symptoms were attributed to
the two psychological etiologies, anger and sadness.)

When one considers that none of the subjects had ever had

any course which directly discussed and attacked their folk beliefs, the results indicate the extent to which they themselves have reconciled the old and the new. When asked what they thought accounted for their greater degree of disbelief in folk concepts, the third-year nurses attributed the change to a course in obstetrics that the second-year nurses had only just begun. General education as well as specialized work which brings the person in contact with modern practices correlates with greater disbelief in the more supernatural and magical concepts. Contact with modern practices does not, however, have as marked an effect on changing those beliefs concerning cause and prevention that we have called "mechanical" as do more advanced theoretical explanations. Those beliefs that are most persistent under any circumstances are those whose psychological or mechanical explanations most closely approximate the modern.

The marked influence of higher theoretical training may well correlate with greater relegation of authority to the modern specialist. In response to a question that asked the subjects to state what they would do in case a mother in a maternity hospital requested a postnatal laxative, the third-year nurses were far more apt to leave the decision to the doctor, while the nurses' aides were inclined to agree with the patient and accept the responsibility for administering it. In general, the folk seem much more prone to consider themselves self-sufficient in medical treatment and diagnosis than the average North American. Where the North American may become nervous at the slightest symptom and run to a doctor, the folk immediately classify or diagnose the symptoms according to their own extensive body of knowledge and beliefs and attempt to cure them by themselves. In the grammar-school class that was asked to designate which illnesses could be cured at home and which by a curer or doctor, the boys showed a greater dependence on the specialist whether he be a curer or a doctor while the girls had more faith in the home remedies they had learned from their mothers.

Social factors are also important in the process of acculturation from folk to modern medicine. Among white-collar and
professional classes in Quito a feeling exists that only people
of inferior status use herbal remedies and go to folk curers.
The "better" people are supposed to rely on drugstore remedies and doctors. A test given to one hundred boys in a public
school attended by children of the white-collar class showed
a much greater reliance on the drugstore and the doctor than
the children of the poorer districts. However, in their concepts
of disease etiology the two groups were much more closely
allied. It would seem that the acceptance of the doctor and
his remedies is related in some degree to prestige, independently of an understanding of modern etiology.

In Bogotá, Colombia, where the author has made similar
investigations, social factors play an important part in public
resistance to free health centers. Although the folk beliefs
themselves do not appear as strong nor as well organized as in
Quito, there is greater hostility toward modern medicine in
the poorer districts. Colombia has been affected by a tremendous urbanization movement that has disrupted the old
class system. "Good family" is not the important social criterion it was formerly, while acquired economic status is
becoming more and more important. The cities have been
flooded by rural immigrants who no longer classify themselves
or one another according to a traditional system. As a result
of the competition to rise socially, individuals with some small
position of authority press their weight on others to force
a recognition of the status they wish to have associated with
that authority. Thus, the nurses and doctors employed in the
government health centers are often overbearing in their
treatment of the public. In resentment, the Bogotá folk freely
voice their hostility toward modern medicine. Common household items are books on folk remedies written with overtones
of spiritualism by nationally famous curers.

The social factors are related to economic ones. If the
"better" people in Quito rely more on the doctor despite a

persistence of folk beliefs among them, this is not only due to the doctor's prestige but to the fact that they are in a better position to afford him. Where modern medical therapy is free, attendance is often greater than the traffic will bear. To judge from their appearance, the great majority of the people who frequented the herbalists at the public market undoubtedly belonged to the lowest economic groups in Quito.

Conclusions

First, let us consider the problem of whether the folk can be said to think differently from ourselves or whether their knowledge is less empirical. In treating this problem we shall make use of concepts employed by Dr. Hans Reichenbach in his *The Rise of Scientific Philosophy*.[5] Dr. Reichenbach states that the essence of knowledge is generalization and that correct generalization is dependent upon the separation of relevant from irrelevant factors. By "relevant" he means that ". . . which must be mentioned for the generalization to be valid." Further, he considers generalizations to be ". . . the very nature of explanation" which is sometimes achieved ". . . by assuming some fact that is not or cannot be observed." He gives as an example the casual explanation whereby the barking of a dog is attributed to the presence of a stranger in the vicinity of the house, an unobserved fact which is ". . . explanatory only because it shows the observed fact to be the manifestation of a general law [that] dogs bark when strangers approach. . . ." Such inductive inference, he claims, goes beyond a mere summary of previous observations and becomes an instrument for predictive knowledge. But we can never be sure that dogs will always bark at strangers. In this vein, Dr. Reichenbach says, "The study of inductive inference belongs in the theory of probability, since observational facts can make a theory only probable but will never make it absolutely certain." Thus, in place of absolute knowledge he speaks of "probable knowledge," a term he does not find self-contradictory because it is based on "frequency interpretation" in which "degree of probability is *a matter of experience* and *not of reason.*" From here we may proceed to his concept of a *posit,* ". . . a statement which we treat as true although we do not know whether it is so." Yet, "we try to select our posits in such a way that they will be true as often as possible." The reason we try is ". . . because we want to act—and he who wants to act cannot wait until the future has become observational knowledge. . . . Posits are the instruments of action where truth is not available; the justification of induction is that it is the best instrument of action known to us."

To what extent is folk belief and knowledge a result of induction or "frequency interpretation"? The material resulting from our study of changing folk beliefs in Ecuador has indicated that for the most part the changes are transpiring on just that basis. In the field of therapy, modern medicine is making demonstrations on such a scale that the folk can readily establish *posits* for future behavior in favor of modern therapeutic methods. Resistance is primarily directed at modern preventive medicine in which the generalizations and explanations involved result from frequency interpretations that are not possible under situations of casual empiricism but are dependent upon the observations of trained investigators. The communication of this type of frequency interpretation to non-investigators takes place most easily under situations of special training as we saw from our testing of student nurses.

If we consider the folks beliefs alone without reference to change, it is possible to encounter many generalizations resulting from frequency interpretations, in other words, correlations made between repetitive phenomena. The concept of bad body humor, for example, is very close to our explanation of contagion. It involves an inductive inference based on past observations of a correlation between the onset of disease and certain situations in which contagion is likely. The explanation also assumes something that is not observable, a substance called bad body humor. However, it leads to predictions of situations in which disease can be contracted or avoided. Bodily cleanliness, for example, is a predictable preventive measure that still holds good under modern explanations of contagion although the prediction that disease may be contracted from a warm bus seat does not. The entire concept of bad body humor is a type of probable knowledge involving posits that definitely aid the folk to take action even though some of its posits are far less probable than others.

According to folk belief, cooked food that has been left to stand may acquire a dangerous quality of "coldness." Symptoms resulting from eating such food sound remarkably like those of botulism or enterotoxin-producing staphylococci. The folk have made a correlation between illness and cooked food that has been left to stand, and their prediction that illness can be avoided by recooking the food and thus removing the "coldness" is valid to the extent that in practice it would lead to a detoxication of the poison. But we must note that the preventive measures of cleanliness and storage that would also help to prevent food poisoning are irrelevant to the folk in view of their theory of "coldness." However, unlike bad body humors, the "coldness" of cooked food that has been left to stand is a part of folk observation. Since food infected by staphylococci or spores of *C. botulinum* does not necessarily change in taste or smell, the modern explanation is beyond the limitations of folk experience. Therefore, we see how the validity of an inductive generalization or correlation may be independent of the validity of its *causal* explanation: a condition that is common knowledge to any statistician and the principal reason why the modern scientist has come to think in terms of probability rather than causality. The modern refinement of this folk explanation has resulted from the frequency interpretations of trained laboratory investigators who have simply *increased* the posits by which we govern our actions to avoid food poisoning.

The folk have also drawn a correlation between the symptoms of intestinal infection and the teething stage in the child's devolopment. In this case the explanations add so little that no prediction is possible except that the sickness is inevitable. Since we know that teething children are more apt to insert objects into their mouths and thereby increase the possibility of intestinal infection (under conditions of folk life almost any object on the dirty floor), the folk correlation or generalization is both relevant and valid. However, it is a very simple empirical correlation. The correlation between the symptomatology and the many diverse activities of the teething child that would be necessary to provide a modern generalization is so complex as to make its empirical observation very difficult on a casual basis.

Let us now consider the supernatural type of explanation. Using a completely hypothetical example, we may take the case of a group of mothers who cross a canyon and stop to give their children a drink of water from the polluted stream flowing through it. Later, when the children show symptoms of intestinal infection frequently classified by the folk as malevolent air, the mothers may make a correlation between the illness and the trip through the canyon. Their correlation may be partly correct despite the irrelevance of their belief in spirits or the fact that they overlooked the relevancy of the stream. We cannot, however, use this hypothetical example as an argument that some empirical correlation invariably underlies all folk beliefs. But, as the testing of the student nurses and nurses' aides would seem to indicate, situations providing greater opportunities for understanding modern frequency interpretations are more detrimental to the supernatural explanations and practices than those for which it is easier to discover some underlying empiricism.

On the side of magical treatment, it is hard to see exactly how empiricism enters into the picture at all when a curer attempts to remedy an illness with "cleaning" herbs or guinea pigs. However, we must consider the fact that not all illnesses are fatal. On the average, success is in favor of the curer. This is not so true in the case of modern classifications of illnesses by which we can appraise the relative danger of syndromes with greater exactness. But the symptoms which the folk ascribe to many of their classificatory terms and etiologies are so highly generalized that they may include both fatal and innocent maladies. As long as the law of averages works in favor of the curer, his results are an empirical demonstration that his methods, as well as the theories and explanations on which they are based, are in general valid though not infallible. Our own reasoning may work along similar lines. Recently a well-known professor of medicine from an American university admitted to me that had he been treating himself with one of the modern "miracle" drugs he would probably have credited it with his recovery from a cold that had unexpectedly disappeared without any treatment whatsoever.

In many cases of "supernatural" illnesses the etiology may be psychological. The kinds of partial paralysis that some informants gave as the symptoms suffered by close relatives who had been bewitched as well as their claims that doctors were unable to find a cause, much less a cure for these cases, sounded very much like descriptions of psychosomatic conditions. Furthermore, curers succeeded in relieving the symptoms in a single magical treatment. Again, this constituted a definite demonstration to the informants that the cure was a proof of the correct diagnosis of the cause as well as the efficacy of the treatment. The similarity between these cases and those of psychological or religious practitioners in our own society almost tempts a comparison. A large part of the influence of psychoanalytic dogma on the social sciences is undeniably due to a logic that accepts a cure as "scientific" proof of the theoretical postulates underlying the method of treatment. This writer wonders if "magic" in its broadest sense can ever be completely divorced from "science." Both provide posits for future action, both may include irrelevant correlations, and both may be based on probable knowledge resulting from frequency interpretations. However, the experiences of the folk cannot provide them with the type or quantity of frequency interpretations that can be derived from laboratory experiences.

If it has been difficult to find any difference in kind between the thinking of backward and "civilized" peoples, to what extent are we justified in claiming a greater dependence on magic and supernatural explanations among the more backward? We feel that this question can best be answered by making use of the distinction between esoteric and exoteric population components. Few persons in the exoteric component of modern society attempt to recapitulate the discoveries of such men as Pasteur and Koch, much less view a microbe through a miscroscope. They accept the authorities belonging to our esoteric component who claim that microbes cause certain maladies that may therefore be prevented or cured in a certain way. During experimental health lectures given to a group of school children in Quito, the children were questioned about spirits and ghosts. None had seen one, but certain authorities such as curers or professional herbalists had. Thus it would appear that the greater dependence on magic and supernatural explanations among backward populations is due principally to differences between their esoteric components and ours. How can we explain this difference between the esoteric components of backward and modern populations?

The answer to our question seems obvious enough. Due to technological advances a far greater proportion of individuals in our society have been freed from direct food pursuits to enter many fields of specialization. Our technological system is therefore capable of supporting an esoteric component within our population that can devote full time to checking our casual empiricism, to expanding our frequency interpretations, and to providing us with a knowledge that is much more probable in comparison with that of backward peoples. This becomes clearer when we consider the fact that even the folk curer is usually only a part-time specialist. The author knows of young doctors who attempted to practice in rural areas and were forced to leave because even what few payments they received for their services were generally payments in produce. It is not difficult to understand why the type of "pure" research which is not even directly related to immediate needs is dependent upon a very complex technological system as compared to that of the folk. Nor is it difficult to understand why a society that cannot extend its opportunities for frequency interpretation beyond the casual-empiricism offered by everyday situations will focus its interests in such a way as to reward its esoteric component for posits that appear to have a strong supernatural basis from a modern point of view. In this way, "backward" groups may come to reward certain types of individual behavior that might be regarded as pathological when occuring among members of our society. Therefore, the difference between what we tend to think of as two extremes, magic and science, is related in large part to the limitations placed upon the esoteric component of a given population by the technological system.

The final problems mentioned in our introduction are concerned with concepts of progress and evolution. The major objections to the word "evolution" among present-day cultural anthropologists are related to the fact that early anthropologists explained all parallels between cultures as dues to a unilinear type of progression, and because they reconstructed culture history by assuming that what was different from Western civilization was inferior and therefore older. Subsequent studies have not only demonstrated differential development but the cultural relativity of values. Objection has also been raised against evolutionary schemes because they did not seem as applicable to non-material aspects of culture as to those that were strictly technological. Yet, if we consider the work of three modern neo-evolutionists, we find we can apply their concepts to such a "non-material" subject matter as magic and science without repeating the mistakes of the earlier evolutionists. Leslie White has seen a progression in culture based on the energy harnessed per capita per year.[6] His evolutionism is primarily technological. While not an avowed cultural evolutionist, Carleton Coon has scaled cultures by levels of complexity on what he calls a quantitative basis. His quantification rests upon the complexity of institutions, the number of institutions to which the average individual belongs, the amount of trade, and the degree of specialization.[7] George P. Murdock, who is more concerned with accounting for similarities between cultures than with systems of progression, explains the development of parallel social systems as due to limitations in the number of variations possible.[8]

By combining the three perspectives above we may arrive at a tentative hypothesis. The amount of energy harnessed per capita per year by the technological system of a society places limitations on the size and the type of its esoteric population component as well as limitations on the range of experience available to that component as a basis for frequency interpretations. This in turn limits the range of a society's probable knowledge and the degree to which its participants can estimate the probability of their predictions. Such limitations do not determine precise historical sequences nor precise regional variations. Within the limitations are such allowable variations as were treated in our comparison of social factors in Quito and Bogotá. Nor does this specialization necessarily imply any change from "worse" to "better." On the contrary, we can speak of an evolution from magic to science that is culturally relative. The relativity of this evolution depends upon the fact that the probability of knowledge is itself relative to the limitations inherent in a given cultural situation, and at no point in a progression is it "better" except as measured by the value system of an observer at that particular point.

Returning now to the disagreement between Tax and Rowe, we find that the conclusions of this paper are in accord with Tax's main thesis. The principal differences between the positions of Tax and the present paper are that we have made no qualitative dichotomy between "knowledge" and "ignorance," have suggested a quantitative difference in degrees of probable knowledge and have employed Reichenbach's distinction between probable knowledge and reason. Except for Tax's failure to stress the difference between rationalism and empiricism, we find nothing in his paper that would justify Rowe's criticism that he was assuming absolute truth and using universal and ethnocentric values. According to Rowe, all ethnographers are faced with ". . . the great dilemma of cultural anthropology: the dilemma of cultural objectivity." Thus, the anthropologist who is striving to be objective, that is, to keep his own cultural values out of his comparisons, has but "two obvious choices": (1) ". . . to accept, in so far as possible, the cultural values of the culture being studied . . ." or (2) ". . . to attempt to set up universal values which we can then apply to all cultures."[9] Rowe admittedly prefers the first choice and ascribes the second to Tax. However, if each culture must be appraised separately in relation to its own "values," cross-cultural comparisons are doomed to rationalistic rather than empirical treatment and cultural anthropology to an anecdotal preoccupation with the minutiae of differences. Is there really no other choice than the two Rowe offers? Is there no other way of guarding against value judgments than to adopt a different set of values?

In Ecuador, the magical treatment of illnesses reaches its greatest incidence among children below the age of five, who, like the old, are considered to be weaker and more susceptible to supernatural causes. However, the illnesses from which these children actually suffer are not a peculiar figment of this culture; they are the same which may afflict children anywhere. The death rate of this age group, furthermore, is over 50 percent of the recorded yearly deaths in Ecuador as compared to a figure of less than 10 percent in the United States. Given these two societies, each of which is endeavoring to apply its knowledge to the prevention and cure of the same illnesses, it is perfectly ligitimate to state that the knowledge of the great majority of Ecuadorians with respect to childhood illnesses, it is perfectly legitimate to state that the knowledge cans. To claim their knowledge is "inferior" would depend on whether or not we consider a lower infantile death rate as "better." But the second proposition is not necessarily a corollary of the first. The first is concerned with the observation of human behavior, the second with a value judgment about that behavior.

References

1. The field data on which this paper is based were collected by the author for the Institute of Inter-American Affairs. I wish to acknowledge my gratitude to Drs. Gomez de la Torre, Wilson Salazar, and Julio Falcony of the *Servicio Cooperativo Interamericano de Salud Publica* in Ecuador for their assistance in arranging for and administering the tests on folk beliefs and to Anibal Buitrón for his assistance in collecting public opinions on the maternity hospital in Quito. Special thanks are due to Mr. Preston Blanks, Chief of Field Party, whose cooperation made this study possible.

2. A. L. Kroeber, *Anthropology* (New York, 1948), pp. 296–300.

3. Sol Tax, *Animistic and Rational Thought* (Kroeber Anthropological Society Papers, no. 2, pp. 1–5, 1950).

4. John Howland Rowe, *Thoughts on Knowledge and Ignorance* (Kroeber Anthropological Society Papers, no. 2, pp. 6–8, 1950).

5. Berkeley, 1951. The quotations in their order of appearance are taken from pages 5–7, 229, 94, 263, 240, and 246. Italics ours.

6. Leslie White, "Ethnological Theory" (in *Philosophy for the Future*, R. W. Sellers, ed., New York, 1949), pp. 357–84.

7. Carleton S. Coon, *A Reader in General Anthropology* (New York, 1948), pp. 612–14.

8. George P. Murdock, *Social Structure* (New York, 1949) pp. 184–259.

9. Rowe, p. 6.

Part VIII

CONCLUSION

Conclusion

Though not concerned with social action in matters of health alone, the works included here reemphasize the following ideas:

(1) Cultural change can best be realized if one (the donor) understands his own culture, as well as the culture of those individuals he wishes to influence.

(2) Cultural change occurs more rapidly when the individuals experiencing the change feel a need for the particular change, realize some advantage in it, and can participate in planning and affecting the change.

(3) Fundamental culture patterns tend to remain unchanged, even though general acculturation is observed.

The work of Adams is of special interest in that it offers three value orientations found among Koreans and reported to exist among other East Asians whose fundamental orientation has been influenced by Confucianism. These were *time* orientation, *man-nature* orientation, and *power* and status orientation.

So, in today's world, effective living and working with people of various cultural heritage require awareness, and application, of the cultural (anthropologist's) approach. To use a phrase from Dr. Mead, ". . . the very use of the word 'culture' implies a democratic approach."

23

The Monkey and the Fish:
Cultural Pitfalls of an Educational Adviser

by Don Adams

Don Adams, Ph.D., is Professor, Director, Center for Development Education, Syracuse University. He has served as Educational Consultant for the UN Korean Reconstruction Agency (1954–55), and Educational Consultant, U. S. State Department, Korea (1957–58). He was a Scholar, East-West Center, University of Hawaii (1965–66). His publications include: Patterns of Education in Contemporary Societies, *McGraw-Hill (1964); (editor)* Educational Planning, *Syracuse (1965); (co-author)* Education in the Developing Societies, *McKay (in press). His article "The Monkey and the Fish: Cultural Pitfalls of an Educational Adviser" is reprinted with permission of the author and of the Society for International Development from* International Development, *Vol. 2 (February, 1959), pp. 22–24.*

There is an old oriental story that accurately depicts the plight of an unwary foreign educational adviser: Once upon a time there was a great flood, and involved in this flood were two creatures, a monkey and a fish. The monkey, being agile and experienced, was lucky enough to scramble up a tree and escape the raging waters. As he looked down from his safe perch, he saw the poor fish struggling against the swift current. With the very best of intentions, he reached down and lifted the fish from the water. The result was inevitable.

The educational adviser, unless he is a careful student of his own culture and the culture in which he works, will be acting much like the monkey; and, with the most laudable intentions, he may make decisions equally disastrous. Using Korea as a case in point, I shall describe some of the cultural pitfalls facing an American working in that country. The description will involve examining some of the basic assumptions, or "unconscious canons of choice" as the distinguished anthropologist Ruth Benedict called them, of the Korean people. This analysis will be made in terms of the behavior promoted by such assumptions in order to indicate how such behavior may appear to be illogical or even unintelligible to a Western adviser. Many of the value orientations described here also appear in other East Asian countries where similar cultural roots may be found. Japan and Korea, for example, were both greatly influenced by a variety of cultural forces emanating from China, the most profound of which has been called Confucianism. But sharply contrasting twentieth-century forces of militarism, communism, and democracy have brought elements of noticeable dissimilarity among Asian countries that make extensive generalizations dangerous.

Time Orientation

The first obvious cultural difference noted by the American in Korea is regarded by some to be an especially important element in differentiating cultures. This is *time orientation*, the perspective with which a nation views the process of time. All peoples must examine problems rooted in the present or past and yet must try to anticipate the future. The differences in the view of time pointed out here are related to the degree of precedence given.

The American, for example, has historically looked with pleasant anticipation toward the future. Tomorrow is expected to be brighter than today, and, with minor exceptions, only things bigger and better can be envisioned for the future. History itself is often viewed as a continuum of progress, with each succeeding generation more advanced than the former. American schools consider that one of their major functions is the examination of the present so that their products may better plan the future.

Contrast this with the Korean culture, which historically has been oriented to the past; where the Good Life has been defined completely in terms of past living; where history has largely been viewed as cyclical, with the future regarded as a mere repetition of some portion of the past and where innovations in terms of things bigger and better may be disrespectful to one's ancestors. The American technical adviser, geared to "getting things done" and "getting things moving," is often frustrated by situations in which his Korean colleagues appear to be acting too slowly or even stalling. Conversely, the American may by his direct approach appear exceedingly rude to the Korean, who sees no reason to be upset over current ills since the good times of the past are bound to reappear.

Historically, then, Korea has not viewed its institutions as developmental to the same degree as is done in the USA. While not adept at operation thinking, however, Korean students often pursue with skill the more purely academic and aesthetic interests. In so doing they exhibit characteristics that make the current-and-future-oriented American often seem superficial, even at times crude. Education in this cloistered setting could not be expected to be dynamic or experimental, and until the Japanese introduced colonial-flavored modern education in the twentieth century, the Korean school system was designed only to perpetuate the best of the past in an unaltered form. From ancient times the prescribed curriculum was the written wisdom of the Chinese sages and constituted what might be called a series of Asian Great Books. From the tender age when he memorized his first Chinese character until many years later when, if exceptionally able, he might pass the royal examination and become a government official, the curriculum of the scholar was the literature of the past. He studied not only the ideas involved but the author's phraseology and his technique of calligraphy. As the ancient texts assumed the proportions of canons, he studied to imitate rather than to exceed, to conform rather than to create. Education that was prized was divorced entirely from the social, economic, and scientific problems of the present.

The Man-Nature Orientation

A second cultural difference lies in the relation of man and nature or what might be called *man-nature orientation*. In America man has increasingly expected to gain mastery over nature and he has watched his wildest expectations come true. Mountains he crossed, tunneled through, or even pulverized. Rivers proved no obstacle to his energy, for these were easily dammed or bridged. In the East Asian culture, man typically has not been so concerned with gaining mastery over his environment as he has been in living in harmony with it. Mountains that might obstruct travel and rivers that might be impassable during certain seasons have not been viewed as merely frustrating inconvenieces. Rather, these are historical facts to which man must discipline himself. The challenge lies not in constructing new weapons for mastery but in developing a higher degree of resignation.

As with time orientation the traditional view held by Koreans with respect to nature has not contributed to a dynamic educational system. If man does not seek mastery over nature, there is little need for the schools to be concerned with the tools and skills for manipulating the physical universe. Rather, schools should be concerned with developing not the active but the passive person, one who seeks to avoid the common, tedious, daily environment by finding and developing problems in a more esthetic realm. The educated man is the man of contemplation who carries about him at all times an air of peace and tranquillity. His view toward the natural environment is shown in many and diverse ways but perhaps is best expressed in his works of art, in which he so often chooses as his subject the essential harmoniousness of the universe and avoids portraying the raucous world of change and discord.

This view of man's relation to nature coupled with his orientation to time has created what Thorstein Veblen once called "a poverty of wants." Until recent years little need was felt among the great bulk of the population of Korea for the fruits of an educatoinal system geared to produce the wide variety of skills and understandings needed to revamp and improve the existing mode of life. This does not mean that the less sophisticated people lack educational drive. On the contrary, individual families willingly make tremendous sacrifice to obtain schooling for their children. Yet these same families exert no pressure toward making the school an economically oriented institution capable of teaching functional knowledge. The urgency of keeping up to date lest history leave you behind or nature overwhelm you is not present to the same extent in the Korean culture as in the American. The goal of Korean education was, until the recent impact of Western culture, adjustment rather than improvement.

The Power and Status Orientation

A third cultural difference could be called *power and status orientation*. The United States has been proud of its decentralization of political and educational responsibilities. Under a system where considerable power is exercised at the state and local levels, every citizen becomes a leader, inasmuch as he has the right to share in decision-making. The town meeting, the school board, and all the trappings of direct and representative democracy have been widely eulogized. Because of these opportunities the American citizen, it has been said, is a more sophisticated voter than his foreign brother, and the American student a more independent learner, as well as a better team man. Obviously there is more than a little jingoism mixed in these interpretations. Nevertheless, the fact remains that Americans are still committed largely to the belief in shared decision-making.

A power structure has existed in Korea that has equated

position with authority while social custom has further equated authority with validity. This hierarchal structure and manner of decision-making are also reflected in the classroom and in the family. The teacher and the father both occupy positions of ultimate trust, respect, power. Their word is law. The obvious difficulty of using modern educational methods within this framework is readily seen. The school in both fostering cooperation and stressing at the same time reliance on the individual's ability to solve his own problems runs into conflict with family and societal tradition. Moreover, it is difficult to break down the school's authoritarian structure because of the fear that the teacher may lose the traditional respect felt for him.

The organization and administration of Korean education reflects the power structure found elsewhere in Korean society. Until 1948 and to a gradually modifying degree since then, Korean education has operated within a framework that was highly centralized. Major decisions emanated from the Ministry of Education. Even though opportunities for local control have been provided, they have not been taken advantage of, and lesser educational officials invariably refuse to take responsibility for decisions clearly within their jurisdiction but prefer the decisions to be made "higher up." The danger, in addition to the perpetuation of authoritarian procedures, is that the bases for determining professional action are largely founded on judgmental evidence as represented by the expressions of a status person rather than on factual evidence.

There are further and widespread educational implications of this lineally organized society. As with individuals in an organization, the schools have a definite order of rank, as do the courses of study within the school. Since academic subjects carry the most prestige, the technical and vocational schools, in attempting to gain recognition, tend to deemphasize the applied parts of their curriculum. There is so much status value attached to abstract and difficult works that Korean students enjoy being immersed in little understood concepts and often rebel in studying subjects within their comprehension.

Language is another major curriculum problem which is rooted partly in status factors. Although a simple phonetic alphabet, Hangul, had been developed in Korea in the fifteenth century, it had never been widely accepted by scholars. Government officials historically have used a written script based on Chinese characters, which has served to create and perpetuate the gulf between the Korean people and their culture. During the latter part of the Japenese annexation, to further complicate matters, the Koreans were required to use the Japanese language on all occasions. After being freed from colonial status, Korea erased most traces of the Japanese language, and the vernacular was not only reintroduced into the schools but also increasingly stressed in all literature.

The net result of this complex language situation is that Korea in 1959 finds itself with very little professional literature appropriate for students at the secondary school and college levels. There are few modern technical or professional books written in Chinese, and the children entering school after 1945 have been receiving only limited work with Chinese characters anyway. Most of the books written in Japanese (and all educated Korean adults are fluent in this language) have been destroyed. Moreover, the generation of Koreans now in school have no familiarity with the Japanese language. And at the present time, in spite of official government urgings, newspapers and most professional periodicals are being made incomprehensible to a major part of the Korean population by the inclusion of a large number of Chinese characters rather than relying on the vernacular. (It is interesting to note that under communism North Korea has made great strides in eliminating the use of Chinese characters, simplifying and refining the pure Korean. It appears that all literature being published in North Korea uses only the simple, practical Hangul script.)

The indirect influences of the West through Japanese colonialism and the direct contacts since 1945 have forced a re-examination of Korean value orientations. The sincere if awkward attempts to industrialize and democratize a nation with a long agrarian and authoritarian heritage have produced a considerable number of inconsistencies within the Korean society. For example, the political party in power one day exalts democratic freedoms, yet on the next may order all students to participate in "spontaneous demonstration" to promote a particular party bias. Police in one section of the country initiate youth clubs to combat delinquency yet themselves may at times use extremely harsh methods. The government through all avenues of propaganda promotes moral education, yet, as in older times, the bribe may often be the easiest recourse for the Korean citizen who attempts to get action through official channels. Such discrepancies indicate not only policy incongruities and personal confusion but also identify a major obstacle to a smooth cultural transition. Unity, loyalty, and morality are well defined and practiced in the family, making this an institution long admired in the West, but these qualities are yet to be raised to the societal level.

The Adviser as Catalyst

The role of the foreign educational adviser in this setting is, then, both sensitive and difficult. His own knowledge and skills are to a certain extent culture-bound and unintelligible or incongruous in new surroundings. Yet it may be precisely his new perspective that is badly needed. The task of technical assistance can obviously not be defined as "teaching them to do it our way." But neither is the counter-alternative, "helping them to do what they wish to do better," completely satisfactory. The former runs the danger of technical inapplicability or of cultural resistance while the latter may involve no substantial progress toward the newer and only partially defined goals. The adviser by his increased technical knowledge sheds light on possible alternatives, but neither through coercion nor through persuasion does he determine the direction of change.

Perhaps the adviser can best be likened to a catalyst. By bringing his knowledge and experience and points of view to the new situation, his role is to speed desirable change. To fulfill this role adequately the adviser must be a student of the culture and metaculture. He must establish guidelines that will determine in broad outline educational priorities acceptable to the host nation. He must face up to the enigmatic problem of focusing attention on grassroots education—for example, increasing literacy, helping the farmer to eke out a slightly bigger yield per acre—or striking out on a broad scale to teach the highly developed skills and understandings needed by a nation moving toward industrialization. Since it is extremely difficult or impossible to change a cultural pattern by attacking its isolated parts, he must answer the question whether the establishment of a few model projects can be justified in hopes that their influence will spread.

Korea is a nation in the throes of a rapid but uneven cultural change. While members of the older generation may still cling to the belief that "the scholar should neither shoulder a carrying pole nor lift a basket," young students are beginning to seek the skills requisite for nudging an ancient culture toward new directions. In Korea, as in any developing country, cultural modification depends primarily on the initiative and drive of the people. Through his minor but vital role, the adviser, by participating from the beginning with the people whose lives are being affected, may be able to lessen the traumatic effects of such change.

24

Understanding Cultural Patterns

by Margaret Mead

Dr. Mead, well-known anthropologist, psychologist, and lecturer, is curator of ethnology at the American Museum of Natural History in New York City. Also, she is chairman of the Social Sciences Division and Professor of Anthropology at Fordham University's new liberal arts college, at Lincoln Center in New York City. She has written for numerous journals and among her recent publications are: Continuities in Cultural Evolution, *New Haven, Yale University Press, 1964;* Anthropology: A Human Science, *Princeton, Van Nostrand, 1964; and* Anthropologists and What They Do, *New York: Watts, 1965. "Understanding Cultural Patterns" is reproduced with her permission and by permission of the American Journal of Nursing Company from* Nursing Outlook, *Vol. 4, 1956, pp. 260–262.*

Understanding differences among the patterns of behavior in peoples of different cultural backgrounds has obvious relevance to nursing. In fact, the relevance is so obvious that it has been taken for granted, to a degree, and has not been treated systematically in the nursing curriculum.[1]

It can be argued that the nurse who is sensitive to the needs of her patient, and who has been trained to interpret verbal protests and outcries and other signs—slight stubbornness, flushing of the skin, tightening of the lips, and clenching or loosening of the hands—as signs of discomfort, pain, or relaxation, will realize that entering a hospital, undergoing a physical examination, having a baby, losing a relative, suffering a long illness, or accepting a permanent physical handicap, will mean very different things to different persons.

Reactions will differ in those recently come from peasant communities in southern Europe or Puerto Rico, and in long-time residents of American cities, in the educated and in the uneducated, in those with a clear religious faith and in those without religion. It can be argued that the nurse will *naturally* take these matters into account.

But the matter is not so simple. To begin with, in order to take into account the cultural background of a patient—or a patient's relative, or another nurse, or a physician, or the medical social worker, or a Red Cross volunteer—it is necessary to have some experience with the kinds of cultural differences which are important. One needs a clear idea of which kinds of cultural difference to look for.

By relevant cultural differences we mean not only differences in language—which, of course, are conspicuous and well recognized—or in religious attitudes which will involve food practices and religious observances, or in dietary practices which may necessitate changes in the routine hospital diets, but many other, less conspicuous, much subtler things. We mean differences in attitudes toward pain, for example. Where members of one culture will maintain stoic self-control, members of another will wail and moan with regularity, and a third will first state how terrible the suffering is, and then bear it grimly.

If the nurse herself comes from a culture which applauds self-control and refusal to "give in" to pain, she will have to allow for her "cultural" tendency to approve the stiff upper lip and condemn the wailing and moaning. But, if she comes from a culture where wailing and moaning are the approved behavior—which means she will respond more easily to such wailing and moaning—then she will have to contend, within herself, with a feeling that those who are obviously in pain and refuse to admit it are in some way rejecting her, refusing the aid and comfort which she wishes to give. In addition, the nurse and the patient will be acting within the particular version of our culture which is represented by the whole practice of the medical arts in American society—with its expectations and rules about what may be regarded as a "reasonable complaint," a "normal" amount of pain and an appropriate response from the private duty nurse, the ward nurse, the public health nurse, and so on. To the extent that patient, nurse, and hospital or clinic all belong to the same cultural background, communication is smooth and efficient. The patient knows what to expect and how to behave; so does the nurse, and, even in situations of sharp conflict, they can express to each other exactly what they mean to express.

Cultural differences among any of the participants in a nursing situation may be regarded as complications which do least harm when they are most articulately recognized. Take, for example, the woman patient on the tenth floor of a hospital facing a park. She objects to having her body exposed for examination or bathing if the window shade is up. If the nurse does not see this as a feeling about exposure which also includes the moon shining in at the window, she may interpret it as a peculiarity verging on the pathological. If she has been more thoroughly trained in psychiatric considerations than in cultural, she may even alert the psychiatric staff. Or, if a Polish patient becomes extraordinarily demanding and loud in his complaints, the nurse who has no knowledge of his cultural expectations of woman's role of extravagant sympathy to a sufferer in order to permit him to show no weakness, may misinterpret his noisy complaints as complaints about his pain.

Patients from some cultures are apt to preserve their self-control better if they see as little of their relatives as possible; patients from cultures with a different family structure will go into depressions unless they are surrounded by a close, warm group of relatives.

A nurse who gives care to patients from varying types of culture may find herself misjudging each as individuals because she takes the contrast in their behavior as an individual matter, rather than a cultural matter.

What can be said of response to pain and attitudes toward relatives, can be said of every other habitual response—attitudes toward reward and punishment; responsibility; money; privacy and exposure; cleanliness; eating, sleeping, and excretion; success and failure; beauty and fertility.

But, if this is so, the nurse, either during her basic nursing education or in graduate courses, already overburdened with the hundred new items on the curriculum, may well ask, "What in the world am I to do about it? In the course of a year, I will probably meet patients, their relatives, or professional colleagues representing twenty or more cultures. They may include American Indians, Burmese, Eastern European Jews, French Canadians, Texans, Scots, Mexicans, and Mennonites." She might add, "Can you give me a handy little compendium in which I can look things up? It ought to have a good index, so when someone bangs a door in my face I could look up their culture and see what door-banging means. Or back-turning, or too much bowing, or overeating, or taking the same medicine twice and not objecting to the double dose. Have you anthropologists got such a compendium?"

This, in effect, was the question put to me ten years ago by a particularly sensitive and aware nurse who was teaching nurses. She got the idea that the section of the curriculum concerned with "the patient as an individual" ought to include cultural differences. So, with characteristic enterprise she came up to the American Museum of Natural History to ask for a "chart" which would show the principal differences between different groups of mankind. After we had discussed the problem a little further, she devoted a year to a most exacting, self-assigned field task. She went back into general-duty nursing to study the response of one cultural group—the Italians—to the nursing situation. Like all pioneer attempts, her study smoothed the way for future students. We no longer have to send a nurse field worker into hospitals to study each cultural group in such an arduous way.

From her studies and from other studies of related types of behavior—responses to pain, to rehabilitation, to plastic surgery, to changes in diet, to school situations, to health education, and so on—we now have accumulated a great deal of illustrative material. We can produce not a "chart," or a simple, well-indexed compendium, but reports which will give the interested nurse an idea about the kind of cultural differences to look for in her patients.

If the nurse is aware that she herself comes from a culture with a full set of cultural attitudes on every subject—from reward and punishment to the exact spot over which one should brush one's teeth—and learns to watch the ways in which she responds culturally (that is, with the same order of behavior as any other woman of her age, class, religion, education, and from her part of the country), this is half the battle.

Watching one's own cultural behavior sensitizes one to cultural behavior in others. If, for instance, you know that you are not being rude or mean in telling another that he owes you fifteen cents, you are better prepared to understand that a member of another culture may think that only a heel would mention a debt under a dollar. If you recognize that your respect for those who "overcome a handicap" is cultural, you will be less moralistic and more understanding of those who face a handicap with depression and despair.

Merely being aware that behavior may be cultural is an enormous help. As the awareness filters through, one gets continual, little, watchful, half-articulated warnings—"Remember she's a Puerto Rican, perhaps in Puerto Rico. . . ." Remember she came to this country only a few years ago from Germany, perhaps the Germans. . . ." "Remember he is a southern, rural Negro, newly come to New York; perhaps he doesn't expect. . . ." "Remember, she belongs to a small religious sect who live communal lives, possibly this situation has. . . ." These are the watchful, protective attitudes in the back of one's mind which permit one to suspend judgment. They help us to question whether behavior is individual or cultural, to allow for whimsies and strange requests without becoming resentful, and warn us to watch for the combinations of circumstances which bring on depression or elation in others. And, in really serious situations, these attitudes lead us to seek expert help from one who knows the cultural patterns in question.

One of the difficulties which is encountered by those of us who attempt to communicate something of this point of view to nurses and students of nursing is most important. We have found that nurses seem to shrink from any recognition of cultural differences as being, somehow, undemocratic. They have grown up in a period which saw Hitler's attempted annihilation of Jews and Poles and Gypsies. They have witnessed the long, uphill fight against segregation in the United States. These events have emphasized the undesirability of the use of stereotypes to describe any people. They have experienced, in some degree, the long battle of the nursing profession for status and recognition. They have been taught that it is not correct to "discuss religion," nor polite to refer to someone's socio-economic class position. How, then, is it possible for nurses to deal with these cultural differences which seem to be so tied up with race and class and religious considerations?

They may meet these objections, to some degree, by recognizing that the very use of the word "culture" implies a democratic approach. The anthropologist treats all cultures, whether that of a small Eskimo tribe or of a great modern state, as comparable wholes, as the way of life of a people—the way of life within which they have married, reared their children, prayed, labored, and perpetuated their group. By emphasizing cultural differences—which are the learned ways of a people and which cut across class, racial, and religious lines—we enhance the dignity of each people, and we mute the types of judgment involved in political and religious differences. We then come to realize that race is irrelevant. We can more easily tolerate religious and political views which are contrary to our own if we do not confuse them with cultural differences which require not toleration, but recognition and discriminating appreciation.

Note

1. This situation is being remedied in some schools. For example, Cornell University-New York Hospital School of Nursing has provided a program for the integration of social science in the curriculum, clinical areas, and research under the direction of Frances Cooke Macgregor.

Bibliography

Abell, Theodora M., and Joffe, Natalie F. Cultural backgrounds of female puberty. *Am. J. Psychotherapy* 4:90–113, Jan. 1950.

Huger, Margaret. *Attitudes of Italian-Americans Toward Nursing Care.* New York, Cornell University-New York Hospital School of Nursing. 1948–1949. (Unpublished manuscript)

Hughes, E. C. Studying the nurse's work. *Am. J. Nursing* 51:294–295, May 1951.

Macgregor, Frances M., and others. *Facial Deformities and Plastic Surgery.* Springfield, Ill., Charles C. Thomas, 1953.

National Research Council, Committee on Food Habits. *The Problem of Changing Food Habits, 1941–1943.* (Bulletin No. 108) Washington, D.C., The Council, 1943.

——— *Manual for the Study of Food Habits.* (Bulletin No. 111) Washington, D.C., The Council, 1945.

Paul, B. D. *Health, Culture and Community.* New York, Russell Sage Foundation, 1955.

Saunders, Lyle. *Cultural Differences and Medical Care.* New York, Russell Sage Foundation, 1954.

World Federation for Mental Health. *Cultural Patterns and Technical Change,* edited by Margaret Mead. (United Nations Educational, Scientific and Cultural Organization, Tensions and Technology Series) New York, Columbia University Press, 1953.

Zborowski, Mark. Cultural components in responses to pain. *Journal of Social Issues,* Vol. 8, no. 4, pp. 16–30, 1952.

Bibliography

Ackernecht, Erwin, H. "Natural Diseases and Rational Treatment in Primitive Medicine." *Bulletin of the History of Medicine* 19 (1946): 467–97.

———. "On the Collecting of Data Concerning Primitive Medicine." *American Anthropologist* 47 (1945) : 227–32.

———. "Primitive Medicine and Cultural Patterns." *Bulletin of the History of Medicine* 12 (1942) : 545–47.

———. "Primitive Surgery." *American Anthropologist* 64 (1947) : 24–45.

———. "Problems of Primitive Medicine." *Bulletin of the History of Medicine* 2 (1942) : 503–21.

———. "Psychopathology, Primitive Medicine and Primitive Culture." *Bulletin of the History of Medicine* 14 (1943) : 30–67.

Adair, John; Deuschle, Kurt; and McDermott, Walsh. "Patterns of Health and Disease Among the Navaho." *The Annals of the American Academy of Political and Social Science* 311 (May 1957) : 80–94.

Adams, Don. "The Monkey and the Fish; Cultural Pitfalls of an Educational Advisor." *International Development Review* 2 (February 1959): 22–24.

Adams, Richard N. "On the Effective Use of Anthropology in Public Health Programs." *Human Organization* 13, no. 4 (May 1954) : 5–15.

Alpenfels, Ethel J. "Cancer in the Situ of the Cervix—Cultural Clues To Reactions." *American Journal of Nursing* 64

(April 1964) : 83–86.

Arens, Richard. "The Tambalan and his Medical Practices in the Leyte and Samar Islands, Philippines." *The Philippine Journal of Science* 86 (March 1957) : 121–30.

Bailey, Flora L. "Suggested Techniques for Inducing Navaho Women to Accept Hospitalization During Childbirth and for Implementing Health Education." *American Journal of Public Health* 38 (October 1943) : 1418–23.

Barnett, H. C. *Being a Palauan: Case Studies in Cultural Anthropology.* New York: Holt, Rinehart and Winston, Inc., 1961.

————. *Innovation: The Basis of Cultural Change.* New York: McGraw-Hill Book Company, 1953.

Benedict, Ruth. *Patterns of Culture.* Boston: Houghton-Mifflin Company, 1934.

Bharara, S. S. "Changing Beliefs—One Method of Doing It." *Health Education Journal* 24, no. 2 (May 1965) : 109–12.

Buchler, I. R. "Caymanian Folk Medicine: A Problem in Applied Anthropology." *Human Organization* 23, no. 1 (Spring 1964) : 48–49.

Chance, Norman A. "Cultural Change and Integration: An Eskimo Example," *American Anthropologist* 62 (1960): 1028–44.

Ch'ih, J. C. "Medical Culture and Philosophy of China." *Delaware Medical Journal* 37 (June 1965) : 140–42.

Currier, Richard L. "Hot-Cold Syndrome and Symbolic Balance in Mexican and Spanish-American Folk Medicine." *Ethnology* 3, no. 3 (July 1966) : 251–623.

Darity, William A. "Some Sociocultural Factors in the Administration of Technical Assistance and Training in Health." *Human Organization* 24, no. 1 (Spring 1965) : 78–82.

Dubos, René. *Mirage of Health.* New York: Doubleday and Company, Inc., 1961.

Erasmus, Charles John. "Changing Folk Beliefs and the Relativity of Empirical Knowledge." *Southwestern Journal of Anthropology* 8 (1952) , 411–28.

Fathauer, George H. "Food Habits—An Anthropologist's View." *Journal of the American Dietetic Association* 37 (October 1960) : 335–38.

Firth, Raymond. "Health Planning and Community Organization." *The Health Education Journal* 15 (1957) : 118–24.

Foster, George M. "Guidelines to Community Development Programs." *Public Health Reports* 70 (1955): 19–24.

———. "Medical Care in India." *American Journal of Public Health* 50 (1960) : 28–35.

———. "Oriental Renaissance in Education and Medicine." *Science* 141, no. 3586 (September 20, 1963: 1153–61.

———. "Use of Anthropological Methods and Data in Planning and Operation." *Public Health Reports* 68, no. 9 (September 1953) : 841–57.

Freeman, Howard E., and Camille Lambert, Jr. "The Influence of Community Groups on Health Matters." *Human Organizations* 24, no. 4 (Winter 1965) : 353–57.

Gelfand, Michael, M.D. "Meet the Nganga." *Abbottempo* 2, no. 2 (May 15, 1964) : 30–34.

Gerlach, Luther P., Ph.D. "Socio-cultural Factors Affecting the Diet of the Northeast Coastal Bantu." *Journal of the American Dietetic Association* 45 (November 1964) : 420–24.

Gideon, Helen. "A Baby Is Born in the Punjab." *American Anthropologist* 64, no. 6 (December 1962) : 1220–34.

Gonzalez, Nancie L. Solien. "Beliefs and Practices Concerning Medicine and Nutrition Among Lower-Class Urban Guatemalans." *American Journal of Public Health* 54, no. 10 (October 1964): 1726–34.

———. "Health Behavior in Cross-Cultural Perspective: A Guatemalan Example." *Human Organization* 25, no. 2 (Summer 1966) : 122–25.

Gould, Harold A. "The Implications of Technological Change for Folk and Scientific Medicine." *American Anthropologist* 59, no. 3 (June 1957) : 507–16.

————. "Modern Medicine and Folk Cognition in Rural India." *Human Organization* 24, no. 3 (Fall 1965) : 201–8.

Grout, Ruth E. "Health Education in Public Health Practice." *The Health Education Journal* 26, no. 1 (March 1967) : 25–29.

Hallowell, Irving. "Primitive Concepts of Disease." *American Anthropologist* 46 (1935) : 365–68.

Hostetler, John A. "Folk and Scientific Medicine in Amish Society." *Human Organization* 22, no. 4 (Winter 1963–1964) : 269–75.

Hunt, Robert. *Personalities and Cultures.* New York: The Natural History Press, 1967.

Jelliffe, D. B. "Social Culture and Nutrition—Cultural Blocks and Protein Malnutrition in Early Childhood in Rural West Bengal." *Pediatrics* 20 (1957) : 128–38.

————, and Bennett, F. John. "Cultural Problems in Technical Assistance." *Children* 9, no. 5 (September-October 1962) : 171–77.

Jocano, F. L. "Cultural Contest of Folk Medicine: Some Philippine Cases." *Philippine Sociological Review* 14, no. 1 (1966) : 40–48.

Kenny, Michael. "Social Values and Health in Spain: Some Preliminary Considerations." *Human Organization* 21, no. 4 (Winter 1963) : 280–89.

Khare, R. S. "Folk Medicine in a North Indian Village." *Human Organization* 22, no. 1 (Spring 1963) : pp. 36–40.

Kiev, Ari. "The Psychotherapeutic Aspects of Primitive Medicine." *Human Organization* 21, no. 1 (Spring 1962) : 25–29.

————. "Beliefs and Delusions Among West Indian Immigrants to London." *British Journal of Psychiatry* 109 (1963): 356–63.

Kimball, Solon T., and Pearsall, Marion. *The Talladega Story.* Talladega: University of Alabama Press, 1954.

Kluckhohn, Clyde, and Romney, A. K. *The Rimrock Navaho:*

Variations in Value Orientations. New York: Harper and Row, 1961.

Knutson, Andie L. *The Individual Society and Health Behavior.* New York: Russell Sage Foundation, 1965.

Koos, Elma. *The Health of Regionville.* New York: Columbia University Press, 1954.

Krush, T. P., et al. "Some Thoughts on the Formation of Personality Disorder: A Study of an Indian Boarding School Population." *American Journal of Psychiatry* 122 (February 1966) : 868–76.

Lieban, Richard W. "The Dangerous Ingkantos: Illness and Social Control in a Philippine Community." *American Anthropologist* 64, no. 2 (1962) : 306–12.

Lipton, E. L., et al. "Swaddling, A Child Care Practice, Historical, Cultural and Experimental Observations." *Pediatrics* 35 (March 1965 Supplement) : 519–67.

Loomis, Charles P. *Social Systems.* Princeton, N.J.: D. Van Nostrand Company, 1960.

Loughlin, Bernice W. "Pregnancy in the Navaho Culture." *Nursing Outlook* 13, no. 3 (March 1965) : 55–58.

McDermott, Walsh; Deuschle, Kurt; Adair, John; Fulmer, Hugh; and Loughlin, Bernice. "Introducing Modern Medicine in a Navaho Community." *Science* I, 131, no. 3395 (January 1960) : 197–207; II, 131, no. 3396 (January 1960): 280–87.

Macgregor, Gordon. "The Development of Rural Community Health Services." *Human Organization* 25, no. 1 (Spring 1966) : 16–19.

MacLean, Catherine M. U., "Hospitals or Healers? An Attitude Survey in Abadan." *Human Organization* 25, no. 2 (Summer 1966) : 131–39.

Mahan, M. B. "Cultural and Social Factors in Mental Health." *Mental Hygiene* 50 (January 1966) : 12–17.

Malina, G., et al. "Indicators of Health, Economy and Culture in Puerto Rico and Latin America." *American Journal of Public Health* 54 (August 1964) : 1191–1206.

Malinowsky, Bronislaw. *Magic, Science and Healing*. Glencoe, Ill.: The Free Press, 1948.

Mead, Margaret. *Cultural Patterns and Technical Change*. New York: New American Library, 1955.

———. "Understanding Cultural Patterns." *Nursing Outlook* 4, no. 5 (1956) : 260–62.

———, and Wolfenstein, Martha. *Childhood in Contemporary Cultures*. The University of Chicago Press, 1955.

Mechanic, David. "The Concept of Illness Behavior." *Journal of Chronic Disease* 15 (1962): 189–94.

———. "Religion, Religiosity and Illness Behavior: The Special Case of the Jews." *Human Organization* 22, no. 3 (Fall 1963) : 202–6.

Middleton, Evelyn. "Bridging the Gap." *Health Education Journal* 24, no. 2 (May 1965) : 88–93.

Minor, Horace. "Body Rituals Among the Nacirema." *American Anthropologist* 58, no. 3 (June 1956) : 603–7.

Minturn, Leigh, and Lembert, William W. *Mothers of Six Cultures*. New York: John Wiley and Sons, Inc., 1964.

Murdock, George P. "Anthropology and its Contribution to Public Health." *American Journal of Public Health* 42 (January 1952) : 7–11.

Nurge, Ethel. "Etiology of Illness in Guinhangdan." *American Anthropologist* 60, no. 6 (December 1958) : 1158–72.

Opler, Marvin K. *Culture and Mental Health*. New York: The Macmillan Company, 1959.

Opler, Morris E. "The Cultural Definition of Illness in Village India." *Human Organization* 22, no. 1 (Spring 1963): 32–35.

Paul, Benjamin D. "Anthropological Perspectives on Medicine and Public Health." *Annals of the American Academy of Political and Social Science* 346 (March 1963) : 34–43.

Paul, Benjamin D. *Health, Culture and the Community*. New York: Russell Sage Foundation, 1955.

Polgar, Steven. "Health and Human Behavior: Areas of Interest Common to the Social and Medical Science." *Current Anthropology* 3, no. 2 (1962) : 159–205.

Rubel, Arthur J. "Concepts of Disease in Mexican-American Culture." *American Anthropologist* 62 (1960) : 795–814.

Saunders, Lyle. *Cultural Difference and Medical Care*. New York: Russell Sage Foundation, 1954.

————, and Hewes, Gordon W. "Folk Medicine and Medical Practice." *Journal of Medical Education* 28, no. 9 (September 1953): 43–46.

Shiloh, Ailon. "A Case Study of Disease and Culture in Action: Leprosy Among the Hausa of Northern Nigeria." *Human Organization* 24, no. 2 (Summer 1965) : 140–7.

————. "Conceptual Progress Toward Structuring the Universal Pattern of Medicine." *The Health Education Journal* 21, no. 1 (March 1963): 47–51.

————. "Middle East Culture and Health." *The Health Education Journal* 16, no. 4 (1958) : 232–342.

————. "The System of Medicine in Middle East Culture." *The Middle East Journal* 15, no. 3 (1953) : 277–88.

Simons, L. W. "Impact of Social Factors Upon Adjustment Within the Community." *American Journal of Psychiatry* 122 (March 1966) : 990–8.

Simmons, Ozzie G. "Implications of Social Class for Public Health." *Human Organization* 16, no. 3 (Fall 1957) : 57.

————. "Popular and Modern Medicine in Mestizo Communities of Coastal Peru and Chile." *Journal of American Folklore* 68 (1955) ; 57–71.

Smith, Alfred G., ed. *Communication and Culture*. New York: Holt, Rinehart and Winston, Inc., 1966.

Spicer, Edward H., ed. *Human Problems in Technological Change*. New York: Russell Sage Foundation, 1953.

Spiro, Melford E. "Ghosts, Ifaluk and Teleological Functionalism." *American Anthropologist* 54 (1952): 497–503.

Waneka, Annie D. "Helping a People to Understand." *The American Journal of Nursing* 62 (July 1962) : 88–90.

Warner, W. L. *A Black Civilization: A Social Study of an Australian Tribe.* New York: Harper and Row, 1941.

Wellin, Edward. "Implications of Local Culture for Public Health." *Human Organization* 16, no. 4 (Winter 1958) : 16–18.

Whiting, Beatrice. *Six Cultures—Studies on Child Rearing.* New York: John Wiley and Sons, Inc., 1963.

Wolff, Robert J. "Modern Medicine and Traditional Culture: Confrontation on the Malay Peninsula." *Human Organization* 24, no. 4 (Winter 1965) : 339–45.

Index

Adair, John, 83, 111, 127
Adams, Don, 435, 436
Adams, Richard, 40
African, Africans, 34, 45, 53, 361, 375, 379. *See also* Bantu, Nganga, Nigeria, South Africa, and Zulus
Aire (disease concept) . *See* Disease
Akernecht, Edwin H., 399, 400
Alpenfels, Ethel J., 25, 70
Alus (ghosts) , 277–287
Amish, 82
Arabs, 59, 60

Bailey, Flora, 82, 156
Bantu, 361
Basuto, 53
Benedict, Ruth, 74
Bennett, F. John, 24, 43
Borfirma (charm) , 46
Buganda, 53
Burgess, A., 271
Burma, 53

Child feeding practices, 300, 301, 306. *See also* Diet and Nutrition
Congenital hip, 127–131
Coon, Carleton S., 430
Cultural changes, 485; agents of, 338; conflict and, 415; Middle East, 373; pitfalls, 437; problems in, 62; role of the advisor in, 443; using caution in, 67, 143, 435
Culture: underlying principles of, 343; understanding and respecting others', 61
Currier, Richard, 212, 255

Darity, William A., 359, 362
Dean, R. F. A., 271
Deuschle, Kurt W., 83, 111, 127
Diet: Bantu, 383; restrictions in illness, 312. *See also* Hot-cold dichotomy
Dietetics. *See* Food and Nutrition
Disease: classification and concept of, 222; concept and etiology of, 211 319; "Situations," 321, 322

Erasmus, Charles John, 401, 402

Fathauer, George H., 25, 59
Folk beliefs: changing, 409; conflict in change of, 415; nature of, 404
Folk medicine: concept of, 32, 411; conflict with western medicine, 409; in western culture, 404; psychotherapeutic effects of, 400; relationship to scientific medicine, 406, 407
Food: acceptance and consumption (Africa) , 391; classification (Bengali) , 308; concepts, 218, 219, 294; cultural aspects of, 63–66; habits, 63, 64; symbolism of, 66; superfoods, 52; suitability of, 52
Food production: practices of, 384; agriculture in, 386; influencing factors of, 390
Foster, George M., 23, 24, 30, 31
Fulmer, Hugh, 111, 127

Gaps: cultural, 32; status (in U. S.

461